PRAISE FOR
NOT LESS THAN EVERYTHING

When it comes to spirituality and life, Turak is as authentic as it gets. Wonderful read!

– Michael Keaton, Actor

This book is a spiritual classic. It's a must-read for any spiritual seeker.
– Jonathan Cook, Editor-in-Chief, LiveReal.com

I absolutely love this book. The ideas fascinated me. The stories gripped me. *Not Less Than Everything* represents a vision of what life can be when it is lived in dedication to something higher. It spoke to me in a way that no other book ever has.

– Kenny Felder, Author, *Modern Physics*

This book is moving and 100 percent authentic. In seeking the transcendent, August Turak finds the utterly personal and profoundly intimate experience of divine love. Read this book and you too may suddenly realize that the God you thought was missing has been calling your name your whole life.

– Georg Buehler, Editor-in-Chief, *Abandoned Text*

This masterfully woven story will take you on a miraculous journey as you become partner and witness to Turak's gripping and deeply personal spiritual tale of transcendence, acceptance, and most of all… gratitude.

– Robert Cergol

I loved this book! The storytelling is superb. Best of all is how Turak heroically perseveres through all the pain and suffering: a heroic struggle that ultimately brings him and his readers to a magical resolution of the human condition.

– Jonathan Reams, Editor-in-Chief, *Integral Review*

NOT LESS THAN EVERYTHING

One Man's Quest for Spiritual Enlightenment

AUGUST TURAK

New Revised Standard Version Bible: Anglicized Edition, copyright © 1989, 1995 the
Division of Christian Education of the National Council of the Churches of Christ in the
United States of America. Used by permission. All rights reserved.

Published by Clovercroft Publishing, Franklin, Tennessee

Interior Design and Cover Layout by Suzanne Lawing

Edited by Robert Irvin

Cover Art by Glenn Harrington

Printed in the United States of America

ISBN: 978-1-954437-99-9

A condition of complete simplicity
(Costing not less than everything)
And all shall be well and
All manner of thing shall be well
When the tongues of flame are in-folded
Into the crowned knot of fire
And the fire and the rose are one.
—T.S. Eliot [1]

DEDICATION

This book is dedicated to my parents. As my first teachers, they instilled the love of learning, coachability, work ethic, and deep respect for teachers that led me to seek out the spiritual mentors who played such a pivotal role in my life.

ACKNOWLEDGMENTS

This book relied on the efforts of many other people. I would like to thank my writing coach, Alex Schnitzler, for his patience, incisive critiques, and constant encouragement. I also owe a debt of gratitude to Glenn Harrington for his cover art, Bob Irvin for his meticulous editing, and my publisher, Shane Crabtree, for steering this book through the countless challenges and deadlines that must be met to bring a book to market.

Most of all I want to acknowledge Melissa Hawks who, as executive director of the August Turak Foundation, has not only cheerfully worn a thousand hats during this laborious process, but been my confidant and guardian angel as well.

CONTENTS

PRELUDE

In 2004, my students at Duke University urged me to enter the John Templeton Foundation's "The Power of Purpose" essay contest. In 3,500 words or less I was asked to answer the question: *What is the purpose of life?* A few days later, only minutes before the deadline, I submitted "Brother John," a story about my poignant Christmas Eve encounter with a Trappist monk. Five months later, it took six strangers on a conference call several minutes to convince me that "Brother John" had just won the $100,000 grand prize.

One day, my brother Chris told me a colleague reacted skeptically to this story.

"You mean to tell me your brother never wrote anything in his life? Then he whips out an essay over the weekend, goes up against ten thousand essays from forty-seven countries, and wins a hundred grand? Man, is he lucky!"

"You don't understand," Chris replied. "Augie has been working on that essay for thirty-five years."

This book is the story of those thirty-five years.

As a young college student in 1971, I was seized by the idea that the mystical state various religious traditions call Enlightenment, Satori, Nirvana, Samadhi, Unio Mystica, Cosmic Consciousness, or the Numinous Experience not only exists but might be attainable by me.

Andrew Sullivan, writing for *New York Magazine,* argues that all these dystopian social ills are merely the myriad symptoms of a single disease: a Spiritual Crisis. In an article called "The Poison We Pick," ostensibly only about the opioid epidemic, he eloquently summarizes this crisis.

> *This nation pioneered modern life. Now epic numbers of Americans are killing themselves with opioids to escape it. To see this epidemic as simply a pharmaceutical or chemically addictive problem is to miss something: the despair that currently makes so many want to fly away.*
>
> *Opioids are just one of the ways Americans are trying to cope with an inhuman new world where everything is flat, where communication is virtual, and where those core elements of human happiness—faith, family, community—seem to elude so many. Until we resolve these deeper social, cultural, and psychological problems, until we discover a new meaning or reimagine our old religion or reinvent our way of life, the poppy will flourish.*[2]

As a young college student in the early 1970s, I too was afflicted by depression, anomie, and the sinking sense that "nothing really matters." This is the story of how, with the help of my teachers and God's grace, I transcended these challenges and became the happy, peaceful, and eternally grateful person I am today. This book shows how I found higher meaning and purpose through authentic spiritual experience, and it is my heartfelt prayer that my journey will help others looking for life's purpose as well.

* * *

Everything in this book is true. Every person is real, and every event, no matter how fantastic, actually happened. As a young man, I found inspiration in fictional works like Somerset Maugham's *The Razor's Edge* and Hermann Hesse's *Siddhartha,* but I decided that if

I was to have any success in remythologizing our dystopic modern view of life, I had to stick strictly to the truth.

However, I did not keep a journal. As a result, I have reconstructed dialogue, scenes, and timelines from memory and therefore I inevitably made errors. But even in these instances I've taken great pains to ensure that the essential aspects are real and not an example of me (like Plato supposedly did) putting my own ideas into another person's mouth for dramatic effect. It is my sincere hope that my effort to be authentic is rewarded, and that you find me to be the credible witness for the incredible I set out to be.

Chapter One

TRAPPED BETWEEN HEAVEN AND EARTH

At the still point of the turning world.
Neither flesh nor fleshless;
Neither from nor towards; at the still point, there the dance is,
But neither arrest nor movement.
And do not call it fixity,
Where past and future are gathered.
Neither movement from nor towards,
Neither ascent nor decline.
Except for the point, the still point,
There would be no dance, and there is only the dance.
—T.S. Eliot [3]

I was brave enough to jump out of an airplane. I just wasn't brave enough to tell a bunch of college kids that, in 1996, at 44 years of age, I was too damn old to be jumping out of airplanes.

My stomach was rising and falling in sync with the tiny plane's gyrations as high winds sent us whoop-de-dooing all over the cold blue skies above the North Carolina countryside.

Minutes earlier, my Duke University students and I, sporting jumpsuits and helmets, were tethered to parachute laden tandem jumpers and herded two by two into the single-engine plane by the jump master like exotic-looking animals being shoehorned into Noah's Ark. I tried to take my mind off my stomach by looking out the window, but the early afternoon sun shimmering off the wing just seared my eyes. I barely had time to blink away the pain before the jump master banged my back and screamed over the roar of wind and engine: "You're up!" Me and my tandem jumper scrambled to the open door, and seconds later he shouted, "Go! Go! Go!"

I can't say I jumped. I can't even say I just let the airplane leave without me. It felt like a recurring dream I've had, where I'm in line awaiting my own execution. Despite my terror and the absence of guards, it never occurs to me to run away. My fate is sealed, and all I can do is passively shuffle forward into the great unknown.

In much the same way, I shuffled out the airplane door.

The free fall was nothing like I imagined. It was disorienting. Utterly disorienting. Rather than the exhilaration I expected, the noisy rush had such a calming effect I slipped into a trance. Time staggered to a stop, and as for space, weightlessness made it seem like I wasn't moving at all. Instead, the earth was moving, rushing toward me at warp speed and all at once. But it wasn't just that checkerboard of newly plowed fields hurtling toward me. With time all ajangle, it felt like my checkerboard future was hurtling toward me as well. A future that, stranger still, seemed to have happened long ago.

All of this took place wordlessly, thoughtlessly, instantaneously, leaving me with the profound sense that life is really nothing like it appears to be. I don't know precisely what folks mean when they say their whole life passed before their eyes, but when I became Eliot's "still point of the turning world" hovering somewhere above Franklinton, North Carolina, I seemed to have all eternity to think about just about anything . . . and so I did.

* * *

I awoke, sat bolt upright, and rubbed my eyes. The achy dent in my back imprinted by the transmission's hump reminded me that I was in the back seat of Bud's two-year-old 1969 lime green Pontiac Le Mans. I'd been sleeping on that damn hump more or less all summer, and I vaguely wondered if that achy dent was now a permanent feature of my 19-year-old back. The sun was well up over the Atlantic, and, with doors locked and windows rolled up, the car was already hot and stuffy.

No, this ain't Nazareth, I thought. *It's Ocean City, Maryland, but I'm still feelin' about half past dead.* I'd been sleeping on those lyrics from The Band all night as well, and, smiling wryly, I decided the song's title, "The Weight," seemed to fit my mood as well. "At least it's not a cop waking me up this time," I muttered half aloud.

Reaching for the driver's bucket seat, I gave it a couple shakes, violent enough to lift Bud from his slumbers. I was so tired, hungry, and disgusted I didn't give him time to come to his senses before I lashed out.

"Bud, you finally gonna' tell me why I had to quit the first decent job either one of us had all summer? Mr. Jackson treated me like his son. I promised to work at his drug store for the rest of the summer, and I barely made my first paycheck. I was making good tips too, delivering prescriptions. By the way, what's with the cloak and dagger stuff? Why'd we leave Wildwood in such a damn rush? I don't even have my toothbrush and . . . "

"Cool it," Bud interrupted. "Your toothbrush and other crap's in the trunk. I got it out just in time. I just didn't feel like talkin' last night. Too depressed. What that rental agent failed to tell me was the house we rented is owned by the mayor. It was bad enough that every hippie in Wildwood came to our party, but when His Honor found out about all the acid, he freaked and told the cops to raid the joint. I got a tip on the street and decided that under the circumstances, an expeditious exit might be judicious."

"Wow, but how is . . ."

"Everybody's fine. No one got busted. It's a shame . . . it was that chick Diane's birthday party." Bud paused. "I hope she has another set of glasses," he said while reaching for a tiger-striped case on the dashboard. "She left these on the kitchen table. Nobody seems to know that freak who passed around all the LSD, but you gotta' admit," he grinned, "it made for a birthday party she'll never forget."

"I won't either," I added, rubbing my back again.

We were back in Ocean City hungry and destitute. The same place we started from a few Yogic yugas and a smattering of incarnations ago and in much the same condition. Or it sure felt that way. One of the things I learned, to my chagrin, during the summer of 1971 is the same kinds of adventures that later make for great bar stories aren't all that much fun when they actually happen.

I shimmied out of the backseat of the two-door Le Mans and noticed with a sigh of relief that no one was parked in front of us. Taking my all too familiar position with legs splayed and hands on the trunk as if I were about to be frisked, I shouted, "OK, let's go! And whatever you do, go easy on that damn steering wheel. Remember, it's a cripple!"

Most folks have their morning rituals. For me and Bud, working around the busted starter in that dodgy Le Mans was ours. I was no stranger to kickstarting cars, but in Pittsburgh the hills do the heavy lifting. The beach was tabletop flat. Besides, the power steering didn't work unless the engine was running, and it was manhandling our ride out of tight parking spaces that finally became too much for the cheap pot metal of the steering wheel. When the wheel finally snapped off, Bud continued to drive one-handed using the center hub left behind, but when the cops took exception to his work-around, we were forced to get the wheel, ever so precariously, braised back on.

Back in May, Bud and I set out from the Steel City for Ocean City in search of adventure and summer employment working on the local crab boats. Unfortunately, these high-paying jobs proved chimerical, and we'd been more or less hungry ever since. We eventually abandoned Ocean City and headed north for the Jersey Shore, only to find that jobs of any kind were scarce. At times we snacked on toothpaste, and I eventually lost 20 pounds. In Wildwood we ate fresh-caught crabs from the bay behind our house along with heaping sides of stale, instant mashed potatoes the previous tenants were kind enough to leave behind.

I started pushing, the stubborn wire wheels reluctantly began to whirl, and when Bud dropped the clutch in second gear that 350-cubic-inch V-8 roared to life once more. We drove around until we found a small coffee shop with a parking lot that mercifully offered me and our starterless Pontiac a slight incline to work with later. I had the check Mr. Jackson gave me for two weeks of stocking shelves, but until we could figure out how to get it cashed, a cup of tea for me and coffee for Bud was about all our collective treasury could underwrite.

I quickly got my tea and sat down in a booth, but as Bud started back from the counter, he veered off and began talking to some disembodied voices a couple booths away. When he took a seat, I walked over and discovered Bud laughing with two young women.

Ann and Nancy were college friends spending the summer at the beach. Ann was a cute, blue-eyed blonde, mischievous and fun-loving, while Nancy was a slender, shy, attractive brunette with long hair parted in the middle and remarkable green eyes. Ann was working at the local Dairy Queen while Nancy worked nights cleaning rooms at a motel. After listening to our two-month tale of mournful misadventure and hand-to-mouth living, Nancy offered to let us bunk that night in the laundry room at her motel. The following day she gave us the key to a room made available when some guests left early without checking out. The day after we moved into their cozy second-story apartment a few blocks from the beach.

By this time Ann and Bud were an item. Bud moved in with Ann, and I got the couch in the living room. Soon we established a routine. Ann worked days, and Bud took his surfboard to the beach. Nancy worked nights, and since I enjoyed her company and wasn't much of a surfer, we spent a lot of time together.

One day we were sitting on the beach watching a couple of frustrated anglers in floppy hats surf casting from a sandbar when I heard her softly sniffling.

"Nancy, what's wrong?"

"Oh, don't worry, it's nothing you said," she said, laughing away her tears. "I just start crying sometimes, and I don't really know why."

I'd learned with Nancy not to pry. Maybe it was because she was so fragile, high-strung, and reticent. Maybe it was because that beautiful, almost spiritual, melancholy that hung around her made me feel protective toward her—protective even from me.

"I've never been with a man, you know," she finally said, giving me a shy sidelong glance as she wrapped her slender arms around both knees.

"It's not that I haven't had opportunities, and it's not even that I'm saving myself for the right guy or marriage or something, though that's part of it."

It was early evening, and several seagulls were tussling over an abandoned hot dog bun a few feet away as I waited for her to go on. Eventually, she did.

"It's something my mother said. 'You know, Nancy, the terrible thing about sex is that if you love somebody . . . I mean if you really *love* somebody, you want to *merge* with that person, but you can't. Sometimes it feels so close, but in the end it's all just a tease.' I know how unhappy my mom is. I know she drinks too much, but I still can't stop thinking about what she said. And it's not just sex, there's something just *wrong* about *everything*."

"I think I know what you mean," I said excitedly while involuntarily squeezing two fistfuls of sand. "I mean, what your mother meant. I dropped acid back in Wildwood, at Diane's birthday party. Not a lot but enough to get pretty buzzed. I eventually wandered out to the end of the dock behind our house. The sky was crystal clear and speckled with about a gazillion stars. It was the most beautiful thing I've ever seen, and suddenly I wanted to *merge* with all those stars. I wanted it so bad I started jumping up and down on the dock trying to zoom up and take my rightful place among the constellations. I wasn't totally zonked. I knew what I was doing. I knew it was impossible and ridiculous, but what I was longing for was dead serious. What life's really all about was *right there,* on the tip of my tongue, but it was still as far out of reach as all those stars."

Nancy unwrapped her tanned arms, leaned back on her palms, and playfully shoveled sand with her painted toes in my direction.

"Wow, it's nice to know I'm not the only one who thinks nutty stuff like that. Ann's like a sister, but I wouldn't know how to talk to her like this."

"No, and I didn't tell Bud about jumping up and down on that stupid dock either," I said, echoing her laughter. "But you know, we're not the only lunatics around. I had this crazy experience just before I left Pittsburgh for the shore, and just like you with your mother, I can't stop thinking about it."

"Tell me about it!"

Slowly rubbing my hands together, I watched the sand trickle through my fingers as I gathered my thoughts.

Charlie was a bus driver who lived next door to my parents, I told Nancy. One day he asked me to play poker with him and his bus driver friends. I'm not much for poker, but I was flattered so I agreed to sit in.

After the game I sat down on the sofa with one of Charlie's friends. He was a bloated, unhealthy looking guy in his early thirties, with a face already ravaged by drinking. He was also a Vietnam veteran, and he quickly had me riveted with one gut-wrenching story of combat after another. His tour ended when a mortar round hit the edge of his foxhole. He woke up in the hospital deaf and blind, and he described what it was like to live for weeks in silent darkness before he finally began to recover.

There was no bravado in any of this, I added, still staring at the little pile of sand under my now empty hands. In fact, I told Nancy, what made it so trippy was his utter lack of emotion. It was like he was reading from the newspaper.

When he finished his story, he picked up his can of beer and sat studying it. Then he took a long pull.

"I miss Vietnam," he whispered hoarsely, his eyes burning. "I'd go back tomorrow if they'd have me.

"You don't get it, do you?" he snorted at the look on my face. "Listen, I was *alive* in 'Nam, man. There's no gray in 'Nam, man, no nonsense. Just you, your buddies, stayin' alive. That's it, man. People talk about intimacy, trust, love . . . bullshit! They're already dead and don't know it. You want intimacy? You want trust? You want love? Go to 'Nam, man. Go to 'Nam.

"Guys who *know* . . . one heartbeat . . . hangin' their asses out for each other every fuckin' minute of every fuckin' day provin' it. And I was one of them, man, I was one of them. There's only one fuckin' thing in 'Nam, man, and every fuckin' thing is that fuckin' thing. No hesitation, no doubts, just a single point of white-hot intensity called *life*. When you're livin' that you're *there*, man, you're *alive*, man, and you know in your gut what life's supposed to be. This," he said, waving his beer can at the walls of the room, " . . . *this* is all nothin' but phony cardboard bullshit."

28

I glanced over at Nancy, worried that the vet's language had offended her. She leaned toward me, her long brown hair now neatly tucked behind her ears. Relieved to see she was still with me, I picked up my story.

The vet suddenly seemed embarrassed by his outburst. He stopped and stared down at his beer can as he slowly crushed it in his hand.

"Look at me now," he continued without looking up. "I'm a bus driver with a wife who loves me. Yeah, she loves me all right. She loves me so much she's sendin' me to beautician school so we can open a beauty parlor. A fuckin' *beauty parlor* for Chrissake. But the joke's on her, man . . . the joke's on her . . . she don't know it, but I been dead for years. I died in 'Nam, man, I died in 'Nam. They just shipped me home without my body bag."

Without another word he drained the last dregs from his misshapen can, hoisted himself out of his seat, and lumbered out the door. I just sat there in a daze until I realized I was overstaying my welcome.

I'd been staring absently out to sea as I relived my story, but returning abruptly to the present, I noticed tears in Nancy's eyes.

"Yeah, I feel sorry for him," I said. "But I envy the hell out of him too. He saw something important. He paid an incredible price, but what I saw in him was the raw possibility of what life could be. What life's supposed to be. Somebody said God's both terrible and fascinating. God's like some terrible train wreck. He's so awful, but you can't look away. That Vietnam vet was awful. He was so terrible, but he filled me with awe. I loved him to death, I wanted to kiss his feet, but he scared me somethin' awful too."

I hesitated, and we sat silently for a minute or two immersed in our thoughts.

"But what's really bugging me," I finally told Nancy, "is wondering why he opened up to me of all people. He was like some kinda' prophet: a half-mad, alcoholic, bus-driving burning bush insisting I *do something* with my life."

I told Nancy that when the mood finally wore off, I was just totally depressed.

"It felt like the last scene in that flick *Easy Rider,* when Dennis Hopper and Peter Fonda are cruising along on their choppers and Hopper yells to Fonda, 'We blew it.' Then they both get killed. The vet left me with this overwhelming sense of just how easy it would be to blow it, to waste my life on nothin' but a lifetime of 'phony cardboard bullshit.'"

"My God, you're not going to Vietnam, are you?" Nancy blurted.

"Absolutely not!" I said laughing. "I just got my lottery number for the draft, and I'm thrilled it's high enough so I won't have to go."

"Then what are you saying?"

"I'm saying there just must be a way to find what he found and know what he knows. A way to live how he lived in Vietnam without going to war and becoming a bitter drunk. Or maybe there isn't, and I'm just jumping up and down on that stupid dock again . . . "

It was almost dark, the beach was deserted, and the squabbling seagulls had long since finished off their bun. Nancy reached over and took my hand. We sat there quietly until the incoming tide forced us to move.

* * *

Nancy's tiny gesture on the beach gave me permission to unburden myself of all the things that had been whirling around in my brain for more than a year. Over the ensuing weeks we took long walks on the beach, and her modest apartment became my private confessional as I told her about lugging my old record player to freshman English class just so I could play an album called *In Search of the Lost Chord* by the Moody Blues and riff on the "meaning" behind the lyrics. I told her about my first LSD trip, my flirtations with radical politics, of participating in antiwar and Civil Rights demonstrations, and about meeting Ralph Nader. Most of all I told her how it all left me feeling so empty and disappointed.

"I know why," Nancy told me one day while she sprawled on the floor as I sat on the edge of the sofa. "You just don't like yourself very much."

Nancy's knack for exposing the man behind the curtain stopped me cold once again. I recalled an incident from my senior year in prep school. Home on Christmas break and unable to sleep, I paced my parents' paneled basement like a father awaiting his first child until I was finally ready to admit how terribly unhappy I really was.

> ## The SDS was really just a haven for the misfits, and they were so desperate to be cool they were ready to turn the whole world upside down just so they could finally fit in.

"Yes," I finally said, "I guess I don't like myself very much."

I told Nancy about attending a meeting of the Students for a Democratic Society (SDS). I listened to their radical agenda until I suddenly realized the meeting didn't have a damn thing to do with politics. Instead, I was actually watching a coven of angry kids venting over never being invited to the cool kids' parties when they were in high school. The SDS was really just a haven for the misfits, and they were so desperate to be cool they were ready to turn the whole world upside down just so they could finally fit in.

"I never went back," I continued, "but even worse was realizing that even though I did get invited to parties, I'm just as big a phony as they are. I used to be for the Vietnam War. Now I'm against it. I even go to demonstrations. Why? Is it the right thing to do? Or is it just cool to be against the war and, God forbid, I might do anything that makes me look uncool."

Once I started questioning my political motivations, I confided to Nancy, my whole life went under the same microscope, leaving me demoralized, unsteady, and unsure of myself.

"That's one reason, anyway, why I don't like myself. I'm a complete phony. I don't have a single damn idea, thought, or emotion I know in my heart is really me. Something I didn't just pick up from my parents, my friends, my genes, a rock band, or a stupid TV set."

"My goodness, you sound like Demian!" Nancy said teasingly.

"Who?"

Nancy got up, and a few minutes later she returned with *Demian*, a book by Herrmann Hesse. She showed me this quote heavily underlined in black ink:

"All I ever wanted was to live in accordance with my own true self. Why was that so very difficult?"[4]

This quote perfectly captured my aspirations as well as my angst, and when I gushingly told Nancy this, she just smiled shyly like a little girl—a girl who is both thrilled and slightly abashed when her handmade present is so warmly received.

Several nights later, Nancy was working. I was going to bed when I noticed a book on the coffee table called *This Is It!* by Alan Watts. The next thing I knew the sun was coming up over the Atlantic Ocean and I'd read it cover to cover. Twice. I knew Nancy left it for me, but when I asked about it all she did was shyly smile.

Watts introduced me to Zen Buddhism and the idea of Satori or spiritual Enlightenment, a state the psychiatrist Richard Bucke called Cosmic Consciousness. Satori seemed to be what I was looking for. A way to experience the vet's "single point of white-hot intensity called life." A way "to live in accordance with my own true self." It was on that warm summer night in 1971 that Watts also reassured me that the same profound, almost supernatural, yearning to "become one with All That Is" that sent me jumping up and down on that stupid dock had been inspiring mystics from all the great religious traditions for thousands of years.[5]

* * *

Labor Day was rapidly approaching, and it was time to head home. Ann and Nancy insisted on accompanying us to Interstate 95 to extend our goodbyes even though it meant hitchhiking back to Ocean City. Standing on the side of a noisy road near the on-ramp, I was just beginning my final goodbye when Nancy threw her arms around my neck, told me she loved me, and burst into tears.

Overwhelmed, the next thing I knew we were speeding along I-95, and Bud couldn't stop laughing at my beet red face. Every time he got control of himself, he would glance my way and go to pieces again.

"How could you be so thick?" he finally managed to gasp. "Everybody in Ocean City but you knew how Nancy felt. Ann wanted to wise you up, but Nancy freaked out about it."

This jibe unleashed a jumble of emotions. Bud, a college friend, was two years older and a consummate ladies' man. I envied his effortless conquests which only added to the sting. Besides, I could hear my highly educated Irish mother asking me yet again why her oldest son, a "tall, good-looking, intelligent young man" couldn't seem to get a girlfriend.

Looking down at my faded jeans, I saw with fresh eyes the painstaking way in which Nancy turned them into bell-bottoms by breaking open the seams and sewing the parti-colored cloth she salvaged from discarded drapes at her motel into the gaps. Then she stenciled the denim with hand-painted "magic mushrooms" along with a psychedelic drawing of my acid-inspired electric hero, Reddy Kilowatt. The evidence was now so obvious that Bud's ridicule was more than deserved. So why didn't I see it?

It wasn't that I wasn't attracted to Nancy. On the contrary, I was very attracted to her and her big green eyes. Part of it was the fact that I found her so attractive I didn't think she could possibly be interested in *me*. But there was more to it. Every time a girl got too close, I seemed to freeze up somehow and go cold. It already happened once that summer with a buxom California girl named Betsy. Worst of all, there was something I couldn't tell Nancy and would never tell Bud. I too was a virgin, and despite the genuine feelings I had for Nancy, deep down I was relieved to be leaving whatever terrible threat her love represented behind.

So much so that I failed to keep my promise to write to her after I returned home.

Chapter Two

THE TEACHER APPEARS

O dark dark dark.
They all go into the dark,
The vacant interstellar spaces, the vacant into the vacant,
The captains, merchant bankers, eminent men of letters,
The generous patrons of art, the statesmen and the rulers,
Distinguished civil servants, chairmen of many committees,
Industrial lords and petty contractors, all go into the dark . . .
—T.S. Eliot[6]

By the time I returned to the University of Pittsburgh, I was certain that, having paid my dues as a starving beach bum, I was now a bona fide hippie, more than a match for Tim Leary or Ken Kesey. Maybe, on a good day, I might even stroll through Haight-Ashbury with Hunter S. Thompson and Jack Kerouac hanging onto my every word. I was lean, deeply tanned, and the business casual look of my freshman year had been reimagined by Nancy's magic mushroom-speckled bell bottoms, a collection of tie-dyed T-shirts, and a pair of leather sandals sporting an obligatory peace sign I picked up somewhere at the beach. My brown hair, parted in the middle, now draped over my shoulders, and in a moment of weakness I gave my new look some faux sun bleaching with a few spritzes of my mother's hair lightener.

It was an exciting time to be in college, and Pitt hummed with spiritual, political, and alternative lifestyle enthusiasms of every sort. Taking our cue from a song by the Fifth Dimension, we all eagerly awaited "The Age of Aquarius" when "peace will guide the planets and love will steer the stars." Even without the aid of that golden drop of Retsyn called LSD, the entire universe seemed to be magically shimmering just a bit in anticipation. Authenticity was at a premium, and we were forever admonishing each other to "keep it real," "tell it like it is," and "let it all hang out." Me and my friends staked out some prime real estate under the clock in the center of the student union. Meanwhile, vigorous discussions about everything from NATO to Plato popped up like more prosaic mushrooms throughout the union.

As a freshman, Russia—with its tortured artists, visionaries, revolutionaries, mystics, martyrs, and madmen—captured my imagination, and I quickly became the protégé of the Russian history department. I'd already taken all the undergraduate courses, so now, as a sophomore, I was taking graduate level courses and learning Russian. While my atheistic professors had me devouring reams of Lenin and Trotsky and writing long papers on why the abortive Russian revolution of 1905 came a cropper, I was secretly devouring everything I could get my hands on about Zen and driving my friends crazy with it. I also decided to abandon all thoughts of a career and instead take only courses I felt would help me get to the bottom of things—by which I meant, mostly, getting to the bottom of myself.

Deep down, what I wanted most was a mission. In the movie *Apocalypse Now*, Martin Sheen's character, Captain Willard, says, "I wanted a mission. And for my sins they gave me one . . . And when it was over, I never wanted another."[7] I wanted a redemptive mission too. I wanted a mission so meaningful and pure I could throw myself headlong into it without any doubts or hesitation. A mission so utterly ennobling and worthwhile that, like Willard, I'd never want another. Yet when I mustered up enough courage to take an honest look in the mirror, I saw only a frustrated young man, plagued by romantic delusions of grandeur, riddled with all the same doubts and hesitations the Vietnam vet so aptly described and so mercilessly derided.

Orysia was one of my Russian history professors. She was actually Ukrainian and her name, she told us, came from the Greek for calm or peaceful. An attractive blonde in her thirties, she shared a two-story brick house just off campus with one of her colleagues. Once a week we met at her house for a graduate-level seminar on the Russian intellectual tradition. We sat around on sofas and comfortable easy chairs in her darkly paneled and dimly lit study as Orysia, belying the etymology of her name, passionately led the discussion. At one class Orysia happened to use the word "anthropomorphic." Unfamiliar with the word, I cleverly asked a question designed to get her to use it again in another context so I could figure out what it meant. Orysia just grinned and said, "Augie, if you don't know what anthropomorphic means, just ask." The room erupted in laughter, and Orysia laughed hardest of all. I was mortified to be called out—especially in front of much older graduate students in such a rarefied setting—but two good things came of it. First, I never tried to hide my ignorance again. Second, I think my boyish attempt to hide my vulnerability drew Orysia to me.

I lingered after class one evening asking questions when she surprised me by offering a cup of tea. I could see she had something on her mind, so I waited, giving my piping cup of black tea a chance to cool. "*Chto delat*, August Augustovich?" she finally said. "*Chto delat*?" My Russian was just good enough to know that, in using my patronymic (my father's name was August as well), Orysia had just asked me, in a formal way, the quintessential Russian question. That burning, all-consuming question every Russian intellectual must answer: *What is to be done?*

Startled by her question and praying it was rhetorical, I continued to wait. "I really don't know what I'm doing anymore," she said, wearily shaking her head. "It just seems as though we're out of ideas. We've tried everything, thought everything, questioned everything, and here we are, like Omar Khayyam, just as empty and confused about life as we ever were."

Deeply flattered to be taken into her confidence, I wanted to suggest Cosmic Consciousness, but I didn't dare. Several weeks earlier I brought up Alan Watts with one of my philosophy professors, a man I admired, only to have him smile indulgently and roll his eyes. Losing my nerve, I played it safe.

"What about that Einstein quote you mentioned? 'No problem can be solved at the same level of consciousness at which it is posed.' What if that's our big mistake? What if trying to solve philosophical questions with philosophy is impossible? It's like trying to lift something off the ground while standing on it. Maybe we need a breakthrough, a whole new level of consciousness, a completely new way of thinking about stuff."

I was instantly embarrassed. What was intended as a thoughtful reply had actually been blurted out in a stream of what sounded, to me, like raw, grade-A, post-adolescent enthusiasm.

Smiling slightly, Orysia arched a bemused eyebrow that wordlessly said: OK, I'll bite. Go on.

Completely flustered, whatever I did manage to say was deeply unsatisfactory, even embarrassing, and I spent the next week or so berating myself for not having the guts to tell Orysia what was really on my mind.

* * *

One week prior to my conversation with Orysia, I'd been visiting some college friends at their off-campus house when there was a knock at the door. The knocker was looking for his younger brother.

His brother was out with the other guys getting beer, but when I said they were expected shortly, he decided to wait. Jay was a good-looking guy, blond, six feet, about thirty, and somehow we soon fell into a serious discussion. Suddenly he sprang to his feet and began pacing up and down the living room floor. He must have paced for several minutes, deeply agitated. Finally, he stopped dead.

"I'm going to tell you something," he said with so much vehemence he startled me. "I'm going to tell you something I've never told anyone. Not even my wife."

He took a few more turns across the floor, sending hectic shadows whirling all over the walls.

"I own the parking concession for some five-star restaurants," he said, continuing to pace. "I hire guys to chase cars and collect tips. They work by the hour, and I keep the difference. One night some guy stuck a gun in my ribs and, before I could give him my cash, he pulled the trigger."

Jay went on to describe what has since become a textbook "NDE" or Near-Death Experience. He watched the medical team working on him from the ceiling of the operating room, heard them screaming, "We're losing him, we're losing him!" and made the journey through the tunnel toward the "white light" calling him "home." But just before he merged with the light, he was reminded of unfinished business and sent back. He later learned that his heart stopped for several minutes on the operating table, and every detail he witnessed from the ceiling actually transpired.

I don't know whether I was more amazed by his incredible story or his remarkable transformation. In a scant few minutes, he went from an affable, relaxed, blue-collar kind of guy to a man who seemed enveloped in a Pentecostal fire that raged without consuming. After his story he resumed his silent pacing among the shadows for another minute or two. When he turned to me again, the fire had been replaced by so much pure anguish I was drawn and repelled at the same time.

"What am I supposed to do?" he screamed. "I don't belong here. I don't want to be here. If I could only tell you what it was like . . . nothing matters anymore. . . . Nothing matters—except for God . . . "

As if amazed at the words that just popped from his mouth, he slowly repeated "Except for God" in a voice that trailed off to a whisper. Then he sat down on the couch and wept.

I'd like to say I comforted him, or tried to, but I just sat there stunned in an old overstuffed chair that one of my friends rescued from a one-way ride to a landfill.

Finally, he looked up and said, "The hardest part is I can't tell anyone. Who'd believe me? They'd say I'm nuts. I can't even tell my wife."

NDE experiences like his were virtually unknown at the time, but I didn't think he was nuts. I believed every word. Despite his agony, or maybe because of it, I was overwhelmed with a sense of beauty and wonder, a supernatural sense of horror mixed with ecstasy. Most of all, I wanted that white light. I wanted to merge with Jay's white light just like I wanted to merge with all those glittering stars back in Wildwood.

I also couldn't help but wonder why, just like the Vietnam veteran, Jay chose *me*, a kid, a perfect stranger, someone he met only minutes before, for his terrible secret. If the vet was a prophetic burning bush, Jay was the ghost of Hamlet's father: a ghost fresh from the Other Side urgently imploring me to remember *why* I was here and what life expected of me. Jay's agonizing question, "What am I supposed to do?" so neatly echoed the question nagging at my own heart it felt like a gut punch.

I really wanted to tell Orysia about Jay's experience. She gave me my opening. She even paved the way by opening up to me first. Then she hit me over the head with Russia's version of Jay's same damn question: *What is to be done?* But just like with Nancy's love, fear once again paralyzed me. I was terrified that, rather than therapeutic, opening up to Orysia would only allow all the chaotic emotions buffeting me to well up and overwhelm my makeshift defenses. Instead,

I told Jay's story to no one, and though his brother and I remained friends for several years, I never saw Jay again.

* * *

What I found so fascinating about Jay and the Vietnam vet is that they had, each in his own way, *seen through life.* They both discovered that behind that phony cardboard cutout we usually take for reality there is something more real, magical, and infinitely more important. I remember lying in my bed in my basement bedroom as a boy staring intently into the pitch-black darkness hovering right above my nose. If I just had a knife sharp enough, I thought, I could slice that inky blackness open, shove my head through the crack, and see what was on the other side. As Captain Ahab says to his first mate Starbuck in Melville's *Moby Dick,* "All visible objects, man, are but as pasteboard masks." For half-mad, Heaven-storming Ahab to "strike through the mask" is the only damn thing worth doing regardless of cost.

Of course, there is a price to pay for seeing through life, and that price is paid in painful disillusionment. The cardboard construct the vet so despised does have its uses as well as its charms: its mind-numbing, ersatz, superficiality provides a wonderful buffer against all the terrible truths about life and ourselves we would rather not face.

At the ripe old age of 19, I was seeing through life as well, but rather than Jay's white light or the Vet's single point of white-hot intensity, I was merely seeing through myself, and these insights were far less spectacular—and about to get much darker.

* * *

I grew up on a one-mile circular cul-de-sac in the suburbs of Pittsburgh. My family lived in one of those 950-square-foot cookie-cutter ranch houses that sprang up all over America after World War II; my parents bought it new in 1954, two years after I was born.

Six brothers and a sister rapidly followed suit, which kept my college educated but chronically underpaid white-collar dad busy buying bunk beds, building basement bedrooms, working second jobs, clipping coupons, and endlessly shuttling back and forth to the grocery store.

As a boy I was a big, gregarious, outgoing kid. I walked to Catholic school, did well in my studies and in sports, and was popular with my teachers and fellow students. At 13 I won a scholarship to an exclusive New England boarding school called The Hotchkiss School. Yet despite the fact that my blue-eyed, rambunctious resemblance to central casting's beau ideal of the "all-American boy" probably helped me get into Hotchkiss, as well as later in life, my own taste in friends often led me to introverts, eccentrics, bookworms, and a string of high-strung, hyper-smart, highly opinionated Jewish deep thinkers.

Chip was an introverted, eccentric, non-Jewish product of our local public high school who turned me on to smoking pot, dropping acid, and the writing of Richard Brautigan, Marshal McLuhan, Buckminster Fuller, Thomas Pynchon, and J.R.R. Tolkien. Small, even slight, he probably only weighed 120 pounds, and his frail body, blue eyes, extremely fair skin, and almost white-blond hair gave him an ethereal, almost diaphanous, look. Extremely artistic, meticulous to a fault, Chip was as visual as I was not, despite his circular wire rim glasses that were so thick they suggested he was probably legally blind without them, which in fact he was.

Introduced by a mutual friend, Chip was three years older, and I soon discovered he was also a self-taught architect, obsessively creating drawings in his parents' basement of Fuller's geodesic domes and the Bilbo Baggins-inspired "Hobbit hole" he intended to inhabit someday. Chip combined all this marvelous eccentricity with a self-deprecating, impish sense of humor that included cheerfully acknowledging that a homemade Hobbit hole was the ideal habitat for a man who bore more than a passing resemblance to an actual Hobbit. Even after I started college, Chip and I remained close. I introduced him to my college friends at Pitt, and when, one year later, in the fall of 1972, Bud and I moved into a five-bedroom house off campus, I was thrilled when he and the others insisted on offering Chip a room.

When I returned from my summer at the beach in 1971, Chip was still living with his parents in another red brick ranch house about a mile from ours. His younger brother was in the Navy, home on leave, and one night Chip invited me to the bachelor party they were throwing for another sailor while their parents were out of town. We all dropped LSD, and Chip's brother put on an X-rated film just to see what watching porn on acid would be like. Soon he had every moveable mirror in the house cluttering up the living room as he bounced the flick from mirror to mirror and from there to the walls and ceiling creating, as he did, quite the phantasmagoric, 3D hologram of pornographic psychedelia.

The overall effect was high frat boy hilarity, and then somebody asked me to call the radio station and request a song. I called but the phone just rang and rang. Then the ringing seemed to move inside my head and become louder, faster, and more insistent. Alarmed, I slammed down the phone—but the ringing didn't stop.

Starting to panic, I went out on the front porch and stretched out on the cold concrete. It started to rain on the aluminum awning above my head, and as the rain pounded harder and harder and louder and louder, it seemed to be just an outward manifestation of that insistent phone ringing in my head. The ringing rain built to a thunderous crescendo until, just when I thought it was about to swamp my sanity, it would reset and start building again. *Something* was insisting I answer this phone, and I was terrified to find out who or what was on the other end of the line.

Staggering to my feet, I stumbled out into the storm and walked for miles through dark, deserted suburban streets, desperately trying to walk off this nightmare. I finally collapsed from exhaustion on someone's front lawn in the pouring rain, only to have the police pull up. The shock of their arrival seemed to straighten me up, and I managed to talk my way out of it. But when I awoke the next day, that same sense of dark, impending doom was still there in the pit of my stomach.

> Rather than give way to these irrational fears, however, I just gritted my teeth and forced myself to adhere to my daily schedule. Of course, true to form, I was ashamed of my weakness.

Over the next six months this darkness would reemerge without warning, and every time it did, I had to fight it off or give way to panic. I became agoraphobic, afraid to go out for fear I would panic in public. Rather than give way to these irrational fears, however, I just gritted my teeth and forced myself to adhere to my daily schedule. Of course, true to form, I was ashamed of my weakness and told no one about these episodes.

I abandoned drugs altogether, and eventually these anxiety attacks tapered off and went away. Yet when they did, they left a dark residue, and I listlessly went through my normal routine with the sense that nothing really mattered. My worldview became an empty, shadowy moonscape without any real substance or meaning. Terrified that the enveloping emptiness that drove me out into the rain would return to swallow me up, my reading on mystical spirituality in general and Zen in particular became obsessive. I was like a man given up for dead, poring over dusty medical journals, looking for a treatment or antidote his doctors overlooked.

One day I was sitting on the sofa reading a book on Zen by Christmas Humphreys. Finishing, I felt the same way I always did. Something utterly magical, that indescribable answer I was looking for, was right *there* on the tip of my tongue—but I just couldn't seem to grasp it.

"That's it," I said to myself in frustration. "I've been reading instead of doing. I have to start doing, and to hell with reading. But how do I begin? Where will I find a teacher?" Then I threw the book against the wall.

If I'd obeyed the first rule of Zen and been paying attention, or the first rule of Christianity and had faith, perhaps I would've noticed what jumped out at me when I came across that same book many years later. There, on the first page, was an inscription, a teaching common to all mystical traditions, which I'd read many times before:

"When the pupil is ready the teacher appears."[8]

* * *

One day I got a call from my friend Ray. "There's some Zen guy speaking at the Theosophical Society on Sunday. Wanna' go?" he said in his almost preternaturally deep voice.

I'd known Ray since first grade. He was my partner in crime in countless boyhood capers, and now we were hot for Zen Buddhism with its mystical tales of Zen masters, Samurai warriors, paradoxical riddles called koans and, most of all, the cosmic experience of Absolute Reality that Zen calls Satori.

For my part, I was captivated by Zen's clean, pragmatic approach to spirituality. Zen takes a dim view of theology, dogma, and rituals. Zen, more a system of self-exploration than a religion, is based on the intuitive argument that the One True Self and Absolute Reality are one and the same. Better still, I thought at the time, even this intuitive argument isn't accepted unequivocally "on faith." Everything in Zen, even the goal of Zen practice, Satori, is merely a working hypothesis. All Zen's concepts are just provisional starting points like the given statements in a geometry proof.

Zen insists that no theological or metaphysical assumption is true until it is validated through experience. The only way we can really understand romantic love, for example, is by falling in love. Similarly, Zen argues that the only way to know whether Cosmic Consciousness or God exists is through mystical experience. Are God and Satori the same thing? To this a Zen master might politely smile and say, "When you reach the Truth, be sure to come back and tell me. For now, I have a question: just exactly *who* is asking me this question? When you answer my question, you will answer your own."

So when Ray called about a Zen lecture, I eagerly signed on. I spent the intervening days disconcerted by an exciting sense of anticipation that, despite my best efforts, I couldn't suppress. I knew I was setting myself up for a letdown, but I was helpless to do anything about it.

* * *

Ray was driving, and on Sunday I rode my barely street-legal dirt motorcycle over to his cookie-cutter red brick ranch house that was almost identical to my own. There, another grade school friend, Steve, met us, and we climbed three abreast onto the bench seat of Ray's old, faded green Chrysler Imperial his uncle gave him. I was sitting at the passenger window with my motorcycle helmet on my lap. Somehow, Ray neglected to get precise directions to the Theosophical Society, and when we reached downtown Pittsburgh, we found ourselves driving around looking for the place.

There were a fair number of people on the sidewalks, and passing a corner I saw two men engaged in conversation. Both appeared to be in their fifties and were neatly dressed in sport jackets, slacks, and open collar shirts. One was short, stocky, and wearing a fedora while the other was tall, bareheaded, and of average build. Without thinking, I pointed at the fedora and screamed, "Stop the car! That's him!" before jumping from the still-moving car in mid-traffic.

Even so I found myself almost a block beyond the men, and in my excitement still carrying my helmet. Reaching the sidewalk, I turned back and began walking. As I closed in on the strangers, they stopped talking and stared at me with such bold curiosity it made me uncomfortable. I suddenly realized I had no hard evidence these men had anything to do with the lecture, let alone that one was the speaker. But it was too late now, and putting on my best face, I walked up and asked a question that would not prove too embarrassing if my intuition was completely wrong.

"Is this where the Zen lecture is being held?"

The tall one nodded, "Yes."

"Tell me something," the stocky man under the fedora said. "Do you think this Zen fellow can help you?"

Suddenly there was a lump in my throat. "I sure as hell hope so."

With that he erupted into a loud peal of laughter, stuck out his hand, and in a gravelly voice exaggerated for emphasis, said, "The name's Rose."

I stared into the most amazing set of clear, ice-blue eyes I've ever seen. It was as if I'd tumbled into a hall of magic mirrors. These eyes simultaneously sucked me in by their warm invitation and pushed me away by the way they were looking straight through me, out the back of my head, and on into God-knows-what.

This push/pull hard on the heels of his personal question and my emotional answer knocked me mentally off balance. I shivered and a spark jumped between us, an electric jolt that stunned me and drained every thought from my head. Startled and afraid, all I could do was just stand there with one of those stupid smiles people get when being addressed in a language they don't understand.

Still a bit shaken, the next thing I remember is sitting next to my helmet, directly in front of the speaker, in an otherwise deserted first row in a large rectangular room full of folding chairs. The room, smelling sweetly of incense, had that Oriental, occult, esoteric feel which has always made me vaguely uncomfortable.

Richard Rose was like a close-up on a giant TV looming just above my head. He leaned nonchalantly on the podium, watching the seats fill, and occasionally met my eyes with a broad grin. He was no more than five-foot-seven, powerfully built, with a round, completely bald head. Even though I later learned he was of German/Irish extraction, his slight paunch and almost Asian folds at the corners of his eyes suggested the Buddha in a cream-colored sport jacket. Since the few lines in his otherwise smooth, round face were obviously etched there by laughter, I decided he looked like a laughing Buddha at that.

He spoke without notes or microphone and started the lecture by leaning both elbows on the podium. With a friendly smile and open curiosity, he began inspecting the audience, happily meeting the gaze of anyone who cared to take him up on the offer. It was as if he was looking for some long-lost relative, and his smile was his way of asking permission to conduct his search. He was in no hurry and so relaxed he could've been snugly situated behind a two-way mirror. As the seconds ticked by, his close inspection seemed to build tension and settle the audience all at the same time.

"Well, I don't know what you folks had to pay to see this circus," he began.

"Two bucks," I blurted loudly, embarrassing myself.

"Wow," he said arching his eyebrows and pursing his lips, "that's indecent. I'm from West Virginia, and back home only the governor commands that kind of money. Hell, the last one's in jail right now for commanding only half that much. In bribes. For two bucks I better deliver. By the way, where's the back door to this joint?"

The audience laughed, me hardest of all. I laughed so hard, in fact, that Rose, looking over my head at the rest of the audience, pointed at me, eyes a-twinkle, and said, "He liked that."

"Anyway," he continued when we all settled down again, "as payin' customers, I guess you got a right to hear somethin' you don't already know. So I'm going to start by sharing a secret. A secret only a few people really know, and them that do paid with their lives, one way or the other, for the privilege."

We all leaned forward, and Rose softly said, "Someday you're all going to die."

The audience tried to titter but, failing to pull it off, fell silent.

"You're all going to die someday," he repeated after a moment or two. "But you think you're going to live forever, and that's your first mistake. You're livin' like sleepwalkers dreamin' you're awake, and despite your pretensions you're driven mainly by instinct—aimlessly bumping your way through life like cattle, oblivious to the fact that all cow paths lead to one place: the slaughterhouse.

"You don't know who you *really* are, where you came from, or where you're goin', and as a result you know nothing. You were pushed off a cliff at birth, and you're desperately hangin' onto all the debris falling around you as if all that debris will make a damn bit of difference when you hit the ground. You think that debris insulates you and makes you safe, and that's your second mistake."

Again he hesitated and, staring down at the podium, seemed lost in his own thoughts. "The real score is you'll never know anything until you know Everything, and you come to Everything by letting go of all that debris, especially the debris you built your life on and cherish most. This kind of debris usually begins with the words 'I believe.'

"Belief and twenty-five cents will get you a cup of coffee where I come from, because the only thing worth real money is what you *know*. Down through history, folks a lot smarter than me came up with a name for letting go of all the BS—for the kind of *unknowing* that leads to the only *knowing* worth a tinker's damn, and they come from all over the world and every religion on earth. They call it dyin' while livin.'

"To die while living is the only thing that matters, and it's a life's work, and if any of this scares you, I'm earnin' your two bucks. Because plain truth is, you're in a tight spot. That clock on the wall is running down, and the older you get the louder it ticks, and whether you want to admit it or not your salvation lies in facing your worst nightmare before that hearse pulls into the driveway. And your worst nightmare is that somewhere deep in your gut you know the person you like to think you are isn't who you are at all. You gotta' let go of all your foolish games, face this nightmare square, and come out the other side. And you gotta' do it right here and right now.

"Anyone with any hope of helping you must remind you of that nightmare as well. So to the best of my feeble ability, I intend to spend my time today tryin' my best to do just that. And with a little luck, for my trouble, you'll send me back to West Virginia with the head I brung still firmly attached."

Nothing about this lecture was what I expected. I expected some impassive Asian guy with an inscrutable smile sitting cross-legged on a raised dais in flowing robes, saying little, and occasionally sipping tea from a tiny Chinese porcelain cup while radiating compassion and gentle acceptance from his beaming brow.

Instead I got the smoldering intensity of a man of unswerving conviction and straight talk. Rose was a ball-peen hammer of a man. A man who knew exactly what he was about and was happily getting on with it, the rest of the world be damned. I never imagined such spontaneity, freedom, raw conviction, and fearless audacity was possible, and here it was all wrapped up in just the kind of irreverent, almost wicked, sense of humor I found irresistible.

> Rose was a ball-peen hammer of a man. A man who knew exactly what he was about and was happily getting on with it, the rest of the world be damned.

Rose was at his best taking questions. With fearless spontaneity he jumped from one to the next. Soon, as if thoroughly rehearsed, the audience wasn't even raising their hands but simply chiming in, one on top of the next. The result was a *bang! bang! bang!* of questions from all over the room that had Rose ratcheting around the podium like some Kung Fu master whirling to parry the lunge of each fresh opponent.

Rose was elaborating on the subject of self-knowledge and its relation to Enlightenment when a man in his late thirties suddenly interrupted. "Do you know who *you* are?" he shouted.

Rose leaned toward the man, seated perhaps three rows away, and quietly said, "Yes."

"Well, who the hell are you, then?" the man yelled in triumph.

"Me?" Rose said evenly and instantly. "I'm the clerk at the Waldorf Astoria."

The room erupted in laughter, leaving the heckler flushed and twisting in his seat. Rose for once didn't join in. He just gazed at the man with almost fatherly concern. The room became quiet, the man squirmed even more, and finally Rose spoke again, this time softly.

"There was a famous Shakespearean actor who specialized in Shylock. He would work himself up to such a fever pitch that when he hit the stage, he damn well *was* Shylock.

"But after each performance he had a heck of a time rememberin' he wasn't Shylock after all. Two stagehands would walk him up and down the alley behind the theatre shouting into each ear: 'You're not Shylock, you're John Brown. You're not Shylock, you're John Brown.' These stagehands kept shouting, feedin' him whiskey, and slapping him around, until by and by he'd wake up and remember who he really was.

"So I'll tell you who I am. I'm nobody. I'm nothin' but a hillbilly stagehand. I'm here, if you'll let me, to walk you up and down all those dark alleys deep in your mind. All the while I'll be screaming in your mind's ear: 'You're not Joe Blow, God's gift to women . . . You're not Joe Blow, chairman of the board . . . You're not Joe Blow, scared, empty, alone . . . You're not Joe Blow at all . . . you're *God*.'"

His final words caught the room flat-footed. A stunned silence descended. Suddenly there were tears running down the heckler's cheeks. Tears he didn't seem to notice or care to wipe away. Rose waited with an almost otherworldly look on his face. Then he whispered: "That ego you're defending is a coward. Let him die."

Then he grabbed the empty chair next to me, turned it around, and sat down. I don't know how long we sat. All I remember is the room seemed electrically charged. Rose finally looked up from his clasped hands and said, just loud enough to be heard, "Words mean nothing."

He stood up, and the lecture was over.

* * *

I remained seated after the lecture, lost in my impressions, watching the others file out. They spoke little and seemed slightly dazed by the mystical mood which still hung heavily in the room. Occasionally someone would walk up to Rose, shake his hand, softly say a few words, and continue on his way. Noticing that Rose was beginning to gather up his things, I jumped to my feet and took his hand. But before I could say anything, I noticed the heckler Rose moved to tears. Intent on avoiding Rose, he was using a little knot of people for interference as he beelined for the door.

Perplexed by this behavior, I turned back toward Rose. Not only was I still stupidly holding onto his hand, Rose was happily enjoying my obvious consternation.

"Don't be too hard on him," he said, still grinning. "He ain't half bad as people go. He just got a glimpse of the chaos. For a split-second he saw how thin the ice under his feet really is. He'll go home, have a couple of beers, and by tomorrow he'll be sure it was all because of somethin' he ate."

I didn't understand this at all, and it must've been written all over my face, because his grin broke into a chuckle.

"Let me tell you something," he said, no longer smiling. "Real spirituality ain't no lark. It's serious business. I've never seen that man before, but I know him to his shoelaces. He's pushin' forty, got three or four kids runnin' him ragged, a big mortgage, a job he hates, and a wife who's all business."

Reaching for his brown, horn-rimmed glasses still on the podium, Rose jammed them carelessly caseless into the inside pocket of his jacket as he continued his critique.

"He came today to be entertained and have his spiritual vanity flattered. When my lecture as much as told him—to his face—he was kiddin' himself, it pissed him off and he took a swing at me. Then our minds locked, he brushed up against what's spiritually possible, and he wanted it more than air.

"But now he also knows what livin' it would cost, and that's why he ran out the door, and is still runnin'. Authentic spirituality means *change*, reordering priorities, flushin' the bullshit, maybe even tellin' off the boss. But that would play hob with his precious normality, so it scares him half to death. Hell, it's like the poor fellow took a trip to the zoo, fell in love with a couple of bear cubs, and just for a moment there toyed with takin' 'em home with him. Then he imagined the look on his wife's face and decided again' it." Rose finished with another chuckle.

What struck me about this little speech, even more than the fact that it was so obviously accurate, was the conversational way Rose delivered it, as if it were common knowledge and nothing special. He reinforced this impression by continuing to gather up his things in preparation for departure.

"How do you know all that?" I blurted.

"A better question might be why don't *you* know all that?" he replied without looking at me. Then, turning to go, he said, "Like the Zen master said to the student who asked him to define Zen: 'Attention!' I just pay attention, and you should too."

Then he was walking toward the door. I hesitated for a second and ran him down.

"Mr. Rose," I said, stammering. "This was incredible, thank you so much. Are all your lectures so intense?"

"Don't mention it," he replied, both pleased and slightly embarrassed by my boyish enthusiasm. "You ain't seen nothin'. Back in West

Virginia this wouldn't even pass for a sideshow. We got some real cir-cuses down there, and they stay at it 'round the clock. As for 'all my lectures,' we'll have to wait and see if they have me back. This was my first one."

"How do I learn more?" I said, fearful I'd never see him again.

"Well, if it strikes your fancy, come down to visit. I live outside of Wheeling. It ain't far, no more'n sixty miles, I'd say."

Chapter Three

ROSE'S KITCHEN

The wounded surgeon plies the steel
That questions the distempered part;
Beneath the bleeding hands we feel
The sharp compassion of the healer's art
Resolving the enigma of the fever chart.

Our only health is the disease
If we obey the dying nurse
Whose constant care is not to please
But to remind us of our, and Adam's curse,
And that, to be restored, our sickness must grow worse.
—T.S. Eliot[9]

The following Saturday, me, Ray, and his old Chrysler set out for West Virginia, taking Interstate 79 South as far as Washington, Pennsylvania, before catching I-70 West for Wheeling. After considerable soul-searching, we gave away our tickets to a sold-out rock concert to accommodate Rose's schedule, and now, we smugly decided, we'd just successfully navigated our first great spiritual trial.

(Steve said little after the lecture and declined to join our Wheeling expedition. Not long afterward I lost track of him. Many years later a mutual friend put us back in touch through email. I couldn't resist asking about Rose and that first lecture. This was his succinct reply:

"We went downtown to a crowded hall with green folding chairs [how's that for memory?], where a tiny Indian man struck a chime and said, 'Mr. Reeechard Rose.' Mr. Rose was frightening, so much so that even though I knew what he said was critically important, I put it out of my mind. I'm not sure what happened next, but one morning I woke up to find a wife, four kids, a house, and minivan that apparently all belonged to me. The rest, as they say, is history.")

When Ray and I reached Wheeling, we took the bypass toward Benwood, where Rose lived. Benwood turned out to be a dilapidated little steel town huddled next to a series of abandoned mills along the Ohio River about five miles from Wheeling. It was heavily stained with the coal soot of better days and wedged tightly between the river and the elevated bypass carved into the face of a mountain. Marshall Street was the main drag, and we quickly found the address we were looking for: 1686. Following Rose's instructions, we parked across the street in the gravel lot of a coal dust-blackened junior high that looked like it predated the Great Depression.

Everything was depressing, so much so that even though it was an incredibly hot summer morning and Ray's car had no A/C, we stared glumly at Rose's house. We saw nothing to cheer us up. Rose lived in a sagging, two-story, asphalt shingle-sided house that needed a coat of paint and just about everything else. The house stood recessed into a hillside that backed up to the bypass and was sitting on a shuttered street-level storefront. The store windows bore the faded scars of a white stenciled sign too sparse to read and were so dirty inside and out that, though we worked at it a while, we could see nothing inside. On the door was a faded poster with a smiling face urging "Sberna for Chief." What kind of chief Sberna was running for the poster didn't say, though by its age I could see the issue was long decided.

We soon realized we were stalling, and we began climbing the concrete steps beside the store that took us in turn to four or five sway-back wooden steps that carried us to the house's front porch. Knocking at the screen door, we were surprised when a woman of about forty appeared.

"What do you want?" she said in a tone so clipped it was almost angry.

"We're looking for Richard Rose."

"He isn't here. He went to sell a car. You can come in and wait if you want."

She unlatched the door and led us down a dark, carpetless hallway until we reached the first door on the right. She gestured us in, saying, "You can wait here." The door closed and we heard footsteps retreating down the hall. Then, except for the sharp ticking of a clock somewhere in the room, silence.

The lofty 12-by-15-foot room was dark, musty, and hot as an oven, and it took a moment for my eyes to adjust. The only window facing the street was shut and heavily curtained, and the fireplace with the ticking clock on the mantle was bricked up and retrofitted with an old-fashioned gas space heater, which mercifully was off. Along the back wall was an old couch with mismatched cushions, and in one corner loomed a huge, darkly stained piece of ornately carved furniture with a full-length mirror attached. Squinting, I decided it was some kind of antique combination fold-down bed and wardrobe. In the opposite corner was a rocking chair facing a small writing table, and next to the rocker a table and freestanding lamp. The only other artificial light was provided by a chandelier hanging by a fraying cord from the high ceiling. Thickly strewn around the room were spiritual books, several open and upside down to mark the page, and on the writing table was an open notebook with a pen in the crease.

The overall effect was spooky, as if we stumbled into the garret of some cranky old alchemist; neglected, maligned, misunderstood, and bitterly blaming the small minds of the modern world for his isolation. Ray and I gingerly took a seat on the couch and sat there intimidated, sweating, and listening to the clock.

Finally, Ray whispered, "Who do you think that woman was?"

"I dunno. Probably his landlady."

"Maybe, but if she is, he must be a coupla' months back on the rent. She wasn't too friendly. Maybe we should've told her we'd just come . . ."

Suddenly Rose burst in. While he obviously didn't expect to find us in his room, his initial surprise soon morphed into a wide grin.

"The hell you say!" he roared and, pumping our hands, said, "When'd you hit town?"

"We've been here about twenty minutes," I said. "Your landlady let us in."

Rose's eyes widened and he began laughing so hard he had to bend over and cross his arms around his belly. "Landlady?" Then, stammering out a pretty fair imitation of a vaudeville comedian, he added, "That ain't no landlady, that's my wife!"

My heart sank. I hate to admit it, but I found this news distressing. I was already well into constructing my mythology around Rose, and while I could work in the crank alchemist, he definitely wasn't supposed to be married.

I didn't have time to think about it much because Rose pulled up a chair, sat down, and merrily began chatting away. It was so hot in that room I could barely breathe, and this made me wonder what the hell Rose was doing in a heavy, long-sleeved lumberjack shirt over a T-shirt. I studied him closely for a sign the heat was getting to him, but finding none I was beginning to despair of getting out alive . . . when he stood up.

"What do you fellas think? What say we pack us a lunch and head out to the farm? I can show you around and we can get some privacy. My 16-year-old son makes me feel like I'm roomin' with a tornado. I'm surprised we've been alone this long. I've never seen such energy," he added, shaking his bald head. "I bought him a bicycle, paid good money for it too, and he ran it to the rims insida' three weeks. I kid you not, three weeks."

At the mention of a farm my heart leaped. This was more like it. Rose led us into the kitchen and introduced us to his wife, Phyllis, who was just leaving for work in her nurse's uniform. Fifteen years younger than Rose, she was of average height and build, and later I learned that her year-round tan and wide nose supporting her glasses came from Cherokee ancestors on her mother's side. She displayed none of the coldness we first experienced and came across instead as a lively, sarcastic, rough-and-tumble country girl. She was inordinately fond of wisecracks and was soon good-naturedly exchanging them with her husband, easily giving as good as she got.

As we chatted with Phyllis, Rose made our box lunch. He started with one of those two-pound loaves of artificially colored and flavored wax that bears a passing resemblance to cheese. It was Chef's Delight. I was familiar with it, and by way of comparison, I considered Velveeta a delicacy. Using a butcher knife, he cut six or eight wide slabs, folded them into single slices of white sandwich bread, wrapped the results in wax paper, and stuffed them into a brown paper shopping bag. That was lunch, and so, in short order, we were ready to go.

Rose led us back to the junior high parking lot, to an old rundown black Oldsmobile with Ohio plates. The back seat was full of tools and assorted junk, and I climbed into the front seat with Rose. Ray decided to follow us out so we wouldn't have to retrace our steps before heading back to Pittsburgh. Rose turned the key, and after a few coughs the car came to life with a roar so loud it startled me. We sat there for a few moments with Rose gunning the engine.

"She ain't much to look at," Rose shouted over the roar, "but I got her for two hundred dollars about two years ago and she's been a good car. The muffler's shot and that's why she makes so much noise, but she's got a big motor and actually ain't too bad on gas."

In the time it took to make these comments, we were already heading up the steep mountain road that led under the bypass and out of

Benwood. Rose kept the Olds floored, and we roared along at a considerable pace. The road snaked around the mountain, had no guardrails, was barely two car widths wide, and when the cliffs were on my side all I could see was air. Though I considered myself something of a thrill seeker, I was rattled by the way he drove. He continually shaved the inside lane on the way into curves and churned up showers of stones from the paper-thin shoulder on his way out.

At first he made me so nervous I had a hard time keeping up with the nonstop stories he tossed out over the engine's noise. Every house, cemetery, country store, and little village we passed seemed to have a tale to tell, and no matter what was bearing down on us from the other side of a blind curve, I was going to hear them all. They were hilarious, and Rose, much to my delight, seemed to enjoy them most of all. Soon, despite his driving, I was too busy laughing to think much about it.

After a thirty-minute ride we emerged on a narrow dirt road redolent with the old motor oil the state road crew sprayed to keep the dust down. We passed one last overgrown cemetery and then a long tangle of blackberry bushes that, to my amazement, were trying to conceal a rusting bulldozer. Just shy of a white farmhouse, Rose pulled into a little grass-covered lot and killed the engine.

"This is my family's farm," Rose said, pointing through the windshield with a stubby index finger. "I got hold of it when my folks passed on. There's 186 acres, but you can see it's mostly hills and timber. The first settlers came from Virginia, George Washington owned land hereabouts, and they took the fertile fields along the river bottoms. When the German and Irish immigrants, my people, got here, all that was left was ridges like this. I got the farmhouse rented. It don't bring in much, but it keeps the local hell-raisers from shootin' out the windows when they're drunk and lookin' for somethin' to do.

"C'mon. I got a trailer parked over there I use when I come out."

We emerged just as Ray pulled up. Luckily, Rose had given him directions because we easily left him behind. Catching my eye, Ray signaled his opinion of Rose's driving by arching his eyebrows and shrugging his shoulders.

Rose's farm was classic West Virginia. The white, two-story, clapboard farmhouse faced the road, had porches front and back, and seemed deserted except for three obligatory old refrigerators on the front porch. It was obviously very old, and the back porch was screened by heavy, corrugated lime-green plastic to protect the denizens from winter winds. On our side of the house in the unfenced yard was a round, stone-lined cistern to capture rainwater, a huge Sycamore shade tree, and behind that an old storage cabin. Beside the cabin was a chicken coop full of cackling chickens, and on the other side of the house a lean-to shed full of so much firewood it was clear the house lacked central heat. Twenty yards in front of us was an old, small, brown trailer with rounded ends precariously perched on flat dry-rotted tires and cement blocks, and beyond that, a concrete block outhouse.

The land sloped away from the road gradually into a tangled field of scrub brush and half-grown locust trees that apparently had once been farmed. In the far-right corner of this field, just shy of the tree line, was a dusty, hollowed-out area harboring fifteen or twenty junk cars, an old road grader missing a front wheel with a spider web bullet hole in the windshield, and several rusting school buses up on blocks.

"Free enterprise, hillbilly style," Rose said following our eyes and chuckling. "That's a half-built racetrack that a couple guys were sure would make us rich. All that's left of them days of delusion and high promise is that gimpy grader, the bulldozer, and this sawmill here. We cut oak trees right off the farm and sawed them into planks for bleachers. They're stacked and rotting away down along the track as something of a monument to human folly. I think they call it being undercapitalized," he finished, grinning.

"What sawmill, Mr. Rose?" I asked.

Rose led us toward the blackberry tangle along the road. There, hidden from view, were the rusting remains of a small sawmill. It was powered by an old car up on blocks with a drive belt wrapped around the right rear wheel rim in lieu of a tire.

The whole place had that neglected, junky, tumbledown feel that inspires so many jokes at West Virginia's expense. But to a city boy and hopeless romantic intoxicated by Rose, it was something completely different. I saw a crumbling, moss-covered Camelot littered with iron-clad knights that a wicked sorcerer turned into car-like statues ages ago. There they were, huddled together on the racetrack, sleeping on their shields, their armor rusting away where they dropped. Around them were not wounded graders and abandoned buses, but their heavy machinery of war, neglected and forlorn. Any minute now Rose would utter the magic words that would awaken those sleeping knights and return Camelot to all its former glory.

Rose led us to the trailer, unlocked the door, and threw the sandwiches on the table.

The trailer was unshaded, and the heat was so intense it took my breath away. But again, Rose in his flannel shirt and felt hat didn't notice, or if he did, didn't mention it. The trailer had such a strong musty odor I wondered when Rose used it last. After offering us a sandwich which we politely declined, Rose opened one and finished it in two bites.

"So," he said with a broad grin, still working his second bite, "what can I do for you fellas? I know you didn't come all this way just to see what all the inbreeding in the hollows around here has unleashed on an unsuspecting humanity, even though, I assure you, it would curl your hair."

This plain indictment of his own set him to giggling, and we couldn't help but join in. I never encountered a human being before or since whose laughter was so infectious. The man was irresistible.

"Well," I said nervously, "I really liked your lecture, and what I really want to know is, how do I begin?"

"Well," he replied, suddenly all business, "the first thing is realizing you can't make a frontal assault on Truth. You don't know what the Truth is. If you did, you'd be there already."

Rose recommended backing away instead from what he described as "nonsense and BS." You do this, he said, by taking a hard look at your life and eliminating what is obviously absurd, counterproductive, and a waste of time. Rose told us to replace the more absurd with the less absurd and "just keep goin'. You'll find 90 percent is common sense—the hard part's doin' it."

He urged us to focus on what is, and not what we'd like it to be, hope it will be, or what someone else told us it will be. Doubt everything, Rose said, "except your ability to doubt."

"Sure," he continued, "some old fart like me might be able to tell you where a few land mines are buried, but until you get to the end of the road, always remember I could be wrong.

"Most people don't want all the work this implies, and so they pay the preacher to carry the load. It's depressing.

"There's more, but that oughta' get you started. What do you say to a hike around the farm?"

Without waiting for a reply, Rose led us outside and locked the door. As he did, I saw our cheese sandwiches still sitting on the table in that microwave of a trailer. I doubted the hike, however strenuous, would do much for my appetite.

For the next several hours Rose led us on a forced march. He was almost three times our age, but he walked us right into the ground. The farm was a tangle of trees and underbrush slashed here and there by old logging roads. With an almost perverse pleasure, Rose repeatedly abandoned these roads, pushing through briars and thickets, over rock ledges, and straight up hillsides in search of some old tree with a date carved into it or a view he wanted us to see.

Most of the time we walked single file, with Rose breaking trail, taking the occasional question, and talking nonstop. I was in the rear, and my height and large frame added to my difficulties. Compounding my struggles, Ray, much shorter, scooted under low-hanging limbs while impishly using his arms to whip them back in my face. But he was soon out of gas, and from then on it was all we could do to just keep up.

What amazed me about Rose, beyond his stamina and the relentless way he attacked everything in life, was the way he jumped from philosopher to naturalist and back again without ever losing his place. He knew every tree, bush, and mushroom on his farm, and occasionally he would pull out some May Apple or Ginseng root and describe its medicinal properties. He was an amateur geologist as well and pointed out the various types of rock we encountered along the way.

Eventually we emerged at a mountainside spring deep in the woods behind the house. The spring had once been housed in concrete, but the encroaching hillside had long since broken the concrete shell into big clammy chunks. Planted in the ruins was a long steel pipe that emptied into an overflowing, four-legged, antique bathtub lined with bright-green moss. We drank some of the best water I ever tasted, and then, mercifully, Rose suggested we "rest a spell." The shade and cold water cooled things off considerably, and we sat down on some old logs and a tattered, nylon-latticed aluminum lawn chair someone left there.

Rose described the geology of the hillside, explaining how the pressure, type of rock, and water table created the spring. Mentioning the water table touched off a jeremiad against digging pits for outhouses.

"Most folks around here dig pits, and they don't give a damn about what that means for the water. That is, until they get liver flukes, cholera, or God knows what. I won't have pits on my farm."

"Wow, Mr. Rose," I said, half sincere and half to keep him from resuming the hike, "you really believe in living in harmony with nature."

"I don't know what living in harmony with nature means," he replied sharply. "Look around. Maybe it seems like beauty, tranquility, and peace, but it's actually a slaughterhouse. Every living thing in this forest is eating its neighbor while tryin' not to get eaten in turn.

You call it harmony because your ears aren't good enough to hear the screaming. Ever hear a rabbit scream when an owl's got hold of it?"

"No. I didn't know they could scream."

"Well they do, and it'll give you the nightmares." Rose paused before continuing. "Everything in nature's a fight. Every breath is an effort, and those liver flukes, they'd love to take a bite out of you too. But luckily you boiled that spring water before you drank it, didn't you?"

He giggled at this remark and so did we, but in spite of myself I tried to recall whether Rose took a drink or not.

If Ray and I wanted "to get anywhere spiritually," Rose told us, we'd have to take a "hiatus" from the strictly "vegetable existence" nature had planned for us long enough to figure out nature itself, and everything else for that matter.

"But when you find what you're lookin' for, you also gotta' be willing to pay nature back—with interest. Just watch my kids," he said, smiling. "You'll see I'm payin' nature back every day. And since I got three kids, the interest I'm payin' is compounded daily."

The spring, over time, cut a deep ravine through the tree-covered mountainside, and we sat quietly for a few minutes, listening to the murmuring spring and enjoying the view of a dairy farm in the valley far below. As we did, I tried to get used to the effect Rose had on me. On one hand I was put off by the stark, uncompromising way in which he looked at life, but on the other, I was thrilled by his willingness to say things I always half suspected but was afraid to admit.

It wasn't just that. It was his intensity, his drive, his enthusiasm, his spontaneity, his fearlessness that thrilled me. His philosophical views, like everything in his life, were only a reflection of this. As we sat by the spring I began fantasizing about becoming his student, but something about that also scared me half to death.

My reverie was interrupted when, still gazing into the valley, Rose began speaking. He spoke as if musing to himself, and there was that same otherworldly thickness to his voice I heard at the lecture when he said, "Words mean nothing."

"You know, if I ever met anyone really committed to reaching Enlightenment, I would drop everything and dedicate my life to helping him find it."

Suddenly, the same scary energy I felt when we first met on the sidewalk was welling up inside me again. Choking it back, I tightly closed my eyes and anxiously waited until my heart rate and breathing returned to normal. Reopening my eyes, I saw Ray and Rose already walking away. I jumped up and followed them down a steep old logging trail that led to a wide stream called Big Wheeling Creek.

Our hike became a blur. My mind raced as I tried to figure out what was happening. Part of me was convinced that Rose had just read my mind about wanting to be his student. Or maybe he didn't speak at all but merely telepathically projected his voice into my head. The other part was terrified that I was taking such mad possibilities even half seriously. Whether Rose had supernatural powers or not, though, he'd answered my question: I now knew what was so frightening about him.

> My mind raced as I tried to figure out what was happening. Part of me was convinced that Rose had just read my mind about wanting to be his student.

It was as if, without even trying, he was putting a demand on me. Or maybe it was more like an invitation, but an invitation with all the force of a voice from Heaven crying, "Thus says the Lord!" Was I imagining things or was something crazy happening? Was my fear legitimate—after all, he said himself he could be wrong—or would fear cost me the magical opportunity I was desperately looking for?

This all came to me, not in full sentences, but in a convoluted stream of half thoughts, recursive loops, and raw, discombobulated emotions. All as thickly braided together as the tangled briars, brambles, and underbrush of Rose's farm.

I was jolted from my musing by a sudden halt and the vague sense that, for some time, Ray and Rose had been chatting without me.

"No need to retrace our steps," Rose was saying as he lifted his hat and wiped the sweat from his bald head with a checkered handkerchief. "I think if we cut up through here, it'll bring us back somewheres close to where we started."

Looking around, I realized Rose had led us for a mile or more down one bank of the winding stream, and now he was heading into an underbrush-choked thicket and straight up the steep mountain we originally descended via the logging trail.

Despite the heat and difficult terrain, I immediately plunged back into thought. The only thing I knew for sure from all my disjointed pondering was my life back in Pittsburgh was in serious jeopardy. Like a hungry, stiff-necked Israelite trudging wearily behind Moses through the desert, my life back in Egypt now didn't seem so bad. I'd assumed spirituality would be an added dimension to my normal life. There were many things I liked about my current situation, and spirituality was supposed to complete, enhance, and fulfill my existing life, not yank it up by the roots. I wanted to *integrate* Rose into my normal life, and something was telling me this might not be possible.

Huffing, puffing, soaked with sweat, we eventually emerged from the woods at the abandoned racetrack. As the late afternoon sun stung my face, I decided that even though it was high time to head home, I had to muster the courage to ask Rose about all this before we left. But as so often before and so often after, fear held me back, and we stood around chatting while I kept looking for a safe opening. A particularly funny Rosean story finally gave me one, and I launched into a little autobiography. I told Rose what I was doing at the University of Pittsburgh and how important my education and plans for graduate school were to my parents.

Rose listened patiently, nodded his head, and even asked a question or two.

"So here's where I'm at, Mr. Rose. I'm blown away by everything you're talking about. You, your hospitality, this farm, everything's so far out. But you seem to be talking about an all or nothin', full-tilt boogie kinda' thing. I also want to help people. I want to go into politics and help people. I'm wondering how that fits in with everything you seem to be saying."

Rose smiled, bent over for a little piece of grass, and began chewing on it thoughtfully.

"Well, since you asked, and I like you, I'll tell you what I think," he finally said as if it were all the same to him. "You don't give a damn about anyone but yourself. When I look at you, I see a cock on a woodpile crowing to the hens. It ain't enough that your parents love you, your brothers and sister love you, and your friends love you. No, you won't be satisfied until the whole damn world loves you, and hey, you're a pretty smart guy, maybe you can pull it off.

"Now, if that's what you want from life, I won't stand in your way. But please, don't come down here feedin' me that bullshit about helpin' people."

My knees buckled. My inner world collapsed into a jumble of four incoherent thoughts spinning feverishly and continually interrupting each other: *My God, it's true . . . I didn't know . . . No, I always knew . . . But how did he know?*

Reduced to a helpless spectator of my own mind, the only thing I vaguely remember after that is staggering to Ray's car.

* * *

By the time Ray dropped me off back in Pittsburgh, I was in a tailspin. For a week I walked around like a shell-shocked soldier sporting a thousand-yard stare. Rose took all the secret doubts about myself and my motivations that I so carefully shared with Nancy and crudely rubbed my nose in them. Disdaining the sterile Q-Tip I was using to gently probe my soul, Rose plunged a bloody knife in up to the hilt, and then cheerfully gave it a twist.

I was devastated, hurt, betrayed, and mad as hell. I desperately tried to forget all about the bastard. But I couldn't because I knew in my bones everything he said was true. All he really did was stick his finger into that ever-widening hole in my soul and make it more obvious. As I cooled off a bit, I even had to wryly admit it was one thing to be dazzled by Rose verbally undressing "to his shoelaces" the heckler at his lecture, and quite another to find my own pants snugly hugging my ankles. Keeping it real, telling it like it is, and letting it all hang out is a great idea, I ruefully decided, until a guy like Rose takes you up on the suggestion.

After a few weeks of fruitless tail-chasing, I impulsively gave Rose a call. He answered warmly, and before I knew it, I made another appointment to see him. I didn't mention the psychological drubbing he gave me at his farm and neither did he, and before long I was spending more and more time in Benwood hoping he'd raise the dead and terrified he just might. I was disappointed on both counts, but I did gradually find out that Rose was not only a spiritual teacher, poet, family man, and violin player, his bona fides as a West Virginia hillbilly were beyond reproach.

Several years earlier Rose "let the air out" of one of the local hell-raisers in a melee he always referred to as "the shoot-out." A reporter, sent for an interview, described Rose as having "piercing blue eyes, and a determined looking aspect that seemed relentlessly in search of a brick wall through which to ram his cannon ball-like head."

This reporter went on to say that he found Rose "sitting in a chair on the front porch of his old farmhouse, guarded by a pair of dangerous looking old refrigerators, in hand-patched leather shoes that didn't match, with one pant leg rolled up higher than the other, drinking coffee from a mason jar."

Rose admitted in the retelling that the depiction was, by and large, accurate. Except for the refrigerators. "I had him buffaloed," he said with mock seriousness and genuine glee. "Those refrigerators were busted beyond repair. My guards had long since crossed over to the spirit world. They weren't dangerous enough to push a dead man off an outhouse." However, he also made no bones about how he felt about "what that son of a bitch of a reporter was implying."

Rose was turning out to be a very colorful man, but spiritually speaking, he put precious little effort into playing the guru. While he always seemed glad to see me and freely answered questions, visiting often meant just hanging around as he went through his normal routine—so much so that I sometimes went home wondering if he was testing my seriousness or just wasting my time.

For the last couple of hours on this particular afternoon, for example, Rose had been sitting directly across from me at his kitchen table seemingly oblivious to my presence. His cheap "store-bought" reading glasses were perched on his broad nose as he pored over used car ads in the *Green Tab* as if they were sacred scripture. The *Green Tab* was one of those local barter sheets that always depressed the hell out of me as I imagined some poor soul sitting hopefully by the phone servicing an ad for a three-dollar "almost new" shower curtain.

From what I could tell, Rose's main line of work was buying old cars he called junkers for three hundred dollars and reselling them for four hundred. Occasionally he got lucky and bought an old school bus. He would strip the tires, wheels, and undercarriage for resale at a profit and perch the shell up on blocks out at the farm as a shed. Rose saved everything (he used his leftover cooking grease for handmade hand soap), and like most West Virginians, his appetite for storage was inexhaustible.

Finally, he took off his glasses, stood up, grabbed his white-painted steel cup that was designed for something else, and went for more of the self-brewed coffee he described as "gasoline" and which he swore was killing him by inches. "I've spent my life tryin' to get a line on people, and I still can't figure it," he muttered midstride as if talking to himself. "Man is an isthmus between two oblivions. There's billions of years before he's born and billions of years after he's dead. Every human being's a tiny chess piece wedged between these two oblivions. Yet folks say they got better things to do than spend what little time they have doping it all out. They're too damn busy to find out what god or devil's runnin' this damn game of life by what rules and to what purpose."

Carrying his coffee back to the table, he larded it with two heaping teaspoons of sugar. He was putting on his glasses again when I decided I'd been extended an invitation and grabbed it.

"I think people are just scared, Mr. Rose. They're afraid we can't know anything for sure, so why start a hopeless task?"

"Do you know *that* for sure?" Rose said over his glasses, neatly switching pronouns and reading my mind. "Because if you're sure you can't know anything for sure, then you're sure about one thing. And if you're sure about one thing, then maybe you can be sure about two, and if two's possible, it stands to reason that maybe you can be sure about *everything*. The agony of life is uncertainty, and the rationalization is uncertainty is certain. What folks really want is the *truth*: something they can take to the bank, something that won't crap out on 'em like wet-bottomed paper feedbags when they got starvin' cattle on their hands. When they're dyin', for instance."

"If everyone wants the truth, what's holding them back?"

"They don't want the truth," Rose said, pausing long enough to grin at the bewilderment spreading over my face. "They're scared, all right, you got that much right. But what they're scared of is not the *impossibility* of finding the truth—that's the excuse—but the possibility they will find it."

"I don't understand."

"They want the truth as long as it turns out to be what they want it to be. Truth is a wonderful thing, in the end it's the only thing, but it don't work that way. What folks is scared of is all the small 't' truths they'll have to face on the way to capital 'T' *Truth*."

"I still don't understand."

Rose reached for one of the gooey store-brand sweet rolls he bought day old and four dozen at a time.

"Think about it," he said, munching away. "There's millions of people out there right now who know they should see a doctor but are too scared to make an appointment. Millions of wives want to know where their husbands were last night, but they're so afraid of the truth they pretend they don't. And you're surprised that people want to invite God into their home but are afraid of the mess he'd find?

"The Truth *will* set you free, but it ain't *your* Truth. You got to want it for its own sake and damn the consequences. Most of humanity just don't have the stomach for that kinda' trip."

Pausing, and without explanation, Rose got up and sifted inconclusively through the top drawer of a large free-standing kitchen cabinet. Then he opened the door and vanished down his dark hallway, only to reemerge carrying the biggest ring of keys I've ever seen. I was astonished both by its size and the memory such an assortment of unmarked keys required. But it also seemed vaguely appropriate that a man who dedicated his life to unlocking the secrets of the universe would have just such a set of keys.

Sitting down, he shuffled through the various members of this exclusive club, obviously looking for one in particular. He eventually came to a long, narrow, old-fashioned skeleton key that he patiently and deliberately removed from the large brass ring. I tried to imagine what "key" to the human predicament, the universe, or me he was about to illustrate. Instead, he inserted the skeleton end into his right ear and, scratching vigorously, picked up just where he left off.

"It all comes down to this. You can either huddle in the prison of illusion and wishful thinking or start tunneling out. You can either live and die like a dog or find out why dogs live and die. People are forever saying they're afraid of wasting their lives on such a project. That's bullshit. They don't know who they are, where they came from, or where they're going when they die. They settle for a lick and a promise in hopes the guy on the white horse will pull up on their deathbeds."

Extracting the key, Rose gave the offending ear a final rub with his thumb while continuing his tirade.

"Folks try on distractions like new suits of clothes forever hoping their latest little pleasure will somehow fill that empty hole deep in their gut or help them forget it's there. They never slow down long enough to realize that empty hole is precious. It's God trying to get their damn-fool attention. As for filling that hole, they have about as much chance of filling that cavity with the produce of Mother Nature as an oyster has of extracting a grain of sand by wrapping it with pearl. It only makes the irritation worse."

Retrieving the saltshaker he inadvertently knocked over with his empty coffee cup, Rose absently passed it from one hand to another.

"By the time they hit forty they're burnt out, dead tired, and it's beginning to dawn on them that Death has 'em in his crosshairs. By now they're finding it damn hard to believe that *anything* will turn the trick. So they settle for drowning out the background noise of nameless regret with booze, blaring televisions, and hoping against hope their children don't end up like them. Even if they turn to religion, they don't want the Truth. They want a Sunday emotion that masks full-time pain with part-time effort. Freud had one thing right. Most folks don't *live*. They're merely *lived* by their passions, fears, and rationalizations. That ain't livin'—it's death propped up in a chair."

Rose suddenly caught himself and, glancing at the wall clock, lurched toward his ancient, coat hanger-adorned black-and-white television perched on the kitchen counter. He flicked it on, turned off the sound, and returned to his chair. Rose, always the gambler, was betting once again that by the time the six o'clock news came on that broken-down tube would be warm enough to produce a picture.

I needed the respite that fickle television afforded. Rose had once again knocked me off balance with his uncanny knack for launching into general rants that ended up hitting me so damn personally. What made him so effective was the utterly flat, matter-of-fact way he delivered his tirades. I was angry at his depressing analysis, or maybe just angry at *him* for making me so depressed. Could things really be that bleak? Besides, what made him so damn sure he wasn't just as deluded as the rest of us?

When these clouds cleared, I noticed Rose staring at me. As I squirmed, his blue eyes began to twinkle. "I know, I know," he began in perfect seriousness, except for those eyes. "I'm a mean and nasty man who can't wait for quittin' time so I can get back to pushin' baby ducks backwards in the water."

Then his lips began to twitch and he burst into a fit of laughter that left him holding onto his belly for dear life. Despite my best efforts, I couldn't resist the bastard, and the next thing I knew we were sending each other into spiraling, round-robin, rollicking bursts of laughter until we were merely laughing at each other laughing at each other as tears ran down our cheeks.

No matter how serious things got, Rose and I always found or created hundreds of excuses for these laughing fits. Later he would tell people the only reason I hung around was for the "heavenly hilarity" of these outbursts. But as he shook his head in mock disappointment, his eyes were always on mine, and I will never forget the deep affection those eyes conveyed.

"Well, well," a slowly recovering Rose finally said, "a few randomly tossed bricks busted a few carefully guarded stained glass windows, I reckon. Can't you see I gotta' give you a headache if I want to sell you my aspirin?"

"What are you selling, Mr. Rose?" I said, thinking he was still kidding around.

"I come to you as a man selling air . . . and you will think twice at the offer and price . . . and you will argue that nothing is there . . . although we know that it is . . . everywhere."

Rose tossed off these improvised lines so spontaneously—as if we'd been rehearsing this skit for ages—that I was stunned. He didn't seem to notice. He hesitated, his face softened, and his eyes took on a dreamy cast.

"Wonderful things," he finally said. "I want to sell you wonderful things." Then his eyes glazed over, and he was far away.

"You know, I was in Egypt once," he softly said apparently to himself. "They told me some guy named Carter discovered King Tut's tomb. Well, he chiseled a hole in that seal deep underground. Then he shoved in a lantern, stuck in his head, and froze. The fellow behind him couldn't take the suspense and got to screamin', 'What do you see? For God's sake, man, what do you see!' Carter didn't move a muscle, but his answer echoed back through that tomb like a voice from the Other Side. 'I see wonderful things.'

"The simple fact is I've seen wonderful things. Things I can't put in words and things you can't imagine. And I'm so damn grateful that the only reason I'm still draggin' this slowly rotting carcass of mine around is on the off chance that I might help a few like you see those wonderful things too."

When his blue eyes again met mine, they were again filled with tears, but this time of a different sort. Suddenly, I wanted to see these wonderful things he was selling. I wanted these wonderful things even if it killed me.

I was stunned by my own reaction, and before I could recover another spark jumped from Rose to me. The mood shifted and, so help me God, something luminous appeared on Rose's face. Here was a different man, or perhaps a vessel for something more than man, and when I realized the direction my mind was taking, I was afraid. All I wanted to do was let go, but instead, like a Hebrew in the desert, I mentally cried out for Moses to veil his face. I clenched my teeth, focused on the teacup I was strangling, and fought like a maniac to maintain control.

In less than a moment it was over. Slowly regaining my precious composure, I gradually lifted my eyes. A normal Rose was now sitting motionless at a right angle to the table, his eyes focused on his stubby fingers loosely interlocked in his lap. He was just sitting, that artless, effortless, kind of sitting that is the achievement of a lifetime and impossible to fake.

Summoning all my courage, I whispered, "What do I need to know? What do I have to do?"

"OK," he said blandly. "Here it is. First, I'll give you the facts and then the formula. Ready? There is a God, or Absolute Truth, and He knows what He's doing. There's a little piece of Him in you, and your reason for being here is to bring that spark of divinity to the surface and become it. It's like the difference between potential electricity and actual. Aspiration is the potential, and realization the actual. I call the realization Enlightenment, but it don't matter, because when God gets you by the hair, you'll know it. It's that drastic. It'll take you to your knees, but that's OK because you'll be just where you need to be to start sayin' thanks. From gratitude will come an overwhelming desire to help a world that first and foremost don't want your definition of help. But you'll try anyway. Even if they kill you for it."

In light of my previous reaction, this remark about killing caught me off guard, but I didn't have time to reflect or entirely take it in because Rose was already moving on.

"Now here's the formula. It's simple to say and hard to do. You attack the gates of Heaven with everything you have. Go after it hammer and tongs like your hair was on fire. Spiritual work by definition is anything that increases your addiction to Truth and lessens your addictions to anything less. Face all those little truths along the way no matter where they lead. Attack those heavenly gates with an axe or anything else handy to the job. But here's the catch—" Then he smiled. He smiled the only really beatific smile I've ever seen.

"You *will* fail.

"You'll fail because those gates don't swing in, they only swing out. You can't force your way in. You're only invited. You need some help from the Other Side, because ultimately you can't do it alone. But in your defeat you surrender, and with your surrender the doors magically swing open. Mystics call it the Magnificent Defeat.

"All human beings want the Truth," he continued as he leaned back in his chair and slowly interlaced his hands behind his neck. "The difference between 'em is whether they realize it, how much energy they put into it, and how efficiently they apply that energy. It ain't much different from startin' a business. You make a commitment, learn everything you can on the subject, surround yourself with like-minded people, burn your bridges behind you, and stop at nothing short of evil to get there. This business called spirituality has only one product, but it comes in three colors: service to others, selflessness, and the longing for That Which Is."

Trying to hide anxiety behind levity, I asked, "Does your product guarantee results, Mr. Rose? Do I get a money-back guarantee?"

"I guarantee nothing concerning Enlightenment," Rose said flatly as he leaned forward on his elbows once again. "What I neglected to tell you is the million and one other parts to this formula that ain't no formula. Let's lump 'em all together and call 'em grace. What I know, and you gotta' find out, is this is God's sandbox, and in the end He's calling all the shots. Believe me, I have no standing with the man upstairs.

"All we do is what every businessman does. Play the odds. We work like hell to increase probabilities. Even the businessman needs grace to turn probabilities into success. He just calls it luck. But they'll all tell you the harder they work, the luckier they get.

"But I will guarantee this," Rose said softly as his features followed suit. "Either way, you'll know you spent your life a whole hell of a lot less foolishly than you would otherwise. You'll know your shoulder's been to the wheel of the most noble undertaking there is. And if you stick with it, this work will transform that guy in the shaving mirror into a good, decent, honest, compassionate human being who can make good decisions, see them through, and damn the consequences. In other words, it'll make a *man* out of you, and that ain't too shabby."

Then his voice softened still more.

"But when you get tired and discouraged and start feelin' sorry for yourself, try to remember one thing. If you think you're workin' hard to find God, you have no idea how hard God is workin' to find you."

The phone in the hallway started to ring, and as Rose hurried away to service a potential customer, I noticed that his soundless, wavy-lined old television had managed to produce a perfect picture just in time for the six o'clock news.

Chapter Four

ROLLING STONES AND HOUNDS OF HEAVEN

For most of us, there is only the unattended
Moment, the moment in and out of time,
The distraction fit, lost in a shaft of sunlight,
The wild thyme unseen, or the winter lightning
Or the waterfall, or music heard so deeply
That it is not heard at all, but you are the music
While the music lasts.
—T.S. Eliot[10]

My mind was racing as I drove my dad's Ford Falcon back to Pittsburgh after my strange visit with Rose. His moving admonition about how hard God was working to find me kept echoing in my head. But as the weeks wore on and subsequent meetings proved far less spectacular, all the doubts I entertained after my traumatic first visit to Rose's farm returned, and with them all my ambivalence. After all, Rose was a hick without credentials: he didn't really belong to any spiritual tradition, didn't have other students, and from what I could gather never even had a teacher. In fact, I knew almost nothing about him or his background. Even his wife thought he was a kook and didn't mind saying so. And while I hated to admit it, his poverty depressed me. Is that how I wanted to end up?

Ray and I even created a running joke about wrapping up our Rosean adventure as ancient, burnt-out, spiritual has-beens living in the Main Hotel down in Carnegie. Carnegie was a blue-collar neighborhood a few miles from where we lived, and though Ray was a big fan of the pizza they served in their small, Naugahyde-veneered dining room, the Main Hotel itself was a little nondescript, wood-framed, three-story, twelve-room affair with a glowing sign overhanging Main Street that always seemed to have a few flickering strands of fuchsia-flavored neon slowly flickering out.

While I'd never been upstairs, I pictured a series of narrow, dimly lit hallways smelling vaguely of the dregs of last night's breakfast cereal supper, still soggy with stale milk. The hotel hallways were lined with wooden doors cracked open to coax a whiff of tired air into tiny rooms kept uncomfortably hot by hissing, non-adjustable, cast iron, hot water radiators clanking away under sticky wood-framed sliding windows. Windows that, more often than not, offered a pristine view of an adjacent brick wall a scant three feet away. In lieu of visitors, blaring black and white televisions piped in the forced gaiety of *The Price Is Right* until it reverberated out the cracked doors and throughout the hotel.

The Main Hotel was not for well-heeled itinerant salesmen and intermittent vacationers. It was where down-at-the-heels, hard of hearing, lonely old misanthropic bachelors rented rooms by the week while they eagerly waited to die. So while Ray and I had endless fun adding elaborate storylines to each other's Main Hotel mythologies, we were also most definitely whistling past the graveyard as we tried to laugh away some real Rosean anxiety as well.

Eventually, I did so much anxious backing and filling I couldn't decide whether the light I saw on Rose's face, the third spark between us, and my intense reaction was something genuine or just the effects of an overdose of caffeine on an overactive imagination.

But I couldn't stay away from the SOB either.

Like a mesmerized moth dancing dangerously around a Rosean candle flame, I kept coming back. As the tension grew, I became angry and argumentative. But my philosophical quibbles were only skin deep. Underneath, I was still trying to force Rose to admit that splitting my time between my "normal" life and my "spiritual" life was a valid approach. Didn't the Zen masters say, "The ordinary life is the spiritual life?" Of course, I was only dimly aware of this at the time. All I remember is a vague sense that my moth-like orbit was slowly degrading, and I was feeling the heat. I was, as I later read in one of Rose's poems about his own spiritual ambivalence, "a charmed lover, fighting the spell and languishing into it."

My fears were exacerbated by the fact that I didn't have a single soul to turn to for guidance. My father, an old school Catholic, derisively referred to Rose as "St. Paul." My well read, free-thinking Irish mother, though more sympathetic, thought I was looking for a father figure to compensate for the heated headbutting that ebbed and flowed between me and my dad. Eventually, I moved into a five-bedroom house with Chip and college friends partly to keep my parents in the dark and off my back. As for friends, it was 1972 and Zen was cool, but beyond that they were not interested in Rose and couldn't see what all the fuss was about.

Even Ray was little help. He remained interested in Rose but consistently argued for caution: arguments I came to distrust because they seemed to largely stem from his own fears of ending up entombed in the Main Hotel.

But there was something else happening in Pittsburgh in the summer of 1972. Something that promised to, at least temporarily, unravel that human koan called Richard Rose or at least shove him firmly to the backburner. The Rolling Stones were coming to town, and I had high hopes the Stones would give me the respite I sorely needed from Rose and his damn gravitational vortex.

Ray and I were *huge* Stones fans, and when we read in the *Pittsburgh Press* they were coming to the Civic Arena, we immediately took a bus downtown to order tickets. When we got to the front of the ticket office line, the agent almost laughed in our face. He pointedly reminded us that the concert was still many months away and that everybody— and that meant everybody—wanted Stones tickets. Seats would not actually go on sale until shortly before the concert.

Embarrassed by our naiveté and stung by the agent's snooty condescension, Ray and I were halfway through the door when a stranger caught my eye and motioned us toward a corner in the ticket office. Dressed like a stylish hippie, he had long hair, a mustache, and looked about thirty. Without introducing himself he whispered, "You freaks want Stones tickets?"

Tickets were $6.50 each, and he told us how to make out the check and where to send it. When we pumped him for more, he brushed off our questions, firmly shook our hands, and was gone. The whole incident was so eerie I couldn't help but imagine that state secrets were handed over in the dead of night with far less clandestine fanfare. Despite obvious risks, Ray and I took the stranger up on his strange offer. Six dollars and fifty cents was a lot of money for college kids in 1972, but we scraped up enough for six tickets, and I sent a check. Two weeks later my check came back with a note: "Limit Four Tickets." Encouraged that our ticket office secret agent was actually on our side, I sent another check, as did my brother and one of my college buddies.

Weeks went by. Then months. Days before the concert the newspaper announced that tickets would go on sale on a first-come, first-served basis the very next day. Instantly, an ocean of Stones fans began camping out. When I saw the burgeoning tent city on television my heart dropped, but the following day an envelope arrived with four tickets to the Rolling Stones concert! In a state of shock, I called the Civic Arena's ticket office to find out where we would be sitting. The agent asked for the numbers on my tickets. Then she put me on hold for a few minutes. When she came back, she said, "You're in the front row."

The real identity of our ticket office deep throat remains a mystery, but not only did he get Ray and me four front-row tickets, my brother and my buddy got four second-row seats as well. My college friends hosted an all-night party the night before the concert featuring nothing but Stones music: The Stones had just released *Exiles on Main Street,* so that double disk was heavily featured. Steve, who accompanied Ray and me to the Rose lecture, got busy hand-painting T-shirts featuring the new Rolling Stones "tongue and lips" logo. Someone sprang for body paint, and I stumbled on a discounted Uncle Sam hat left over from the Fourth of July that summoned to mind the Stones' most recent "Get Your Ya Yas Out!" tour when Mick Jagger wore a similar hat.

The night of the concert two garishly body-painted facsimiles of me and Steve gathered once again at Ray's house where his faded green Chrysler stood faithfully at the ready to ferry us to our latest fandango. We picked up Chip along the way and took the Parkway West freeway toward downtown. As we sped through the tunnel under Mount Washington and onto the Fort Pitt Bridge, I wondered whether Pittsburgh, with her crown of sun-dappled skyscrapers glistening while the Golden Triangle's three rivers lapped obediently at her feet, was always this dazzling or whether a Stones advance team had just gussied up the old Steel City with a coat of paint so that visiting royalty like me, ennobled by a front row ticket, would not see anything disagreeable on such a special night.

Soon the Civic Arena, with the last rays of the evening sun radiating off its stainless steel skin, appeared. The Civic Arena was an iconic landmark which Pittsburghers invariably referred to as "The Big Igloo," not merely because the Pittsburgh Penguins played hockey there, but because it looked exactly like a silver igloo. The Arena was originally designed for Pittsburgh's Civic Light Orchestra, and the great acoustics and limited seating (only 13,800 tickets for the Stones concert were sold) made it an ideal venue for concerts.

I saw The Allman Brothers Band before the untimely death of Duane Allman in Pittsburgh's Syria Mosque, a much smaller venue where the Pittsburgh Symphony performed. Nine years later my job in New York City as a founding employee for *MTV: Music Television* gave me entrée to a melting pot of Rock royalty, but nothing compares to the electric excitement that crackled through the Civic Arena on that twenty-second night of July 1972. The legendary rock critic, David Marsh, wrote that the Stones' 1972 tour was "part of rock and roll legend" and the "benchmark of an era." I felt like I was looking through a magical kaleidoscope where even the tiniest twist of my completely sober head revealed yet another swirl of ecstatic voices, sounds, and sensations all dizzily woven into the incandescent atmosphere of what turned out to be, with temperatures well into the 90s, one of Pittsburgh's hottest nights ever recorded.

The stage was on the ground floor at one end of the circular arena and, dazed by our mixed drink of good fortune and overstimulation, we made our way through a sea of people until we discovered four folding chairs a few scant inches from the stage that, *mirabile dictu,* did, after all, belong to us. (Superfluous chairs as it turned out, since it never occurred to anyone in the Arena that night to sit down.) My brothers and college friends were in the second row, and though they were theoretically proximate, the heaving, interstitial throng of hysterical Stones fans meant they might as well have been in Altoona.

I'd barely gathered my addled wits when a roadie strolled to the front of the stage, dropped to one knee, and through a heavy British accent said, "Mick wan's to wea' your 'at." Mick Jagger, yes, The Mick himself, apparently wanted to wear *my* hat! The same hat I picked up as a two-dollar cardboard tribute to the *real* Uncle Sam hat Jagger wore on their previous tour.

Starstruck and weak at the knees, I eagerly forked over my red, white, and blue topper, and the roadie tossed it on the electric piano a few feet away where Nicky Hopkins, the Stones' keyboardist, was warming up. There it sat during Stevie Wonder's opening act, an act that, despite being a fan, I impatiently endured.

Then the booming, disembodied, baritone voice I later learned belonged to the Stones' lighting director, Chip Monck, made an announcement that reverberated like a clap of thunder through the arena, a godlike pronouncement made utterly unforgettable by his calm, understated, matter-of-fact delivery: *"Ladies and Gentlemen, the Rolling Stones."* (Monck's six-word, adjective-bereft, deadpan performance proved so iconic that the Stones named the documentary of their 1972 tour after his laconic intro.)

Monck's introduction was still hanging feverishly in the air when a flash of blinding light from his array of 40-by-8-foot Mylar mirrors backlit by a row of spotlights behind the stage slowly revealed to our bedazzled eyes the bouncing, bounding figure of Mick Jagger wearing *my* hat. Jagger wore my all-American stovepipe on and off throughout the concert, and at one point planted it firmly on Hopkins' head as he pounded away. I was so delirious with joy it seemed like the entire concert was just a fantastic accompaniment, a moving, personal, triumphant tribute to me and my glorious hat. I was so ecstatic, in fact, I didn't really mind when, during an encore of "Jumpin' Jack Flash," Jagger sent Uncle Sam's cardboard topper spinning over my head and into the crowd where it was instantly torn to pieces. I didn't mind because Mick Jagger wore *my* hat.

After the concert, as we slowly fought our way to our car through a tide of fans with much the same idea, it seemed oddly appropriate that the Stones' second encore, "Street Fightin' Man," was still echoing in my now hatless head. But when I finally did take my window seat in Ray's car amid the first real silence I'd heard in two days, a funny thing happened: I was disappointed, even let down. I mentally poked at it for a while, but no, it wasn't just fatigue. It was that same depressing

sense of *Now what?, Is that all there is?,* and *Where do I go from here?*
that I tried with only limited success to convey to Nancy, that same
sense of empty disappointment that for almost two years had been
poisoning everything in my life.

Watching the Stones from the front row with Jagger wearing my
hat was supposed to *mean something.* I was supposed to be a new
person, magically transformed, permanently elevated to a whole new
level of consciousness by the experience. Instead, as a slowly receding Pittsburgh seemed to turn back into that sad, slipper-less, cin-
der-streaked Cinderella she once was, I knew nothing had changed.
I was still the same old me, wrestling with the same old problems,
mired in my all-too-familiar frustrations, fears, and insecurities.

I felt like a guest at a magnificent
wedding. The only guest who knows
that the groom is already cheating
on his beautiful, blushing, ecstatic
bride. It was profound sadness seasoned by helplessness. *Chto delat?
Chto delat?* As I lay in bed that night
with my ears still ringing, Orysia's
quintessential Russian question was
also ringing endlessly in my head.
But what is to be done in such a tragic situation? Tell the bride and spoil
it for her and everyone? Or keep qui-
et and live the lie? But isn't living the lie the very thing that spreads its
poisonous shadow ever wider until it eventually envelops everything?
And I was living the lie.

> I felt like a guest at a
> magnificent wedding.
> The only guest who
> knows that the
> groom is already
> cheating on his
> beautiful, blushing,
> ecstatic bride.

Only a few days after the concert, I read a "tell all" article in *Rolling
Stone* magazine written anonymously by a former groupie. She coolly,
almost surgically, ticked off her bedroom escapades with a who's who
of rock legends. But each fresh fling left her thinking: "That was great,
but it wasn't Mick Jagger." Then she finally managed to bed Mick

Jagger, only to think, "That was great, but it wasn't Mick Jagger"—an admission that sent her spiraling into deep depression.

Rather than that star-strewn sky back in Wildwood, this time it was a rock star who tempted me, just like Jagger tempted that groupie, with his "Sympathy for the Devil"-like promise of *something more*. But instead of delivering on his promise, this diabolic star left me jumping up and down once again. Only this time in front of a stupid stage rather than on a stupid dock. I was nothing but the ridiculous butt of a fiendish joke, endlessly jumping up and down in the vain hope of reaching that palpable, indescribable, glorious *something* that always remained maddeningly just out of reach. After yet another whiff of Heaven, I was once again buried to my nostrils in the rich, redolent manure of Mother Earth. Worst of all, I was beginning to sense, albeit through a glass darkly, that eager anticipation followed by bitter disappointment might very well become the pattern of my life.

* * *

Rose and I were very loose about timing my arrivals. While the day was always fixed (usually a Saturday), the exact time quickly took on an "I'll expect you when I see you" characteristic, and I never knew what to expect when I pulled into Benwood. About ten days after the Stones concert, I arrived one morning and found Rose playing dominoes at his kitchen table with his chain-smoking neighbor, Carl. Carl was about 40, lived with his mother, and was severely handicapped physically and verbally by cerebral palsy. It was not unusual for one of his laborious, cane-abetted walks to wind up in Rose's kitchen, so we were already acquainted.

When the game ended, Carl and the dominoes went their way and Rose suggested a walk to the 7-Eleven convenience store in McMechen for a Coke. McMechen was Benwood's twin, a tiny, tattered, old steel village smelling faintly of sulfur, snuggly tucked along the Ohio River about a mile or so directly up Marshal Street toward

Moundsville. McMechen's sole claim to fame, as far as I could tell, was its aforementioned 7-Eleven. As soon as we left the house, Rose began coughing violently, and I realized our amble had far more to do with Carl's smoking than with any desire for a cold drink. I found it fascinating to see Rose, an avid nonsmoker who assiduously avoided anything that smacked of pure amusement, playing dominoes with a chain-smoker, so when he finally stopped hacking, I asked about it.

"Do you like playing dominoes, Mr. Rose?"

"No. Besides, he cheats, but I let him get away with it."

"Why do you do it, then?"

"We're supposed to visit the sick, ain't we?" he managed to wheeze before he resumed coughing.

This quick-witted, inside baseball allusion to one of the Catholic Corporal Works of Mercy I'd dutifully set to memory as an altar boy cracked me up, but I was also struck, yet again, by the contrast between how remorselessly critical, even cynical Rose could be toward humanity taken in aggregate while still displaying so much compassionate kindness toward any suffering individual like Carl he happened to meet along the way.

Rose was always a brisk walker, and before long we reached the outskirts of McMechen. But well short of the 7-Eleven, Rose detoured onto a side street where he showed me the old wood-framed house where the California hippie serial killer, Charles Manson, was raised by his aunt and uncle. Apparently, the convenience store was not McMechen's only claim to fame, even if in this case infamy would probably be the better fit. Rose knew Manson as a young man and acidly dismissed him as a "two-bit punk and car thief" who had "slid downhill" from even "them meager achievements." Rose told me West Virginia's governor at the time, Arch Moore, also had ties to McMechen and was born in Moundsville. As I painfully discovered on my first visit to his farm, Rose had even less regard for politics and politicians then he did for other vainglorious human activities, and his perfunctory prediction that the governor was a "corrupt SOB who belongs in prison" actually came to pass when Moore eventually pulled a three-year bit behind bars for bribery.

Eventually we got our Cokes as well as a newspaper, and about halfway back Rose was accosted by a washed-out, raggedy young hippie who heard of him somewhere and was intent on vetting him as a speaker for some tiny cult he was starting (probably to attract chicks). After a brief conversation, this wannabe guru brushed the stringy hair out of his eyes, pumped up his narrow chest, and officiously opened formal negotiations by saying, "Yeah, you'll probably do. I think you're heavy enough."

"Heavy enough?" Rose quipped. "What are you, a group of weightlifters?"

Picturing Rose as a human barbell reduced me and Rose to tears laughing, and while I don't remember what happened next, apparently Rose wasn't "heavy enough" after all because, as far as I knew, the lecture never did come off.

Irritated by the hippie's arrogant attitude and suspicious of his motives, as we continued on our way, I blurted out, "Mr. Rose, why do you bother with a guy like that?"

"Why do I bother with a guy like you?" Rose retorted sharply. "It is not for me to decide. When I'm asked for help, I do my best to give it."

When we got back, Rose bustled around the kitchen for a minute or two looking for something. When he finally found his reading glasses in the pocket of his beige jacket hanging from a doorknob, he picked up his convenience store copy of the *Wheeling Intelligencer,* sat down at the kitchen table, and intently began to read. Even though he couldn't afford a subscription, Rose was an avid newspaper reader, and he especially liked local news. He knew just about everyone living in the Ohio Valley around Wheeling, and most of the dead, and no wedding, funeral, traffic violation, want ad, fender bender, lost dog, or man-bites-dog story failed to elicit his undivided attention and, not uncommonly, his often-hilarious commentary. Rose refused to take money for his teaching and accused those who did of "eating off the altar." The only form of compensation I could ever get him to accept was the occasional copy of the *Intelligencer* I pretended I bought for myself.

As Rose was memorizing his newspaper, I was hiding behind the dregs in my empty Coke bottle trying to decide whether to bring up my Rolling Stones letdown. It was a delicate issue. I doubted Rose knew who the hell the Rolling Stones were, and either way I was sure he would take a dim view of "spending damn good money" on such an utter waste of time—a point he would almost certainly accentuate with a couple of his very best zingers at my expense. (I was still smarting, in fact, from the zinger I just collected for egotistically asking the wrong question on our return from McMechen.) Not ready to risk his further disappointment with or without zingers, I was trying, without success, to steal fire from the gods by coming up with a more anodyne way of broaching the issue without having to cop straight up to all the garish body paint.

However, as Captain Ahab would put it, the real problem requires "a little lower layer." Just like with Orysia, I was afraid that sharing my weakness and vulnerability with Rose would not bring the healing release I was seeking. Instead, it would only trigger all that chaotic energy that seemed so determined to well up and overwhelm me. This energy was strongest and at its most threatening whenever one of those electric sparks jumped between Rose and me. So far I'd been able to emotionally "clamp down" in the heat of battle and maintain control, but these high-voltage surges were getting stronger and my defenses weaker.

To make things more convoluted, even outright maddening, it was the whispered promise of something magical and utterly marvelous that seemed to be lurking within these energy surges that kept bringing me back to Rose in the first place, despite my trepidation. I was mired to my hair follicles in a classic Zen koan, a solutionless puzzle I obsessively couldn't stop trying to solve. I couldn't ask Rose about the scary thing that was really on my mind for fear that asking him would trigger the scary thing that was really on my mind. In effect, I was hanging around hoping one of those energy surges would overwhelm me while desperately hanging back for fear one of them just might. And true to form, consciously and (even more so) unconsciously I beat myself up mercilessly for my Hamlet-like hesitancy and cowardly weakness.

All of this tangled, self-strangulating, multi-leveled muddle is what I really wanted to ask Rose about, but at the time I didn't have the words, the self-awareness, the confidence, and most of all the courage to go through with it. All I really knew, as I used my Coke bottle for interference, was that I was finding it impossible to come up with anything that felt safe enough to ask Rose.

Just then Rose looked up from his paper, over the rims of his glasses, and straight through my Coke bottle defense. "You know," he said almost wistfully, "you remind me of the boy with the burning feet. I'm afraid you're destined to just keep running and running until you're just too damn wore out to run anymore."

This dismal prophecy out of nowhere and apropos of nothing stunned me, and apparently it showed. Rose disappeared for a few minutes only to reemerge with a book of poetry. He opened it to a poem called "The Hound of Heaven" by Francis Thompson. He began reading aloud.

I FLED Him, down the nights and down the days;
I fled Him, down the arches of the years;
I fled Him, down the labyrinthine ways
Of my own mind; and in the mist of tears . . .

From those strong Feet that followed, followed after.
But with unhurrying chase,
And unperturbèd pace,
Deliberate speed, majestic instancy,
They beat—and a Voice beat

More instant than the Feet—
'All things betray thee, who betrayest Me . . . '

As Rose continued, his eyes filled with tears. (Later he refused to read this poem aloud because he said it took too much "tuck" out of him.)

Still with unhurrying chase,
And unperturbèd pace,
Deliberate speed, majestic instancy,
Came on the following Feet,
And a Voice above their beat—
'Naught shelters thee, who wilt not shelter Me.

Looking up, Rose, the tears now streaming down his face, finished the poem from memory.

Whom wilt thou find to love ignoble thee,
Save Me, save only Me?
All which I took from thee I did but take,
Not for thy harms,
But just that thou might'st seek it in My arms . . .
Ah, fondest, blindest, weakest,
I am He Whom thou seekest!'[11]

It was now late afternoon. I was too upset and Rose too moved to delve further into the issue of my burning feet, let alone my scary suspicion that Rose had once again read my mind. The Stones had played my favorite song, "Gimme Shelter," but as I drove home to Pittsburgh, Thompson's poetic "'Naught shelters thee, who wilt not shelter Me," as well as Rose's impromptu prophecy, clearly suggested the shelter I was seeking was beyond the ability of even the greatest rock n' roll band in the world to deliver.

In Melville's *Moby Dick*, Captain Ahab admits that he knows not whether the white whale is merely the "agent" or is in fact "the principal," or source, of that inscrutable, supernatural, force slowly driving him mad.[12] Similarly, I still couldn't decide whether Rose was merely the "agent," or messenger, of some heavenly hound hard upon my heels or—like Ahab's mesmerizing hold on the Pequod's doomed and starstruck crew—Rose was some hell-bent, half mad, hellhound determined to drag me down to the fiery depths with him.

Chapter Five

BUS RIDES AND RETROSPECTIONS

Or say that the end precedes the beginning,
And the end and the beginning were always there
Before the beginning and after the end.
And all is always now.
Words strain,
Crack and sometimes break, under the burden,
Under the tension, slip, slide, perish,
Decay with imprecision,
Will not stay in place,
Will not stay still.
Shrieking voices
Scolding, mocking, or merely chattering,
Always assail them.
The Word in the desert
Is most attacked by voices of temptation,
The crying shadow in the funeral dance,
The loud lament of the disconsolate chimera.
—T.S. ELIOT[13]

I don't remember why I took a Greyhound bus to Wheeling to visit Rose in the late summer of 1972. Ray was probably otherwise occupied and my dad was probably holding his car keys over my head in exchange for some concession in our grinding war of attrition I was unwilling to concede. I did have my Yamaha DT-1, 250cc dirt bike, but though the license plate tethered to its plastic fender by two bits of rusty wire made it technically street legal, just thinking about going as far as Benwood on a two-stroke motor, propelling a knobby rear tire, painfully distorted my delicate posterior.

My derriere instead was just taking its window seat on the bus when I remembered why I hated buses so much. My seat was cramped, the worn-out seat cushion worn flat, the detachable head rest missing, the retractable seatback broken, and the A/C either inoperable or absent altogether. The bus was chockablock with crying babies and their chain-smoking mothers, and I knew from harsh experience that opening my window would merely mean ingesting a heady dose of headache-inducing diesel fumes. It was depressing, and I soon found myself reliving an even bleaker bus ride: a trip from New York City to Pittsburgh over Thanksgiving break in 1967 when I was a 14-year-old prep school kid. It was a dismal ordeal that soured me on buses forever and, metaphorically at least, actually began on a high note: my full scholarship to an exclusive New England boarding school.

Long before I knew what it meant, my philo-Semitic Irish mother used to smile proudly and tell me I had "chutzpah." When I was 10, I badgered the high school kid who had the *Pittsburgh Press* newspaper route in our neighborhood until he gave it to me. At 13, the paper boy newsletter said some exclusive, all-boys, boarding or "prep" schools were looking for scholarship candidates, and the paper would be facilitating this opportunity for their carriers.

Apparently, these schools considered a pool of Pittsburgh boys with enough entrepreneurial chutzpah to handle a newspaper route a good starting place to tease out some geographically diverse scholarship prospects. The schools were waving their standard application fees, and rather than insisting that candidates interview on campus, they were sending admissions officers to Pittsburgh instead.

I instantly wanted to go, and I convinced my parents, especially my dad, to back me. I was already in eighth grade, and it was too late to apply to enter as a freshman, so I decided to attend my local Catholic high school for a year and go as a sophomore. After a battery of interviews with an assortment of schools, we filled out some applications, and I took the Secondary School Admissions Test, the high school version of the Standard Admissions Test (SAT). Then in March of my freshman year, letters arrived from five schools offering full scholarships. Overjoyed, my father and I quickly narrowed the list to two Connecticut rivals: The Hotchkiss School in Lakeville and The Taft School in Watertown, only 35 miles from each other. To facilitate a difficult choice, my dad loaded me and my brothers Jon and Tom into our 1965 Country Sedan Ford station wagon, and we drove to New England to visit the schools.

We were more than impressed; we were blown away. While my parents were college-educated and we considered ourselves "middle class," we didn't have any money. A family of ten, we lived in a 950-square-foot, three-bedroom, single-bath ranch house with a tiny "kitchenette" in lieu of a kitchen. We *never* went out to eat or to the movies. My immigrant grandfather, a Pittsburgh steelworker from Slovakia, resoled our shoes and cut our hair. My Slovak grandmother patched our jeans, darned our socks, and stitched patchwork quilts for our beds. My poetry-loving, Latin literate mother canned vegetables from my dad's garden, sewed bespoke Halloween costumes, rinsed buckets of smelly cloth diapers by hand, honed her first-aid skills on the medley of medical emergencies collected by her seven sons, and, while waiting for her bottomless cache of clothesline-strung laundry to dry, furiously ironed her life away. (When my mother came home from the hospital with my brother Jamie, her fifth consecutive son, my dad surprised her with a brand-new clothes dryer, and I will never forget how ecstatic she was when she saw it.)

I occasionally wore hand-me-downs from my cousins and next-door neighbor and never gave it a thought, and while we never went hungry, I remember asking for bread or milk as a very young boy only to have my mother say, "We have to wait until payday." A summer pass to the only swimming pool around was, at twelve dollars, a far too expensive proposition. (On sweltering days my mother occasionally let us play with the garden hose until an out-of-place patch of dark green grass in a sea of brown tipped off the old man that, once again, we were conspiring to pack him off to the "poorhouse" by profligately "wasting water.") My hardworking white collar father's idea of a vacation was a chance to paint the house, and the only vacations I knew as a boy were sleepovers with relatives. The first time I saw the ocean was when Bud and I hit Ocean City, Maryland in 1971.

Things like air conditioning, a private, non-party line phone, air travel, color TV, gym memberships, and even a cookie jar always magically overflowing with cookies were not just beyond our means, they were unimaginable luxuries reserved for the super rich. My brother Jon told me all he wanted from life when he grew up was "all the orange juice I can drink," and by that he meant the condensed, frozen version not fresh squeezed! My dad did splurge on a new Ford without a radio every ten years or so and, addicted to sports as well as economy, he listened to Pirates baseball games on the cheap transistor radio my mother bought him for Christmas propped up against the windshield. Much to my poor mother's grief, however, when at 40 she finally began learning to drive in a city with more than its share of "clutch burning" steep hills, my dad ordered even our heavy station wagon with a "three on the tree" standard shift to save money. But we never felt poor or deprived because, after all, our middle-class neighbors, relatives, and schoolmates all lived much the same way.

So when we arrived in Connecticut it was like four Pittsburgh parvenus suddenly awoke in Shangri-La. Hotchkiss and Taft had golf courses, hockey rinks, indoor swimming pools, and clay tennis courts. The spectacular Hotchkiss campus with its gorgeous Georgian brick buildings encompassed more than eight hundred acres including hundreds of acres of woods replete with trails and log cabins for cross-country skiers and campers. The school boasted a boat house full of canoes and kayaks near its private beach on the southern shore of Lake Wononscopomuc—a beautiful, pristine 348-acre body of water. Rather than the forty students or more I was used to, class size at Hotchkiss and Taft was closer to ten. I was already a confirmed bibliophile (I got hooked on reading, especially history, in third grade), and both schools had spectacular libraries. Taft's library in particular caught my imagination: its high ceilings and cast iron, Gothic, spiral staircase reminded me of Europe's great private libraries. The Hotchkiss library was named after Edsel Ford, and we soon learned that all the Fords were Hotchkiss men to their fingertips.

We came home overwhelmed but no closer to our decision. My father leaned toward Hotchkiss, while I favored Taft. Primarily because I was dying to have unlimited access to a library with a super cool, cast-iron spiral staircase. With deadlines looming, my father prevailed, and in the fall of 1967 I metaphorically parachuted into a whole new world, a world I fully expected to be a wildly entertaining cross between a twenty-four-hour amusement park, a luxury resort, and a country club for gazillionaires.

Within weeks however, as Abe Lincoln would put it, the bottom was out of the tub. I was way over my head and failing miserably at *everything*. As a ninth-grader at my Catholic high school, I was popular, a class officer, a good student, and captain of my freshman football team. Now I was a football disappointment, couldn't make friends, and was failing most of my classes. My first Hotchkiss English composition came back with a note that was instantly seared into my memory:

> *This is puerile. In lieu of a grade (which would be "F"),*
> *I will give you a chance to rewrite it.*

Shell-shocked and fighting back tears, the first thing I did was look up "puerile" and "lieu."

As the weeks wore on, it became clear that none of the strategies I brought with me from Pittsburgh were working in this strange new exotic aquarium. School had always been easy, and my study habits and self-discipline were woefully inadequate for the enormous amount of homework Hotchkiss required. My football prowess was built around being the biggest on the team, and my Hotchkiss teammates were bigger and better. I always used wit and humor to make friends, and now all I got for my efforts were quizzical looks. In fact, I was soon the butt of the joke instead. I found myself comically associated with the cartoon character Augie Doggie and tagged with the unflattering moniker "the Dog." I was tuning in to the soul music of Motown groups like the Four Tops and Supremes. Meanwhile my classmates were "turning on" to the psychedelic sounds of Iron Butterfly and Vanilla Fudge. In Pittsburgh, the primary high school sports were football, basketball, and track. At Hotchkiss, they were soccer, hockey, and lacrosse. I was a "hawk" supporting the Vietnam war while my classmates were "doves" against it. I met my first atheists and saw my first long hair at Hotchkiss, and perhaps worst of all, the guys with the most annoying Boston accents were always the ones who found my Pittsburgh accent ripe for ridicule.

As for all the country club amenities, the academic workload combined with the strict regimen meant I barely had time to use the bathroom let alone play golf or go canoeing. We awoke at 7 AM and went to school six days a week. Meals, chapel, and afternoon sports were mandatory, and I had to be in my room studying from 5:30 to 6:30 and 7:30 to 9:30. We had to be in bed, lights out, by 10.

The net effect was Hotchkiss very quickly went from my shining city on a hill to a dark, subterranean version of William James's blooming, buzzing confusion. I became deeply depressed, desperately homesick, and determined to blame Hotchkiss for my difficulties and freshly minted inferiority complex. Each dormitory had a pay phone in the basement we were only allowed to use between 9:30 and 10 PM, and I was soon burning up the line, my father's phone bill, and his patience with collect calls tearfully begging for commiseration and, more so, for permission to come home.

This was the beginning of my deteriorating relationship with my father. Rather than sympathy, he always offered practical advice, and this advice was invariably a slightly more articulate version of: man up, buckle down, keep your chin up, bear down, grit your teeth, work harder, tough it out, and above all, stop feeling sorry for yourself. (I found this endless litany especially infuriating because, deep down, I suspected he was right.) What hurt most was the anxiety in his voice, the clipped way he spoke, his constant admonitions to write more and call less, and his eagerness to put my mother on the line—all of which meant he was more worried about his damn phone bill than about me. My mother, of course, was far more sympathetic, and she would sometimes speak sharply to my dad when, sotto voce from the wings, I could overhear him urging her to "hurry it up and get the hell off the phone." But while my parents could hotly disagree about the phone bill, they spoke with a single ice-cold voice in rejecting all my pleas to return home.

Wednesday, November 22, 1967 was a dreary, windy, unseasonably cold day in Connecticut with a drizzly mixture of icy rain and snow flurries. It was four years to the day since the assassination of John F. Kennedy, and that made the day even more somber for those of us who lived through it. It was also the day before Thanksgiving, and I was heading home for a few days' respite from my Hotchkiss ordeal. My father couldn't afford a plane ticket, so I was taking a bus from Lakeville to the Port Authority in New York City and another from there to Pittsburgh. I was excited to be going home, but even as I settled into my seat my trip was already tinged with disappointment. I would be getting in very late that night, and since I was heading back to New York at first light on Sunday, best case, I would be riding a bus for two days to be home for barely three.

Even this dismal prophecy proved wildly optimistic. When my bus from Lakeville reached the outskirts of New York, traffic was already backed up, and by the time I boarded my jam-packed Greyhound to Pittsburgh it was absolute gridlock. Literally hours passed as we slowly crawled through Manhattan toward the New Jersey Turnpike. The bus radio was tuned to WABC, one of those Top 40 AM stations that seemed to redundantly replay the same five records. I listened to The Cowsills, "The Rain, the Park and Other Things," and the Linda Ronstadt-fronted Stone Poneys' "Different Drum" over and over and over as we sat motionless—until I hated both.

When we finally did reach the turnpike, things were no better. Traffic was like a mournful bumper-to-bumper funeral procession inching toward Philadelphia, and the westbound Pennsylvania Turnpike toward Pittsburgh was just a longer version of the same agonizing exercise. Squirming silently, sleeplessly, uncomfortably hour after hour on a bus inundated with headache-inducing cigarette fumes, surrounded by cranky kids, snoring men, and nattering women did nothing to lift my spirits or dampen my sense of isolation. I didn't roll into Pittsburgh until 8:30 Thanksgiving morning. What should have been a ten-hour trip took more than twenty-two hours to complete, and I tottered off the bus utterly exhausted.

But what really took the edge off my eagerly anticipated homecoming was knowing for a certainty that all the arguments I was endlessly rehearsing in my aching head for not returning to Hotchkiss were destined to fall on deaf ears and that, come Sunday, I would be boarding an identical bus, full of identical people, for a return journey to an identical situation.

* * *

In the ensuing months, as the invisible band around my head grew ever tighter, Hotchkiss became my boiling cauldron, my fiery furnace, my very first Zen koan. My parents were the irresistible force pushing from behind while Hotchkiss was the immovable object in front, an object I could not appease, avoid, or overcome. I felt like a wounded soldier stranded in no man's land unable to advance or retreat. Meanwhile, my only communication with the outside world—the pay phone in the basement—was about to be cut off by my fastidious father. And though I ranted and raged against Hotchkiss and my stubborn parents, deep down I blamed my own weakness and despised myself for it.

It was at Hotchkiss that I first encountered that dark, billowy, all-encompassing cloud called depression. That palpable, almost visible, inky black apparition that, like one of Stephen King's voracious, time-eating Langoliers, was relentlessly dogging my every step intent on sucking me down and gobbling me up. It was depression's onslaught that chased me out into the rain at Chip's acid party, and the depressing sense that nothing really mattered that lurked behind my Rolling Stones letdown. It was empty, lifeless, purposeless depression that Rose's boy with the burning feet was desperately trying to outrun. And it was surrender to overwhelming despair that I suspected was really hiding behind those Rosean energy surges. Again, I had no idea whether I was being pursued by the Hound of Heaven or merely increasingly at the mercy of some inept, hillbilly hellion about to (perhaps solely by accident) conjure and release all those wild, chthonic dogs I kept barely at bay in my fragile psychological basement. First and foremost, it was critically important to keep all this a secret—from Nancy and Bud and Orysia and Chip and Ray and, of course, Rose . . . but most of all from myself.

* * *

I awoke with a start, and it took a moment or two to remember I was on a bus to Wheeling and not still trapped on that sad bus to nowhere from New York. I'd slipped into a unique kind of dream I had once in a while where a reverie about an actual event gradually becomes ever more ethereal until, as I begin to doze, I step into the scene, forget it's just reverie, and relive it as a dream. Apparently, a nasty bump on a washboard-warped section of I-70 had rudely yanked me from my dismal past and deposited me back in the jarring present. Somewhere on the bus a radio was playing "McArthur Park" by Richard Harris, and I ruefully recalled that during some of my darkest times at Hotchkiss, this dirgeful song seemed particularly, even masochistically, appropriate because I loathed it.

Someone left the cake out in the rain
I don't think that I can take it
'Cause it took so long to bake it
And I'll never have that recipe again
Oh, no![14]

When I got off the bus Rose was waiting and, after greeting me warmly, he suggested a bit of sightseeing around Wheeling so I could "stretch my legs."

As we headed out of the station and up Market Street, I was impressed yet again by Rose's encyclopedic knowledge of the flora and fauna of his immediate surroundings. Only a few blocks from the bus station, I especially remember Rose showing me the Capital Theatre, home of *Jamboree USA*, a live country music show almost as famous as Nashville's *Grand Ole Opry*. Despite my guide's best efforts however, it was clear that Wheeling had fallen on hard times. Once nicknamed The Nail City for its now shuttered mills, the city never recovered from the Great Depression, and the streets were pockmarked with empty lots and shuttered storefronts.

I don't remember how the conversation shifted. Maybe the sad remnants of a once thriving city gradually affected Rose. Maybe he just picked up on the somber, bus-induced, retrospective mood I brought with me.

"I spent the better part of my childhood walkin' these streets," Rose said. "Many's the time I was just hungry, cold, and tryin' not to think about it. We never had any money, and I was the dreamy, romantic type who never got the hang of hell raisin'. So I just walked all by myself," he added while jabbing an index finger at a long line of coal-laden barges slowly inching their way down the nearby Ohio River.

"The habit came in handy later when I was wanderin' the country lookin' for answers. I did most of my philosophical pondering wearin' out shoe leather, and I still maintain more good thinkin' gets done at a brisk walk than in a lotus position."

Rose then began reminiscing about his early life. He spoke quietly, and I felt like he was talking as much to himself as he was to me . . .

Rose was born in Wheeling in 1917, the third of four brothers in an impoverished family. His family was so poor that in early childhood he and his younger brother often lived in an orphanage. His mother was a devout Catholic, and he traced his spiritual yearnings back to her. His father, a plumber, a Catholic in name only, worked when work was available and supplemented his meager income raising cattle on the family farm. One story Rose related demonstrated that he got his pugnacious audacity, almost heroic sense of honor, and bulldog determination from both sides of the family.

His mother was on her way home from early Sunday Mass with Rose and his younger brother when a drunken man began harassing her with lurid sexual innuendos. Returning home, she told her husband. Without a word, Rose's father walked into town and shot the man dead on the spot. His father went to prison, and his destitute mother traveled the two hundred miles to the state capital, Charleston. She camped out in front of the governor's mansion determined to secure her husband's pardon or die right there on the steps. The governor pardoned her husband.

Rose felt called to a spiritual life from childhood, and at 12 went away to become a Capuchin priest. He got a reputation as a troublemaker for asking too many questions, and three years later he left, taking with him a lifelong distaste for authoritarian—or what he called "the Lord told me to tell you"—religious traditions.

Disillusioned by religion, he studied physics and chemistry in college only to be further disappointed by the limitations of science. But his interest in spirituality persisted, and he hitchhiked around the country investigating spiritualism because, as he put it, "I figured that if I wanted to know what happened when I died, I would just ask some dead people about it."

> He hitchhiked around the country investigating spiritualism because, as he put it, "I figured that if I wanted to know what happened when I died, I would just ask some dead people about it."

Most of what he found were hucksters and hoaxes, but in Columbus, Ohio he finally encountered what he called a "genuine materialization."

"Me and a couple other guys spent hours riggin' the medium's basement before the performance so we couldn't be bamboozled. We even dusted the floor with cornstarch so if the 'spirits' were really cheesecloth shills we'd see footprints."

Soon after the medium disappeared into his "closet," a grotesque, manlike little creature emerged and began bouncing around the room. It was about three feet tall and began goading Rose, referring to him as "Baldy" because he was already losing his hair. Eventually this "familiar spirit," according to Rose, settled down and began summoning other spirits. Most of those in attendance met dead relatives, but Rose encountered several eyeless priests and nuns dressed in habits. Rose was initially impressed. He'd said nothing about his religion or time in the seminary, but when he spoke to these entities in Latin, they were unable to answer.

Moreover, none of the "spirits" were able to answer specific metaphysical questions beyond vague generalizations. As a result, even though these "spirits" eventually vanished straight down through his powder-dusted concrete floor without a trace, Rose was unconvinced.

"I don't know what the hell they were, but they weren't dead people," he told me. "And if they were, then Ecclesiastes is right: the dead know nothing."

Rose decided that spiritualism was not only a waste of time but dangerous as well, and he resolved to have no more to do with it.

By the time Rose finished exploring spiritualism, science, and conventional religion he was 21, disillusioned, and depressed. "But what drove me on in the face of disillusionment was disillusionment," he wryly said. "I was damn angry and planned to stay that way. I felt undefined, and it drove me nuts. I was determined to get answers or die trying. Sometimes I think the purest motivation a seeker can have is just getting sick and tired of the BS and deciding to do something about it."

Eventually, he discovered Eastern spirituality and got hooked on the Yogic idea of spiritual transformation. "I didn't buy everything I was readin'," he said, "but I decided to accept certain things provisionally, give 'em a try, and see where it took me."

For Rose, provisional faith and healthy skepticism didn't mean provisional effort. Becoming celibate and a vegetarian, he spent long hours meditating and doing yoga while traveling the country looking for groups and teachers. "I found damn little, and what I did was usually some self-anointed guru looking for money, sex, or God knows what. That's why I promised that if I ever did discover anything, I'd share it no strings attached."

Using his college chemistry, he made his living in various cities as a metallurgist, and he bought 165 acres near the family farm back in West Virginia. He usually wintered there as a hermit, reading and meditating in a ramshackle old farmhouse without heat, running water, or electricity. When he wasn't fasting, he would cook a big pot of vegetarian stew on Sunday and eat it cold all week long.

"I lived that way for seven years," he said. "Say, thinkin' about all them boiled beans makes me hungry. How's about a fish sandwich?"

I was so absorbed in Rose's story I didn't notice that he'd led us to what soon became my favorite Wheeling landmark. Coleman's Fish Market was founded in 1914 and was famous for its fish sandwiches. Even though it was well past noon, the queue stretched out the door and down the sidewalk. The line moved quickly, however, because 99 percent of the customers ordered the same thing: two pieces of fried fish between two slices of ordinary, white sandwich bread wrapped in day old newspaper with sides of fries, coleslaw, and iced tea. Rose, always the contrarian, ordered two standalone fish sandwiches while conspiratorially whispering that the sandwich was "the best deal" and that sides and drinks "ain't worth the money."

We took a seat at an old wooden picnic table, and Rose instantly tore into his first sandwich. I soon discovered why. Despite its simplicity, Coleman's fish sandwich is delicious, and I rarely visited Wheeling after that without stopping in, usually with Rose.

The only downside to our fishy feast was Rose seemed so intent on the task at hand I was afraid he would forget his story and leave me hanging. After what I considered a dignified interval, I decided to give him a nudge.

"Wow, seven years, Mr. Rose. That must have been tough, especially the celibacy," I said, fastening on a subject of critical importance to a 20-year-old male.

"Actually, those were some of the happiest years of my life," he said as we started back to his car. "I discovered the freedom and power of self-control. I could set my mind to just about anything and follow through no matter what. Always remember: the first step to a spiritual life—hell, any kind of life—is gettin' control of yourself. If you lack self-control, you'll always live with shame.

"In retrospect it wasn't what I *did* that was critical but what I *didn't* do. I was in a state of bliss most of the time. I felt like I was dialing Heaven."

"So that's how you found what you were looking for?"

"Hell no!" he roared, making me jump. "I looked in the mirror and my hair was fallin' out and my teeth were fallin' out. I looked like a potato stickin' out of a shirt, and believe you me that ain't the transformation I had in mind. I was nothin' but a fat-headed fool, bloated with self-importance, arrogantly looking down my nose at all the spiritual pygmies huddled at my feet. I was using spirituality as a crutch, a way to feel like somethin' special. At 28 I realized I was nothin' special. I was a corpse in the makin' headin' for the compost heap just like everybody else."

"What did you do then?"

"Nothing," he said with disgust. "I'd been at it since I was 12, and sixteen years later I had nothin' to show for it. I decided to give it all up. I could see…

"Let's go!" He suddenly shouted, interrupting his story.

By the time I could react, Rose was already halfway across the street and headed full tilt toward an altercation a block away. A young man, with a girl huddled between him and his car, was yelling and waving a tire iron as four men slowly and silently pressed in on them from three sides. But when they saw Rose and me coming on the trot, the men broke off and hurried away. Without even making eye contact with the couple he just rescued, Rose recrossed the street and continued walking briskly toward his car.

The whole incident lasted barely two minutes, but my heart was still pounding with leftover fear as I waited for an explanation for our latest adventure. While I admired this fresh demonstration of high-minded audacity, I couldn't square it with the way he continually cautioned against getting caught up in humanity's pointless "games." Games he largely dismissed as "the mindless machinations of deluded human lemmings desperately searching for the closest cliff." When it became apparent that no Rosean exegesis was forthcoming, I shyly ventured one of my own.

"Why did you do that, Mr. Rose? You risked your life for perfect strangers. Why not just yell for the cops?"

The key was in the ignition of his worn-out Oldsmobile when Rose abruptly turned and looked me straight in the eye. "The streets must be safe for women and children," he said flatly. "Someday you'll marry and have children of your own. Then you'll understand."

Then he turned the key and, with a roar, we started off toward Benwood.

* * *

My ambivalence, my fascination, and Rose's spiritual bona fides finally came to a head late that same evening. I was staying the night, it was very hot, and the only trace ventilation in that large, square kitchen was coming from the screen door leading to the back porch and the open transom over the hallway door. Rose was sitting at the kitchen table with his back to his white four-burner gas stove without a pilot light. The stove was adorned as always with a big box of wooden kitchen matches, his grease-coated cast iron frying pan, and the dangerous-looking old pressure cooker he invariably used when his wife was pulling her frequent and interminable hospital shifts. By this time I'd sampled a potpourri of Rose's home-cooked concoctions, and I came to the conclusion that "cook the living hell out of it" was the secret ingredient common to all his recipes, just as it was for life itself.

Rose was as indifferent to the taste of food as he was to heat, cold, sleep, sex, music, sports, alcohol, TV, movies, romance, and anything else that might be called "creature comforts." While he was the most opinionated person I ever met, I can't recall a single instance when he deigned to mutter even a trivial comment about something he was eating or would like to eat, and the only food he ever seemed to enjoy was that occasional fish sandwich from Coleman's.

Since returning from Wheeling I'd been patiently waiting for Rose to pick up the story he'd spontaneously put on pause in favor of the rescue mission. It was obvious that despite his despair he didn't give up on spirituality, but it was now getting late, the heat was making me groggy, and there was still no indication he intended to go on. In fact, I sensed a real reluctance on his part which made me, in turn, reluctant to bring it up.

Then, during a lull in the conversation, Rose absently related an incident with his wife. He asked Phyllis what she wanted from life. "Well, I'd like to have grandchildren," she replied. "And if I can't have that, then a nice house full of antiques."

"Funny," Rose mused, "all I ever wanted, even as a boy, was the Truth. And if I couldn't have that . . . if I couldn't have that . . . say, can I fix you another cup of tea?"

I was stunned by this fresh off-hand demonstration of his mono-maniacal sense of purpose. For Rose there was no Plan B, backup plan, contingency plan, fallback plan, consolation prize, safety net, hedged bet, insurance policy, runner-up trophy, or hanging on to his day job: it was always all or nothing right down the line. Without thinking, I blurted out the question I'd wanted to ask since we met. "Mr. Rose, how did you find the Truth?"

Rose looked at me steadily. "Listen," he said, "I know you been me-anin' to ask me that for a while, and I don't want you to think I been duckin' you. But it takes all the sap outta' me just thinkin' about it, let alone talkin' about it."

Without further elaboration, he picked up his story . . .

. . . Even though, at 28, he decided to turn in his badge as a spiritual seeker, he discovered it wasn't that easy. Intellectually, he gave up on a hopeless project only to discover that the habits of sixteen years had taken on a life of their own. Rose had irretrievably become a seeker whether he liked it or not. The next two years were living hell.

"I wanted to quit spirituality with all my might," he said, "but I was like a drunk who's forgotten how to live without the bottle. I was a runaway train with sixteen years of steam behind it, and by the time I realized the bridge up ahead was out, it was too late to throw on the brakes."

At 30 he hit bottom and, betraying all his principles, decided to marry a woman for her money. He took a bus to Seattle, Washington where she was living—but couldn't go through with it. Instead, he reverted, kicking and screaming once again, to spiritual practices. One night he was meditating when he experienced an excruciating pain at the top of his head. Convinced he was having a stroke, his last conscious thought was wondering how his destitute family would find the money to ship his dead body back to West Virginia.

The next thing he knew he was in another dimension. "I was witnessing creation itself," he said. "I saw everyone who ever lived or ever would and all their darkness and despair was heartbreaking. The love, compassion, and sorrow I felt for humanity's plight just tore me apart.

"Then I thought, 'If everyone's down there, where's Rose?' Instantly I saw myself, and I was nothing but one more member of that endlessly striving tide of foolishly deluded mankind. I saw how ridiculous and egotistical all 'his' illusions were, and how futile all 'his' efforts. I knew 'he' would never see 'me' as I now saw 'him'—never know what 'I' now knew—and the pain of this was unbearable. Everything—I mean *everything*—I ever thought of as 'me' just melted under the strain.

"Then I was hit by a question: If that's 'me,' then who am 'I'? If 'I' is gone, what's left? Who is witnessing all this? And with this realization I groped for my limits and found I had none. I was everywhere and nowhere. Like the mystics say, I'd stumbled into that infinite sphere whose center is everywhere and whose circumference is nowhere, and this final shock hit me so hard I lost my balance altogether and fell into the Void, or Darkness of God."

These last words caught in his throat. Rose was visibly shaken, but when I couldn't take the suspense any longer, I selfishly whispered, "What did you find in the Void, Mr. Rose?"

"Everything and nothing, or no-thing," he said flatly. "Even what I just said about dimensions, visions, questions, and plunging—all happening along some neat, progressive timeline—is nothing but a bunch of half-assed metaphors, more lies than truth. Believe me, there's no time, no thoughts, no questions, and no 'I' to have them. There's nothing but the Absolute Eternal Now. There are no words. Hell, I've had twenty-three years to describe it to myself, and I'm no closer now than I was then."

Rose looked away, and when he looked back his face was painfully contorted. "You see," he whispered hoarsely, "what I can never hope to get across is the *totality*. My God, the *totality* . . . "

With this, Rose staggered to his feet, awkwardly muttered something in my direction, and left the room. The look on his face as he fled was one of physical pain. I was more than moved. I was shocked by the beauty, the eternity, the agony permeating his whispered last words: "the *totality*."

I sat for some time, my heart racing. Eventually something—either the ticking wall clock over the single-tub sink or its dripping faucet—pulled me from my reverie. I noticed a heaviness hanging in the room. I dismissed it as something engendered by the late hour and that stuffy, silent old house.

It wasn't only that.

Even though I was utterly convinced that Rose had been to God and back, I was also sorry for him. Rose lived without a single human being who could look him in the eyes and say those two simple words: "I understand." Like Moses, he tottered under a heavenly mandate, a Burning Bush that left him equally tongue-tied and without even a brother like Aaron to speak for him. Rose had a wife and three children, none of whom had the slightest interest in his Enlightenment experience or a shred of compassion for the anguish its volcanic pressure produced. Instead, they indulgently tolerated him, and he never asked for more.

It was that night that I first encountered the unspeakable loneliness that was also Richard Rose.

But I was too wrapped up in my own concerns to admit it. Perhaps I didn't want to think my hero could be lonely; or maybe I didn't want to face the possibility that I would find myself in the same place, living in the Main Hotel, someday; or maybe if I did acknowledge his anguish, I would have had to reach out to him, something I didn't know how to do.

So, like a disciple at Gethsemane oblivious to Christ's agony and overcome with fatigue, I locked the kitchen door, tightened the dripping faucet, and headed upstairs to bed. When I reached the second floor, the furnace-like heat was suffocating. Entering the spare bedroom, I couldn't open the windows because Rose had nailed them shut against winter drafts. Lying in soaking sheets I sweltered for a while before finally falling into a fitful sleep.

I dreamed I was in a place so dark I couldn't tell where I ended and the darkness began, and like a child hiding even from himself in a cozy closet on a rainy day, this utter anonymity felt safe and comforting. A door opened and Rose appeared, his familiar silhouette framed by the sunlight pouring in. He began walking toward me, his hand outstretched. His demeanor wasn't threatening, but I was terrified. I began backpedaling, but Rose slowly backed me against a wall and then firmly grasped my wrist.

Like the Greek sea god Proteus, I suddenly realized I could change into any shape I wished. Desperate to get free, I morphed into hundreds, then thousands, of monstrous shapes, but Rose, his eyes locked on mine, calmly held my wrist until, exhausted, I resumed my human form. No longer capable of resistance, Rose led me out the door to a three-rung railing running along a high, room-lined corridor of what appeared to be a cheap hotel. This hallway faced the ocean, and the sun ricocheting off the water created an eye-stinging glare.

With Rose still holding my wrist, I awkwardly climbed the banister's metal rails until I was precariously weaving back and forth on top. Then Rose telepathically ordered me to dive into the ocean. Far below, the deserted beach stretched out for hundreds of yards before reaching the ocean. I was certain that if I dove, I would die. But there was no fight left in me, so I dove.

Miraculously, I began to soar. I traversed the beach, sped out over the ocean, and plunged headfirst into amniotic water so warm there was no shock of entry. Reaching the bottom, I pushed off and shot to the surface. Instantly the sun, the crystal blue sky, the warmth of the water, and my exhilaration and relief coalesced into a boundless sense of joy and peace . . .

. . . Awakening, I noticed the sun was coming up. I lay quietly for a while basking in the warm afterglow of my dream. The meaning was clear. It was time to leave my dark and comfortable cocoon, stop all my monstrous and ineffectual arguing, trust Rose, and take the plunge. So I got up, dressed, and went downstairs to the kitchen. Just as I expected, Rose, always the early riser, was already drinking coffee and going through his mail. He greeted me in a friendly way, offered a cup of tea, and then went back to his mail. I sat staring at my tea for a while and then, summoning all my courage, I blurted out.

"Mr. Rose, I want to be your student."

Rose peered at me over the rims of his reading glasses for a few seconds, and then, arching his eyebrows, said, "OK," and resumed his work.

Minutes passed and it eventually dawned on me: that was it. Months of buildup, his Enlightenment story, my dream—all leading to this anticlimactic moment. I felt utterly drained. I pouted for a while waiting for him to notice, but he didn't, or didn't let on he did. Finally, I couldn't take it anymore.

"What happens now, Mr. Rose?"

"Well," he said, pushing back his chair and removing his glasses, "I guess we put first things first. You're going to have to go back to Pittsburgh and build yourself a community of like-minded people."

My heart sank. This was the last thing I expected. What I was expecting I couldn't say, but it was supposed to be something mystical, magical, otherworldly, an initiation ceremony, a Vulcan mind meld . . . *something*.

"What do I need a community for, Mr. Rose?"

"Did it ever occur to you that it's what you can do for them that matters?" Rose said acidly. "What were you expecting?"

"I don't know," I sputtered, flustered. "I was reading about trance meditation and altered states of consciousness and I thought—"

"Trance meditation?" he roared. "What the hell do you want with that? Believe me, you're so deeply entranced now you're hazardous to yourself and other living things. As for altered states of consciousness, each desire or priority is a different state of consciousness, and all these conflicting voices keep you divided against yourself. This work is not about adding more states of consciousness, it's about simplifying your life until the Truth is all that's left.

"But let's cut the nonsense," he continued. "What's really botherin' you is you want to be the center of the universe. I'm supposed to keep you eternally entertained while never lettin' on that I use the bathroom like everyone else."

"No, no, it's not that. It's just . . . well . . . *you* never had a commu—"

"And that's just why you have to have one," Rose interrupted. "I spent eighteen years spinnin' my wheels because I didn't have other people to help me out. We all have blind spots, and the guy with his zipper down is always the last to know.

"That brings us to the next point. There are two kinds of spiritual communities. The first is full of folks who won't tell you when your zipper's down. These people think gettin' along and not makin' waves is the most important thing in life. They don't want pressure, and it never occurs to them that the only thing that's going to crack the toughest substance known to man, ego, is maximum pressure.

"Instead, you need a community of people who push each other through beneficial criticism, peer pressure, and honest confrontation.

Most groups attract too many people lookin' for others to lean on. The community degenerates into a mutually modulated conspiracy of mediocrity hiding behind some rubric about compassion and acceptance: I'll buy your nonsense if you buy mine.

"Now don't get me wrong," Rose continued, absently tugging at his right ear. "I never turn away anyone sincerely looking for help. But it's one thing to help someone over the bar and another to lower the bar. You need a team of individuals, not sheep, or the next thing you know you're runnin' a slumber party instead of an adventure. This ain't no book-of-the-month club. We're talkin' an Everest climb.

"There's another reason why you need a community. You need to teach, and you might as well get started. There's no better way to learn than by teaching."

Rose suddenly became thoughtful. "There's something else," he said almost tenderly. "Community isn't about you or what's in it for you."

Rose told me he had a brother two years older. His name was James, and Rose named his son after him. "I don't think I've ever been closer to anyone," Rose said. "And truth is, James was the better human being." One day the family got a telegram: a German U-Boat sank James's merchant ship off the coast of Florida. His body washed up on the beach three days later.

Rose was devastated, and he took a vow in his brother's name. He swore that if he ever discovered anything spiritually, he would do whatever he could to give it away. "I was spiritually dead in the water until I made that promise," he said.

"You got to learn how to give without expecting anything, and I mean *anything*, in return."

Rose stopped and stared at me until I squirmed under his gaze. "I know you don't understand what I'm sayin'," he said sadly. "You're just like I was. You're takin' the elevator to Heaven, so you can't be bothered with folks you think are takin' the stairs. You need that fire in your belly, but you also need compassion, and your problem is you have no compassion. And I'm afraid it's going to take something like someone in your family dying to finally teach it to you."

I wish I could say Rose was wrong, or that his speech hit home and opened my heart. Instead, I saw the need for other people as a nuisance. A side trip that would cramp our style and indefinitely put off "the good stuff." I was ready to go to sea, and Rose insisted we build a bigger boat and stock it with tourists first. It never occurred to me that building and stocking ships and going to sea are one and the same exercise. I also refused to admit I did want to be the absolute center of Rose's attention. What I felt most of all was unappreciated. I was a remarkable specimen, making an incredible sacrifice, and Rose was taking me for granted. Instead of being celebrated I was criticized, and my feelings were hurt.

His comment about my lack of compassion stung deeply, but only because I wanted perfection. One of my blind spots was I couldn't see the difference between gregariousness and compassion, and since I had plenty of the former, I assumed I had all the latter I needed. All in all I walked away from the whole conversation with a classic "What about me?" attitude.

* * *

However, without further argument, I returned to the University of Pittsburgh, founded a student organization called the Zen Studies Society, and began looking for members. Whatever else was lacking, I was coachable and took my commitment seriously. But I also couldn't understand what Rose was talking about. In fact, I thought he was wrong. Since Rose and his teachings were going to be the focus of our Zen Studies Society meetings, I wondered, in darker moments, if I'd been shanghaied into serving Rose's larger ambitions.

But I did what he asked anyway.

Many of the true tests in a teacher/student relationship revolve around the issue of coachability. If we have blind spots—and we do—

then by definition there will be many times when what the teacher asks of us initially makes no sense. Often these directives will be as scary and counterintuitive as diving headfirst off a multistory railing in hopes of reaching an ocean hundreds of yards away.

Chapter Six

THE KUNG FU REVOLUTION

Time present and time past
Are both perhaps present in time future
And time future contained in time past.
If all time is eternally present
All time is unredeemable.
What might have been is an abstraction
Remaining a perpetual possibility
Only in a world of speculation.
What might have been and what has been
Point to one end, which is always present.
Footfalls echo in the memory
Down the passage which we did not take
Towards the door we never opened
Into the rose-garden.
—T.S. Eliot[15]

The University of Pittsburgh is located in the Oakland section of the city, and its campus sprawls over 145 acres of busy urban streets and neighborhoods. The Cathedral of Learning, the campus centerpiece, is a forty-two-story Late Gothic Revival skyscraper, the tallest educational building in the Western Hemisphere. Rose agreed to a kickoff lecture at Pitt and to come up to run our weekly meetings, and the Zen Studies Society was quickly approved as an official student organization. Ray was not a Pitt student, but he offered to help, and we photocopied some simple black and white posters at an office where he worked evenings as a janitor. (Ray jazzed them up a bit by hand stenciling the words "Zen Lecture" so they looked like they were lettered in bamboo.)

It was still a magical time on college campuses in 1972. Anything having to do with mystical spirituality was guaranteed a crowd. I booked a large room for Rose's lecture, across the street from the Cathedral, at the chandelier- and marble-encrusted student union, which was once the famous Hotel Schenley, a Pittsburgh landmark. We had a full house, and Rose electrified the crowd with his humor and no-nonsense approach. I beamed with pride as I watched a gaggle of students ply him with questions afterward. Rose satisfied them all, and then walked over to where I eagerly awaited my well-deserved pat on the back.

"Well," he said with a tired smile, "I reckon I didn't lay too big an egg."

"I think it went great, Mr. Rose."

"Good. How many names did you get for your group?"

My stomach dropped. With all the excitement I forgot to pass around a contact sheet for those who might want to attend weekly meetings. Sheepishly, I informed Rose. At first he looked disgusted, but something in my face caught his funny bone and he ended up laughing until tears came.

"Well," he finally said, "looks like this is going to be tougher than I thought. We'll just have to do it all over again."

* * *

Next time I collected a bunch of names, and we began meeting with twenty to twenty-five students at 7:30 on Thursday nights on the third floor of the student union. Each week Rose made the 130-mile round trip to Pittsburgh in his old Oldsmobile on worn-out, previously owned tires he called "baloney skins." His dodgy transportation meant he always set out with a full complement of mechanic's tools, two spare tires, a fresh fan belt, four gallons of radiator water, and, like a man wearing suspenders and a belt, jumper cables and a backup battery. True to his word, he asked for no compensation beyond the few dollars in gas money we garnered by passing the hat. Any money collected beyond his fuel went into our treasury, and Rose insisted I appoint a secretary and a treasurer from among the students and keep a strict set of books open to anyone who might care to examine them.

Meetings, like everything with Rose, were unstructured, impromptu affairs. We sat in a big circle of folding chairs as Rose lectured, took questions, and told stories while continually poking and prodding us with questions and personal observations designed to "stir up thinking." This lack of structure and specific spiritual "practices" frustrated those looking for a step-by-step approach, and Rose's freestyle, idiosyncratic take on Zen cost us members. Zen for Rose, however, was essentially spontaneous, and he believed that highly structured spiritual systems, disciplines, and practices merely reinforced the "mechanical thinking" and "sleep walking" that he was constantly trying to upend. Or, as he put it more colorfully, "My job is jamming popsicle sticks into the gears of mechanical thinking." Rose's approach neatly echoed Nietzsche's "To make people uncomfortable, that is my task."

Rose was, of course, controversial from the get-go. His in-your-face methods, to put it mildly, were not appreciated by everyone. But what really made folks squirm was his insistence that, spiritually speaking, "results are proportional to energy applied." For Rose, reaching Enlightenment had far more in common with the single-minded effort required to become a successful entrepreneur, elite athlete, or famous artist than it did with an innocent hobby we practice in our spare time to "round out" our lives and give us "peace of mind." As he liked to say, "If it's only peace of mind you want, you don't need me. Just sit back and wait. You'll get a whole damn eternity of it in the marble orchard."

"Listen," he often said, "don't flatter yourself. We are animals, and nature don't take too kindly to specimens that wander away from the zoo and start questioning their animal programming. You gotta stay awake and on guard, because Mother Nature is a beautiful Siren, forever singin' her seductive song, tryin' to lure you back to the only thing she really cares about: reproduction."

On one occasion, an angry student testily countered that he was intent on "relaxing and going with the flow" instead. Rose drily responded, "Well, you go with the flow if you want. But I've followed up a few flows in my time and they all ended up in the same place: the sewer. We drift into nothing. Except death."

Another time Rose was talking about the benefits of vegetarianism. This had all the vegetarians nodding and smiling, but when one devotee made a comment designed to win some incremental Rosean approval for his culinary predilections, Rose had a quick reply.

"Oh, I don't know. I got a lot of my best insights while fasting, and if you think about it, fasting is a diet of nothin' but meat."

Rose continually undermined the "belief structures" we egotistically lean on as psychological crutches. Rose never answered a question; he always answered the human being hiding behind the question, and his unerring ability to go directly to the heart of his target is what kept people—albeit with some anxious trepidation—coming back week after week. In fact, one of the most poignant examples of Rose at his best actually happened to me.

At the beginning of each meeting I would give a short overview of our group for new people, bring up any incidental business, pass the treasury hat, and then introduce Rose sitting next to me. One time I introduced Rose, but instead of picking up the ball as usual, he quietly continued to gaze at his hands folded placidly on his lap. Seconds ticked by, then minutes, and still Rose remained motionless. Alarmed by this vacuum and the tension it seemed to engender, I ventured a question to break the ice.

"Mr. Rose," I said, "what do you think about prayer?"

Slowly Rose raised his head. "Make your whole life a prayer and it will be answered instantly." Then he became meditatively quiet again.

In one sentence Rose seemed to answer my question generally, answer me and my fears personally, and mildly rebuke me for being unable to sit quietly and pray with him a while. This triple jolt was so effective I found myself "praying" on this koan for days, and I've returned to it periodically ever since.

Half the semester went by this way, and I was beginning to relax and enjoy myself. I always liked people, and once I got over my initial hurt, I appreciated having others around. Besides, I enjoyed being able to channel my competitive spirit into filling the room for Rose each week. Now that we had our community, I amused myself wondering what Rose planned to do with it.

Then one week, before Rose could begin speaking, Nancy, our treasurer, raised her hand and stood up.

"Mr. Rose, we all got together and decided we want to learn Kung Fu."

I was caught flat-footed. I was not invited to this meeting, nor did I have any inkling it took place.

"I don't teach Kung Fu," Rose said quietly.

Nancy repeated her demand, and the edge to her voice told me that whatever was inspiring her was something far more visceral than the then-popular television series *Kung Fu* starring David Carradine.

"I don't teach Kung Fu," Rose repeated quietly but firmly.

"That doesn't matter," she said, tossing her head. "This is a student organization and a democracy, and we want to study Kung Fu." As she finished, our secretary, a young man, backed her with a nod.

"Well, this is the first time I've heard of patients prescribing for the doctor," Rose said, "but if that's your decision, I'll be on my way."

Nancy said nothing, but she was now so openly hostile that, as the Russians like to say, there was enough tension in the room to hang an axe on. Rose slowly and deliberately put his notes for the meeting back in his satchel, picked up his fedora, and started for the door.

As all this unfolded, I was too shocked to move, let alone speak. As Rose reached the door, he turned and said, "Are you coming, Augie?"

Hearing my name broke the spell. I sprang to my feet and followed him out the door. As we walked to the parking lot, I was so depressed I just absently plodded along. All my months of work just went down the drain. Finally giving vent to anguish, I moaned, "Well, Mr. Rose, I guess we just lost our community."

"Why do you say that?" Rose asked with arched eyebrows and genuine surprise. "You're here, aren't you? What else matters?" He told me that only sincerity and purity of purpose really matter, and if I found the courage to live this way, it would pay off in magical ways. This felt like falling back on feel-good superstition in the face of abject failure, and blaming him for the debacle, I just mentally rolled my eyes.

Rose suggested decamping to the five-bedroom, off-campus house I now shared with Chip, Bud, and two other Pitt students to have a cup of tea and plan our next move. I was more inclined toward wound licking than strategic planning, but I was too depressed to say so, and we drove to the house. No one was home, and as I put water on for tea, Rose was completely relaxed, jocular even, which I dismissed as merely an effort to mollify me. We sat in the living room, and I sullenly waited for my tea to cool and for whatever postmortem Rose would offer.

Before he could speak, there was a knock at the door. Peering through the window shades, I saw several shadowy figures milling around on the porch. Flicking on the light revealed a small group of students fresh from our meeting. A young man said they heard that Rose was here and asked if they could come in. Utterly amazed, I dragged in some chairs and put more water on to boil. I was just about to sit down again when another group of students magically appeared. So it went, until my oversized living room was jammed with everyone but Nancy, the secretary, and one other student. There were even a half-dozen people I'd never seen before, including two married couples in their mid-twenties. I was so gobsmacked by this turn of events I was grateful to stay busy answering the door, ransacking the house for chairs, and boiling pot after pot of tea.

When I finally rejoined the meeting, Rose darted a gentle, other-worldly "oh you of little faith" smile in my direction. In little more than an hour I'd watched our community vanish and then magically reappear, and Rose's beatific smile was like a cock crow triggering waves of shame for my selfish despair, for doubting him, and for forcing him to call me out by name before I was willing to follow him out of the room. But there was something more to that smile. It came wrapped in an eerie sense that something supernatural working through Rose had set all this up on purpose to dramatically drive home Rose's contention that faith and purity of purpose lead to magical outcomes.

All these realizations were transmitted in an instant through that Rosean smile, and suddenly the same energy that jolted me when I first met Rose, then at the spring on his farm, and still later in his kitchen, welled up from that same black box deep inside. Once again I found myself momentarily disoriented and fighting for control. Confronted yet again with this fresh indication that Rose might just be capable of bringing the magic I was supposedly yearning for, my only reaction was horror and abject terror.

I never did ask those people how they knew Rose would be at my house, or how they even knew where I lived. I still don't know. We met at my house for a few weeks until the Kung Fu group collapsed. Then we quietly reoccupied the room at the student union. I never saw Nancy—or our treasury balance—again, and I've often wondered if the $18.26 was her take for so admirably playing the role she was scripted to play by that hillbilly front man for fate, Richard Rose.

* * *

Despite all the energy I was pouring into our nascent community and my sincere commitment to being his student, I was still keeping secrets from Rose. For one, I was no closer to asking about these energy jolts even though Rose often spoke about what he called "voltage" and the role it played in spiritual development. An important part of Rose's teaching focused on the ability of a Zen master to "transmit" mystical knowledge by harnessing this voltage or psychic energy and using it to "open up the head" of his student. He said this "mind to mind" transmission could trigger spiritual epiphanies that would "abridge years of work on the part of the student." Years later I encountered this quote about mystical transmission from the great ninth-century Chinese Zen Master, Huang Po.

> *Mind is transmitted with Mind and these Minds are identical. Transmitting and receiving transmission are both a most difficult kind of mysterious understanding, so that few indeed have been able to receive it.*[16]

Transmission, according to Rose, required mastering the fine art of "betweenness" or "a knack for running between raindrops without getting wet." Betweenness is a sort of psychic slipstream running halfway betwixt all earthly opposites; a mystical space where logic stumbles, paradox rules, and miracles happen; a magical spot that T.S. Eliot, in Four Quartets, poetically calls "the still point of the turning world."

> *At the still point of the turning world.*
> *Neither flesh nor fleshless;*
> *Neither from nor towards; at the still point, there the dance is,*
> *But neither arrest nor movement.*
> *And do not call it fixity,*
> *Where past and future are gathered.*
> *Neither movement from nor towards,*
> *Neither ascent nor decline. Except for the point, the still point,*

There would be no dance, and there is only the dance.
I can only say, there we have been: but I cannot say where
And I cannot say, how long, for that is to place it in time.[17]

Rose had an entire physics surrounding this psychic energy or voltage, how it was created, conserved, "transmuted" or refined, and ultimately used. In light of these teachings, it seems incredulous that I continued to hide my experiences from him. My ongoing deception, however, merely demonstrates how terrifying these energy surges were. Even more terrifying, in fact, than entertaining the preposterous notion that Rose was conjuring spiritual communities into and out of existence purely for my spiritual edification.

Meanwhile, throughout the fall of 1972 these little jolts continued intermittently. Five years older than me, Rob was a graduate student in biology who joined the Zen Studies Society. His bespectacled, bearded, soft-spoken, professorial demeanor was such a dead-on foil for his deadpan, madcap sense of humor that, like Chip, I soon added him to my collection of introverted, book-loving, eccentric friends.

Rob was working late nights at his lab unraveling the mystery of how frog hearts work, and he had an oversized refrigerator stocked with shelves of hibernating frogs stiffly lined up like soldiers on three-dimensional parade patiently awaiting dissection to prove it. However, much to the chagrin of his thesis advisor, his impatient girlfriend, his epileptic dog, and perhaps even a smattering of those half-frozen frogs, research had ground to a halt as Rob secretly redirected his dissections into books on mysticism under the mind-altering influence of his faithful lab assistant: weed.

One day Rob and I were sitting in the kitchen kicking around various theories about life after death while Rose clattered away on his ancient manual typewriter somewhere else in the house.

"The problem with the whole concept of life after death," Rob was saying as he pressed the last dregs of tea out of his soggy tea bag, "lies with the word 'after.' If time itself is an illusory construct, then concepts like before and after become meaningless."

"Yeah," I added, "if eternity is happening all at once, how can . . . "

Rose wandered in for some coffee and took it all in on the fly. "You guys got it all wrong," he interrupted while raising the cup to his lips. "Life and death are just two sides of the same coin—a coin with no sides." It was as if the man I knew began that sentence and a voice from the Other Side finished it. Once again, I found myself fighting for control as Rose ambled out of the room. As for Rob, he sat bug-eyed for a full thirty seconds before he finally shivered and said, "Whew!"

Another time I was sitting next to Rose on a couch underneath the big wall clock in the lobby of the Pitt student union. Besides being an obscenely early riser, Rose was fanatical about being on time and, probably anticipating car trouble as well, always arrived two hours early for our Zen meetings at Pitt. Catching on, some of the more eager students began showing up early for an impromptu session under the clock as we waited for our room to become available at 7:30.

Rose was often at his best at these spontaneous gatherings, and on one occasion he was fielding questions and storytelling when a thin, scraggly haired and bearded young man foppishly dressed like some latter-day black magician, with dark-painted fingernails and a long flowing cape, floated by. Rose stopped dead midsentence and stared intently at this young necromancer until this ostentatious apparition blithely exited stage right. Then, without comment, Rose picked up just where he left off. A few minutes later this mysterious sorcerer reappeared, and Rose repeated the exercise until he dematerialized again, this time stage left. When this same wannabe thaumaturgist took center stage yet again for his encore, a transfixed Rose suddenly exclaimed, "That guy's givin' me koans. Someone lend me an axe!"

His audience erupted with laughter, but while they were preoccupied, Rose leaned over and whispered in my ear.

"You know, sometimes I want to just jump inside your head and shake the livin' hell out of you. But you're too sensitive, so I don't do it." Then he picked up the conversation just where he left off. It wasn't just the scary and unexpected nature of Rose's message that sent my mind reeling. It was the compassion in his voice as well.

Eventually, Rose didn't have to say or do anything at all. At the oddest moments I would be sharing the same room as he was frying an egg or reading the paper when suddenly I would feel this same energy surging inside me. My heart would race, and I'd become disoriented. Then I'd clamp down fiercely until whatever was welling up decided to settle down. Since these experiences never lasted more than a moment or two, I would immediately begin explaining them away. But though I wanted, very much, to ask Rose about them, I never did.

The second secret I was keeping from Rose, and to a large degree from myself, was a beautiful girl named Sara.

The second secret I was keeping from Rose, and to a large degree from myself, was a beautiful girl named Sara. I first saw Sara at one of Paul's parties. Paul was a sinewy, six-foot-six, blond-haired, blue-eyed, mechanical genius and motorcycle fanatic with a striking resemblance to central casting's take on a California surfer. He worked in rehab at a local hospital and quickly became an integral member of my college crowd. Our mutual interest in road trips and dirt motorcycles brought us even closer together.

Anything but an introverted, eccentric bookworm, Paul was the loud, boisterous, high energy, hell-raising, beer-loving, all boy, life-of-the-party type I've always had a soft spot for— probably because, in Rosean parlance, when I "took a notion," I could be much the same way. (Rose laughingly told me one time, "The only reason you hang around is you figure if me and you was ever to take a notion we could hit the road and stir up some real trouble!") Paul and his roommate had a sweet deal on a sprawling single-story house with a swimming pool in the Castle Shannon suburb of Pittsburgh, and they were famous for perpetual parties where people wandered in and out at all hours, helped themselves to the bottomless keg invariably on tap and, if they over-imbibed and happened to "take a notion," they just plopped on a couch and got back at it the next morning.

I was swimming in Paul's pool when I first saw Sara. She was checking out the pool in shorts, a halter top, and a pair of sandals. Her hair, adorned by the sunglasses propped on her head, was a sun-bleached dirty blonde worn in a shag. Even from my safe distance I was dazzled by her big blue eyes. One of my favorite bands is the John Sebastian-fronted Lovin' Spoonful, and my first reaction to Sara was right out of one of their songs:

> *She's one of those girls who seem to come in the spring.*
> *One look in her eyes and you forget everything you had ready to say.*
> *And I saw her today.*[18]

Sara left me so tongue-tied, in fact, I don't think we even met at that party, but somehow over the fall of 1972 we became friends. Sara was a Pitt student majoring in physical education, and she lived in a campus dormitory. Unlike Nancy, Sara didn't have a serious bone in her body, and she was as outgoing and vivacious as Nancy was shy and reserved. Sara had an impish, teasing, wonderful sense of humor that made you feel special to be the butt of her joke. She effortlessly kept me in stitches by remorselessly teasing me about my interest in Rose and Zen, interests she collectively nicknamed "Augie and his buddhas." For my part, I made no attempt to turn her into one of my buddhas or even to share my serious side, as I did with Nancy. In fact one of the things I prized in Sara was having a lighthearted antidote to a heavy-duty Rose and all the contradictions, fears, and frustrations constantly whirling around him.

Before long, and long before I was ready to admit it, I was madly in love with Sara. But though Sara was nothing like Nancy, there was one fundamental similarity: my inability to profess my feelings and romantically "make a move." Of course, the usual suspects were in play. Fear that my feelings would not be reciprocated and my terror at losing control and exposing my vulnerability. While I treasured Sara as an antidote to Rose, like Nancy and later Orysia, she also represented a potential catalyst that would usher too many chaotic emotions to the surface. Besides, my romantic still-under-development script for myself as the mythical Zen warrior/monk didn't have a part for a leading lady.

In short, I was in love with a girl who also represented a weakness, a weakness which belied, contradicted, and embarrassed my recent commitment to go, as Rose would put it, "whole hog" for him and his teaching. My relationship with Sara was my latest attempt to "have it all" by somehow combining my spiritual yearnings with a "normal" life. Deep down I knew this, and I despised myself for, as Rose would put it, "still playing games."

I consciously coped with all these potential and actual difficulties by rationalizing my relationship with Sara away as just a friendship and harmless flirtation that didn't have anything to do with Rose and, therefore, was nothing he needed to know. Of course, I could only maintain this convenient fiction as long as I refrained from romantically making a move.

One day I was at Trees Hall, Pitt's gymnasium, leaning against the wall and patiently waiting for Sara to emerge from the women's locker room. I was so besotted that, for the first time in my life outside of formal sports, I was working out regularly with her, trying—without success so far—to swim 500 yards in ten minutes. A feat Sara did easily.

When she finally emerged from the locker room she instantly sang out "Au-gie!" like she always did, and I echoed "Sara Bean!" like I always did. (My mother had a baby sister named Sarah, and my father affectionately called her, for some unknown reason, Sarah Bean, or just Beanie.) Then we both began laughing, apparently in pure delight at nothing more than the sound of our own names, again, just like we always did.

"I don't know how you guys do it," she finally said. "I don't even take the time to dry my hair, and you're still out here ten minutes before me."

I just smiled because I didn't mind waiting for Sara one bit.

Trees Hall was perched on the highest point on Pitt's hilly campus, and I always walked Sara down the hill to her women's dormitory.

"It's almost 5:30," I said in the dorm's elevator on the way to her floor. "I got to meet Rose at the Union for our meeting."

Sara feigned a pouty face and then, as the elevator doors closed behind us, her blue eyes lit up.

"Don't leave yet," she said. "I have a surprise. It'll only take a minute."

In a trice, she had all the other girls on her floor out of their rooms and lined up in the hallway. Then, as I sat on a chair in the doorway to Sara's room, the girls proceeded to do a coordinated dance set to the theme from the movie *Shaft*—just for me.

The whole number was terrific, a perfectly executed cross between a tongue-in-cheek amateur sendup and a well-rehearsed professional performance. When the show ended, I clapped with delight, the girls were breathlessly giggling, and somehow Sara was comfortably ensconced on my lap. She laughingly nuzzled my neck before putting both hands on my shoulders and looking straight into my eyes.

"Au-gie, Au-gie," she softly lilted in a little girl's sing-song voice. "Don't run away to the buddhas. Stay here with meeeeeeee!"

We both collapsed in laughter at her well-timed and expertly delivered joke, but suddenly a cold chill went up my spine. For the first time since we started our community I didn't want to "run away to the buddhas." I wasn't a bit anxious to see Rose. I wanted to stay with Sara instead.

As I made my way from Sara's dorm to the student union, I became confused and deeply upset. Once again, a Rosean prophecy had come to pass. I just didn't expect my encounter with Mother Nature's beautiful Siren to be so explicit!

My God, I thought. *Sara was even singing her damn Siren's song!*

A song that, just like the Siren's Song from Homer's *Odyssey*[19], I was finding increasingly irresistible. It was unnerving. When I got to the Union, Rose was sitting under the clock sipping a McDonald's coffee from a paper cup. I felt guilty for wanting to be with Sara rather than him, but I just papered it over with an open-ended apology for being a few minutes late, an apology he seemed, with a shrug, to accept.

So, despite my best efforts to safely insulate myself, Sara quickly morphed from a casual Rosean antidote into yet another tangled koan I could neither unravel nor abandon. Sara, like Rose, was a candle flame I was dangerously circling, another brick in my mounting wall of frustration that, like Hotchkiss, precluded either advance or retreat. But the most important reason I didn't dare tell Rose about Sara was fear that, as he had so savagely done to my political ambitions at his farm, he would force me to choose between him and Sara, a terrifying choice I didn't want to make.

A few minutes later, as hungry students began arriving for an Early Bird Special extra helping of Rosean wit and wisdom before the meeting, it dawned on me that Sara might become a far more dangerous threat to our group and my commitment to Rose than Nancy and her cadre of Kung Fu revolutionaries ever were.

Chapter Seven

STARSHIPS AND TRUCK TRIPS

The chill ascends from feet to knees,
The fever sings in mental wires.
If to be warmed, then I must freeze
And quake in frigid purgatorial fires
Of which the flame is roses, and the smoke is briars.
—T.S. ELIOT[20]

During Christmas break Rose invited me to accompany him on a trip out west to visit two old friends, a married couple, from his own days as a spiritual seeker. I was providing the transportation, and fortuitously for his Rosean rear end, by this time I'd sold my Yamaha and reinvested the proceeds into one of two used 1963 Ford Econoline vans that Paul and I bought at auction from the telephone company for a hundred bucks apiece. In classic hippie fashion, with Paul's help, I faux wood-paneled the walls and ceiling, and particolored the floor with a couple dozen discarded carpet samples I scrounged for fifty cents each. I painted the exterior a mind-bending Day-Glo green, and topped it off with a circular, bubble top, flying saucer-like sky light that my uncle, a roofer, salvaged from a church. The only thing missing was the obligatory "Don't Laugh Your Daughter's Inside" stenciled prominently on the back. A decoration, in deference to my mother's sky-high standards for what passed for good taste, I decided to forgo.

It was 5:30, Rose's usual starting time, on a cold, dark December morning, and I was just coming up his front steps to pick him up. My van was parked across the street, and according to his careful instructions, was loaded with enough tools, extra tires, and spare parts to rebuild it on the fly if necessary. And since the gas gauge didn't work, Rose also insisted I stock it with three five-gallon cans of gasoline as well.

Before I could knock, a shadowy apparition, backlit by the hallway light, burst through the door. Rose wore about five layers of clothes over his short, stocky body, and over his bald head to his short thick neck was one of those ridiculous fur-lined, black vinyl hats with a fur-lined flap that fastens to the front. The chin straps, which no one who owns one of those silly hats ever seems to snap, hung loosely to his shoulders. In his hands were two rope-handled paper bags brimming with enough turkey drumsticks, hard-boiled eggs, and bananas to feed us both for a year. This unvarying menu was his way of saving time and avoiding restaurant expenses on the road. But what really caught my attention were his outlandish calf-high boots which I am convinced were one of a kind, and which are beyond my powers to describe.

Sensing the question behind my slack-jawed look, his blue eyes lit up with a twinkle.

"Yeah," he chuckled, "I got my mukluks on, and I'm ready. I've rid' these stagecoaches before. That van of yours got no heat, no seat belts, and drives like a greased pig. But I reckon I'm more than a match for it. Give me ten square feet to land on, and I'll bring you home OK."

* * *

I was about to find out if he was as good as his promise. We'd barely arrived at our destination when an emergency phone call from his family cut short our trip, and now Rose was barreling back to do what he could. It was a black, bitterly cold night and we were racing home in white-out conditions down the mountainous section of Interstate 70 just before it reached Wheeling. There were several inches of icy snow on the road already, and Rose was driving way too fast for me and that rickety old van. He had the little six-cylinder engine under a sheet metal-encrusted hump between the seats wound so tight I couldn't hear myself think, and everywhere I looked I saw only imminent disaster.

The windshield wipers barely worked under normal conditions; if the blades had ever been replaced it wasn't by me. All I could see was the fuzzy red glare of what I surmised were taillights swirling around even faster than the snow. The howling wind, gusting continually, was pushing the top-heavy van, with its high center of gravity, all over the road. Then, with a loud *shloomp*, a huge bucket of slushy snow suddenly splattered the windshield. Involuntarily recoiling, I jerked my head toward my passenger-side window and found myself staring straight into the wheel hub of a tractor trailer. The truck was intent on passing in the right-hand lane and was spewing big clumps of snow onto the windshield as it did. The wheel was getting closer and closer, and, hypnotized with terror, I just watched it inch up. Then, with a whoosh, the truck's back draft hit, bucking the unstable van left toward the face of the mountain that, looming huge in the headlights, seemed like the mythological monster Scylla leaning over to grab us.

In a stone panic I ratcheted my head toward Rose and saw that he was desperately working the wheel as he tried to turn out of the slide and into the truck's buffeting back draft all at once. I'd purchased the van with a broken frame, and though I had it welded, now the front didn't quite line up with the back. Worse, the steering linkage was old and tired, leaving the wheel with way too much play. This, combined with the snow, wind, the truck's buffeting, and the nonexistent visibility had Rose frantically whirling the wheel first one way and then the other, faster and faster until, like some cartoon character steering a storm-tossed ship, he seemed to meld into a blur of head, hands, elbows, and steering wheel. The only thing needed to complete the cartoon comparison was the wheel coming off in his hands altogether.

Rose managed to pull us out of the slide, but now he was relying on the steady push of the truck's draft to keep us from sliding under the wheels.

My mind was racing. All I could think was: *What the hell are we doing in the passing lane? My God, why doesn't he just slow down and let the damn truck pass?*

But slowing down just wasn't in Rose's nature, and despite my terror and his comical gyrations, I was struck by the bat-out-of-hell determination etched into Rose's face glowing slightly red from the semi's running lights. It was a face that had made a habit of staring down life and grown to like it. Rose never looked back, and the purposeful expression on his glowing face seemed to light up the van, making him seem larger than he really was with his seat pulled so far forward that he loomed over the steering wheel.

After what seemed like an eternity, the truck finally passed, and the vacuum this created literally picked up the van and sucked it toward the cliff on our right. Somehow, we didn't go over but reverted to wobbling along at what passed for normal in that crazy van on that crazy night.

Suddenly I lost it; I snapped. I was scared stiff, and an hour or so of this nerve-wracking exercise was all I could take. Trying unsuccessfully to catch my breath, I heard a voice in my head screaming, *How did I get into this mess? What was I thinking? Who is this guy? This can't be happening.* Then I heard the gasoline sloshing around in the cans behind my seat, and I decided I had to make my move before the next big rig bore down on us.

"Mr. Rose, don't you think we oughta' cool it?" I said, shocked by the contrast between my firm intentions and the plaintive plea squeaking from my constricted throat.

"What?" he shouted over the whining motor.

"Don't you think we oughta' cool it?" I repeated loud enough for him to hear, and followed it with a furtive glance in his direction.

I was about to mention the gasoline, but his face, contorted with concentration, swung around and fixed me with those amazing blue eyes. An instant later, taking it all in with a glance, all the tension drained from his face as it moved from amusement to a grin that grew wider and wider until all five layers of clothing, goofy hat, and mukluks besides, began shaking with laughter.

"What's the matter, Oogie, scared to die?" he shouted with mock seriousness, trying desperately to stop laughing. "If you are, ride the roof, my boy, ride the roof! From there you can jump off any time you want. You told me you wanted adventure. Here I am riskin' my neck to deliver, and you're busy pumpin' Hail Marys out one end so you don't make a mess at the other. I know how it is: this Zen stuff's fine for a nice, sunny day, but when things get tight, call in the cavalry."

Apparently, this was too much for him, and he went off into another fit of laughter.

The little blood I had left in my extremities went rushing to my head. I *had* been saying Hail Marys, but when I started, and how many I said, I couldn't say. In fact, if he hadn't mentioned it . . . But how did he know? Had I been praying aloud? But the noise . . . we were shouting just to be heard, and it was too dark to read lips.

When I recovered a bit, I noticed something had changed. He was still a whirling blur at the wheel, but when he looked over, he had the look of someone genuinely concerned.

"Listen," he finally said in a voice so soft it was almost feminine. So soft, in fact, that amidst all the noise I couldn't tell whether he actually spoke or just projected his thoughts into my head. "Everything's all right. Everything's got a purpose and everyone a destiny. I don't know exactly how things between me and you are supposed to play out, but I do know this: they ain't going to play out tonight. You'll see. We'll be home soon. Everything is all right."

It was as if an invisible hand reached out, stroked me gently, and pushed me back into my seat. I took the first real breath in what seemed like days, shut my eyes, and watched with fascination as my racing heart returned to normal without my help.

Suddenly I wouldn't have traded my seat on that 1963 Ford starship with anyone, and the next thing I knew we were pulling up to his house, back in Benwood, safe and sound.

Chapter Eight

ISIS UNVEILED

I said to my soul, be still, and let the dark come upon you
Which shall be the darkness of God.
As, in a theatre,
The lights are extinguished, for the scene to be changed
With a hollow rumble of wings, with a movement of darkness on
darkness,
And we know that the hills and the trees, the distant panorama
And the bold imposing facade are all being rolled away.
—T.S. ELIOT[21]

One day in January 1973 I arrived in Benwood unannounced only to find Rose engaged in the last thing I thought him capable: decorating. Strictly speaking, he was hanging a plaque in the kitchen. In all the time I knew him this was the only attempt I ever saw him make to spruce up his surroundings.

Phyllis let me in, and as I walked into the kitchen Rose glanced over his shoulder and, evincing no surprise, said, "The hell you say," and continued hanging the plaque. It was called COMMITMENT.

Until one is committed there is hesitancy, the chance to draw back, always ineffectiveness. Concerning all acts of initiative (and creation), there is one elementary truth, the ignorance of which kills countless ideas and splendid plans: That the moment one definitely commits oneself, then Providence moves too. All sorts of things occur to help one that would never otherwise have occurred. A whole stream of events issues from the decision, raising in one's favor all manner of unforeseen incidents, meetings, and material assistance which no man could have dreamt would come his way. I have learned a deep respect for one of Goethe's couplets:

> *"Whatever you can do, or dream you can, begin it.*
> *Boldness has genius, power, and magic in it."*
>
> – W. H. Murray[22]

Responding to my quizzical look, Rose launched into an exegesis on his plaque. "Commitment is the most important thing there is on a spiritual path. Most folks are all hot to learn some prayer or meditation technique. Hell, it ain't the prayer you *say*. It's the prayer you *live*. And this life as prayer starts with a commitment.

"You read how spirituality is all about waking up to what's important. Sure, every human steer raises his straw-matted face from the feeding trough once in a while just to sniff the air and take a look around. But it ain't enough to wake up; you gotta' stay awake. This means a commitment to changin' the way you're livin.'"

While delivering his homily, Rose led me out the kitchen door to his garage. Everything with Rose was unique, and his forlorn, stand-alone garage was no exception. Like a landlocked ship stranded miles from the beach by an errant tidal wave, there was no driveway, and the sliding door opened directly into the grassy hillside behind the house. Dilapidated and covered with ivy, Rose's garage became an inaccessible orphan when, using its power of eminent domain, the state commandeered the alley and an additional lot behind his house for the elevated four-lane bypass that now loomed over his truncated backyard. This high-handed expropriation rubbed Rose so raw that I always tiptoed around the subject rather than risk one of the endless, expletive-riddled jeremiads that invariably ensued when the issue came up.

Producing his massive key ring once again, Rose unlocked at least three separate locks of various sizes, opened the door, and grabbed some shears. Then we walked across the yard to his backyard grape arbor.

"Folks want to be constantly inspired," he continued while vigorously pruning the vines. "They figure they can work spiritually only when they *feel like it* and let magic, karma, fate, the guru, or God-knows-what take 'em the rest of the way. What you need is *character*, the ability to act on principle and to hell with negative feelings. You gotta' be able to force yourself even when you're not inspired. And that power comes from commitment. You need a back-against-the-wall mentality, and until that's in place, there's no use talkin' about the next step."

"How do I get to that point, Mr. Rose?" I asked as I began gathering up the grape cuttings. "What does 'living the life' look like?"

"Make decisions that put spiritual stones in your shoe if you want to stay awake," he began. "Every religion in the world uses the same word for these stones: they call 'em sacrifices. The more sacrifices you make the more committed you become, and the more committed you become the more sacrifices you're willin' to make. That's why I keep preachin' irritation. Hell, that's all I'm good for. I'm no teacher. I'm a damn spiritual nuisance."

Rose quit pruning and grinned widely. It took a moment to catch on, but I soon grinned back. He'd noticed my head bobbing and was grinning at two equally plausible explanations: I was either agreeing generally or just agreeing that he was a first-class pain in the ass.

"It ain't grace that's in short supply," he said. "It's just sleepiness and forgetfulness is in over-supply. It's the nature of the human beast to sleep, and forgetfulness is the number one obstacle to the spiritual life. If you ain't careful you end up like Rip Van Winkle. You forget and sleep the best years of your life away. Then one day you wake up again, all right. But this time you wake up screamin.'"

* * *

One invaluable trait I got from my father and immigrant grand-father was the ability to hustle. As a boy, besides my paper route, I mowed lawns, shoveled snow, pulled weeds, and went door to door collecting empty bottles after Christmas for deposits to make a little money—money my dad cheerfully expropriated and set aside "for college." I even leveraged the scouring skills I earned on my knees at the knee of my mother into a flourishing floor scrubbing business for the women in our neighborhood at two bits a kitchen. (I can still hear my mother: "Don't forget the corners. Wrap a butter knife with a rag to get the corners!")

At 12 I hustled up my first full-time job by nagging the maintenance manager at my Catholic grade school until he agreed to take me on for the summer as a professional floor scrubber and toilet cleaner for the dollar-an-hour minimum wage.

During high school I worked summers, Christmases, and spring vacations from Hotchkiss on a survey crew for a civil engineering company: a crew where I met the madcap friend who later morphed into the Academy Award-nominated actor, Michael Keaton, of *Birdman, Beetlejuice,* and *Batman* fame.

I underwrote my college tuition by shlepping heavy furniture for a moving company, boiling hundreds of hot dogs under the stands at Pitt football games, filling potholes on a state road crew, raking big clumps into little ones as a landscaper, loading trucks for UPS in 100-degree heat from 5 PM until 4 in the morning while still attending classes, and busting my butt as a creosote-stained "gandy dancer" laying track for the B&O railroad.

All of this gritty, blue-collar work paid off handsomely when I became a business executive and later an entrepreneur. I met many businesspeople who were smarter and more talented, but none who could outwork me.

* * *

It was several weeks after my conversation with Rose about commitment, sleepiness, and staying awake, and my brother Tom and I were dead tired as we pulled up to our last job for the day. Now that I had my own truck, I'd added carpet installation as a subcontractor to my repertoire of hustles, and with Tom as my helper, I was defraying college expenses by working sporadically during the school year while planning to go full-time during the summer.

> All of this gritty, blue-collar work paid off handsomely when I became a business executive and later an entrepreneur.

It was already getting dark on this cold, dreary, winter evening, and as I double-checked to make sure we had the right address, I regretted letting the store manager talk me into one extra job and another late night, and I could see Tom felt much the same way.

It was hard to say what was going on inside of Tom. Four years younger, he was as mechanically gifted as I was not, and he picked up carpet installation so quickly I soon considered him indispensable. Though he was as shy and introverted as I was loud and extroverted, we were very close.

Initially, Tom was interested in Rose and asked a lot of questions, but then, without explanation, he stopped coming to meetings. Months later I asked about it, and he smiled shyly.

"Ever see one of those big steel balls they swing from cranes to knock down buildings? Construction guys call them headache balls.

Rose kept hitting me with headache balls—too many headache balls." With this his voice trailed off, and we never discussed Rose again.

The brown sandstone house in one of the nicest areas of Pittsburgh was very old, and it straddled that invisible line between decidedly upscale and a full-blown castle. The huge lot was covered with trees and tangled undergrowth, and the ivy climbing the walls had reversed course in places, overgrowing the mold-blackened brick walk. The chocolate trim needed a good coat of paint, and the overflowing gutters coughed an occasional shower of dead, windblown leaves.

The gathering dusk, the cold wind, and the gloomy condition of the glowering house created a spooky feel, but overall it was a familiar scene for a carpet installer: an old and neglected house gets new owners, and they remodel the inside before moving in while leaving the exterior and yard for later.

Grabbing our tools from the back of the truck, Tom and I headed up the long walk, but before we could knock a man in his late fifties opened the door. He was medium height, with fair skin and thinning gray hair, and, though not really overweight, he was soft all over. I took an instant dislike to this man. His eyes were small, gray, crafty, and the searching way they darted around looking for a comparative advantage exposed the tight smile on his face for the mask it was. It was one of those smiles that Rose said really meant: *Hold still while I bite you. Or put the bite on you.*

He turned out to be the owner, home alone, and he insisted we tour his castle while he told his story. He was from Prague in what was then Czechoslovakia. He emigrated to the United States, married, made his fortune, and was damn proud of that big Mercedes parked in the driveway. It wasn't so much his bragging but his condescending attitude toward Tom and me that left a bad taste in my mouth. When I told him my grandparents were immigrants from Slovakia, he managed to subtly convey the haughty disdain my grandfather said the Czechs always display toward their provincial poor relations, the Slovaks.

Finally, he let us get to work.

Two hours later I finished stretching, trimming, and tucking the carpet in one room, and picking up my knee-kicker and wall trimmer, I headed for the next. This large, gothically ornate room with an arched ceiling, stained oak paneling, and hand-carved crown molding was the library. Since the furniture would not arrive until after the carpet was installed, it was empty except for a massive, immovable, mahogany grandfather clock that must've come with the house, four wall-mounted, old-fashioned, cast iron, hot-water radiators, and row upon row of book-lined walls.

The room was dimly lit by a single chandelier, and the steady ticking of the clock made me realize just how eerily quiet the house had become. Tom, who had already stripped, padded, and laid out the carpet lapping the walls, waiting to be installed, was nowhere to be seen. I paused for a moment, listening for the sound of Tom's work somewhere else in the cavernous house. I heard nothing but the clock.

Before settling down to work, I indulged in a bad habit I could never resist: I began rummaging through the library's collection of old hard-bound books. In light of the owner's unctuous personality and overt materialism, what I found surprised me. Most of the books were religious: not only theology and philosophy, but also Yoga, Zen, Jewish Kabbalah, and Christian mysticism. But what really caught my attention was a smaller section dedicated to the category that Rose referred to as "occult" or "esoteric."

I ran my fingers over the spines, reading titles until I came to a large volume more aptly described as a tome. Though the red leather was dark with age, I was able to read the faint words *Isis Unveiled* and, underneath, "by Blavatsky." Under the author's name, etched into the spine, was what I assumed was the Egyptian goddess Isis, naked, cross-legged, and sitting side-saddle on a crouched sphinx. Wearing a headdress made of the head and skin of an animal, she held a spear balanced on end, its tip in the air.

Rose often spoke of Madame Blavatsky, the nineteenth-century Russian mystic and founder of the Theosophical Society, the same organization that sponsored the lecture where I first met Rose. He said that Mme. Blavatsky's teachings, which helped introduce Eastern philosophy and meditation to the Western world, were some of the few sources of inspiration and instruction available when he was a young seeker wandering the country in the 1930s and '40s.

Unable to resist this Rosean connection, I pulled the book from the shelf and began reading at random, the musty smell of the yellowing pages adding to the forbidden pleasure of snooping. I felt like I was sneaking a look at Rose's diary from his early life, searching for the juicy stuff.

About such men as Apollonius, Iambillichus, Plotinus, and Porphyry, there gathered a heavenly nimbus. It was evolved both by the power of their own souls in close unison with their spirits and by the superhuman morality and sanctity of their lives, and was enhanced by their frequent interior ecstatic contemplations of God...

These words, the dark-paneled room, and the ticking clock in an otherwise silent house made for an eerie mood. Fooling around, I began softly reading aloud:

Such holy men only pure spiritual influences could approach...

The sound of my voice enhanced the mood, and I imagined I was reading from the mystical Book of Life, a book I spent countless incarnations tracking down. I searched for it relentlessly, braving trials too numerous to mention, only to find it by accident, here in this gloomy castle just where I left it, eons ago. Now, by reading these magical incantations, I was breaking the spell that cloaks our memory of previous lives, and with my circle now complete, I was remembering it all.

Radiating all around them was an atmosphere of Divine Beneficence that caused evil spirits to flee before them...

As I continued to read aloud, my imagination took a different turn. I started thinking of Rose as a young man, wintering in that hovel of a farmhouse he bought with his earnings as a wandering metallurgist, and the solitary months he spent reading, fasting, meditating. The house had no heat, insulation, electricity, or running water, and Rose rarely lit a fire. He would cook a pot of beans or vegetarian stew, enough for a week, and eat it cold. He sat for hours, cross-legged on his cot with a blanket draped over his shoulders, the steam from his moist breath the only motion in his tiny, self-contained universe.

I pictured Rose on his cot, reading this very copy of *Isis Unveiled*. As in a dream, I stepped into the frame and stood there watching him. He wasn't the young man he should have been, but the older Rose I now knew, and he was reading the very words I was reading, and I was reading along with him.

> *. . . Not only is it impossible for such evil spirits to exist in the aura of these holy men, but these spirits cannot even remain in the body of an obsessed person if such a thaumaturgist exercises his will against them . . .*[23]

Raising his head, Rose noticed me watching him. His lips began to move . . .

"Are you interested in the spirit of God in man?"

These words, directly in my ear, startled me from my romantic reverie, and I whirled around. The face of both the owner of the house and *Isis Unveiled* was only inches from my own. He was completely changed; there was no sign of the man who met us at the door. His gray eyes were now crystal clear and staring easily into my own.

I was shocked, embarrassed, ashamed. Shocked to find him standing there, embarrassed because he'd been listening to me ridiculously reading aloud, and ashamed of being caught red-handed rifling through his possessions.

I fumbled for words. "Uh . . . uh . . . yes, I am. Are you?"

"Yes," he said, pausing for a second. "That is, when I was your age. When I was your age, it was everything to me. But I wanted to be somebody. Forty years are gone now, and they're nothing but a blur of late nights at the office, dry cleaning tickets, and plans for dinner."

He paused again and tried to smile. "Somewhere along the way I forgot what's important in life. I got so busy I forgot why we're here. I lost my way and now it's too late for me." He paused for a few seconds before echoing, "It's too late for me!"

Something—maybe the tears running down his face or the look on mine—brought him around and, flushing with embarrassment, he rushed from the room.

I stood staring after him completely flustered. This man's sudden appearance and what he said were even more eerie than what I'd been reading. Remembering the time and how much work there was yet to do, I returned to my labor, grateful to have something to occupy my mind . . .

Several hours later, Tom and I wrapped up the job. It was time to get the customer to check our work and sign the work order. I had not seen the owner since he rushed from the library, and I expected an awkward scene. However, the man had regained his composure, and without the slightest trace of familiarity, he meticulously checked our work. Satisfied, he signed the work order and disappeared again.

We finished cleaning up and repacked the tools. Tom grabbed the cases containing our seaming iron and electric staple gun and headed out the door. Preparing to follow, I bent over to pick up the toolbox and half-empty box of tack strips when I felt a touch on my shoulder.

Turning, I was face to face with the owner. He was changed once again and holding *Isis Unveiled*. "Here," he hissed insistently, "please take it. I want you to have it." Startled more by his urgency than by his gift, I automatically reached for the book, but he stunned me once more by firmly holding onto it.

"Promise me something first. Promise me you'll do more with this book than I did.

"Promise me you'll never forget."

Overcome, I nodded. He wheeled and walked away. The next thing I remember is being at the passenger window of the van asking Tom if he'd drive.

As we drove down the street, Tom noticed the book and how preoccupied I was. He asked if I was all right. I told him I was. He accepted it, and we drove on. Actually, my nerves were all ajangle. I felt like God had spoken to me through this man. I looked down at my lap several times just to make sure *Isis Unveiled* was still there. It took a physical effort not to tell Tom to turn around and go back: I half-expected to find Rose in a hard hat paying off the owner for his command performance while his rank-and-file crew of sprites, elves, and pixies were deftly disassembling the make-believe house.

* * *

Over the next week or so, all I could think about was *Isis Unveiled,* Blavatsky, the Theosophical Society, Rose, and the promise the man extracted from me—and how all these interlocking pieces might pertain to my future. Try as I might, I couldn't write it all off as a coincidence: first, Rose lectures me on forgetfulness, and a few weeks later a complete stranger dramatically makes me promise to never forget.

Then, about two weeks later, something happened that only deepened the mystery. Tom and I were on another job. It was a small apartment in Pittsburgh's suburban Dormont neighborhood, rented by a young married couple. I was kicking in carpet on my knees in the living room while the couple huddled in the adjacent kitchenette crammed to the ceiling with their furniture.

The door opened and . . . the man who gave me the Blavatsky book strode in.

Amazed, I said nothing, and he walked right past me without a glance. Based on snatches of conversation, I surmised he was the owner of the building and discussing some business with his tenants.

I was almost reabsorbed in my work when I felt a tap on my shoulder. Looking up from my kneeling position, I found myself for the third time only inches from the landlord's face. In a gentle, matter-of-fact way, he said, "You know, every person I've ever met who was serious about spiritual work had eyes just like yours." Without waiting for a reply or even a reaction, he ambled out the door.

* * *

As I write these words, almost fifty years later, his copy of *Isis Unveiled* is sitting on the table in front of me. It is perhaps the only completely precious thing I have ever owned. I am embarrassed to admit how many times over the years I have gone to it just to make sure it really exists. I also use it to jog my memory. I use it as a talisman for what I want my life to be about. I pray the good his book has done for me somehow helped the man who gave it to me and brought him peace. And I pray that he would be proud of that young man in whom he saw something. A young man who told him with a nod he would do his very best to faithfully fulfill a promise. A promise to never forget.

Chapter Nine

ZIGGY MEETS
THE ZEN MASTER

The tolling bell
Measures time not our time, rung by the unhurried
Ground swell, a time
Older than the time of chronometers, older
Than time counted by anxious worried women
Lying awake, calculating the future,
Trying to unweave, unwind, unravel
And piece together the past and the future,
Between midnight and dawn, when the past is all deception,
The future futureless, before the morning watch
When time stops and time is never ending
—T.S. ELIOT[24]

Sara was a part-time waitress at The Portfolio, a restaurant near Pitt's campus. Her colleagues threw her a birthday party, and I was thrilled when she invited me. The party was a late afternoon affair, before the restaurant opened for dinner, and I was flattered even more when I realized I was the only non-employee in attendance. Five or six rectangular, linen-layered tables were lined up end to end with a special seat of honor at the head for Sara Bean. As an outsider, I discreetly took a seat well down the makeshift dais from the birthday princess and her provisional throne.

Sara was in fine form, effortlessly playing doyenne while trading humorous anecdotes with her colleagues that, due to their inside baseball nature, were largely lost on me. Soon the good-natured bantering settled on Sara's age. She was turning 21, and her coworkers were apparently convinced that Sara now had, as my father would say, "one foot in the grave and the other on a banana peel."

"Hey, how does it feel to be as old as I used to be?" said one old crone who was clearly pushing 25. "Don't buy any green bananas."

Sara took it all in stride. "I guess my dreams of being an Olympic gymnast are over. Olga Korbut can finally take a deep breath!"

She then broke into a marvelous parody of the Walt Disney character Jiminy Cricket, singing "Enjoy Yourself (It's Later Than You Think)," a familiar tune right out of the songbook of *The Mickey Mouse Club* TV show we all grew up watching in the 1950s.

You work and work for years and years, you're always on the go
You never take a minute off, too busy makin' dough
Someday, you say, you'll have your fun, when you're a millionaire
Imagine all the fun you'll have in your old rockin' chair!

Enjoy yourself, it's later than you think
Enjoy yourself, while you're still in the pink
The years go by, as quickly as a wink
Enjoy yourself, enjoy yourself, it's later than you think

You're gonna take that ocean trip, no matter, come what may
You've got your reservations made, but you just can't get away
Next year for sure, you'll see the world, you'll really get around
But how far can you travel when you're six feet underground?

Enjoy yourself, it's later than you think

Enjoy yourself, while you're still in the pink
The years go by, as quickly as a wink
Enjoy yourself, enjoy yourself, it's later than you think . . .[25]

Sara's take on Jiminy jamming away was so spot-on and her sing-ing so infectious that all her faithful courtiers were soon laughing and shouting the refrain "It's later than you think!" at the top of our lungs. But as the revelry grew in volume and enthusiasm I was struck by a realization: wow, they're right. She's 21. Sara's not a *girl*. She's a *wom-an*. I don't have a *crush* on a *girl*. I'm *in love* with a *woman*."

It's later than you think . . . It's later than you think . . . I abruptly stopped laughing as the chorus ricocheted around in my head. I sud-denly felt isolated as if I was watching the party from inside a sealed glass case. Then, more ominously, the refrain morphed into the voice of the man who gave me *Isis Unveiled* endlessly moaning, "It's too late for me . . . it's too late for me." The louder everyone laughed the more self-consciously "out of it" I felt. It was a flashback to Chip's acid party when that damn phone wouldn't stop ringing in my head, and once again I longed, metaphorically at least, to rush out into the rain so I could, in the argot of the era, "get my head together."

The Portfolio was opening for business, and the party was break-ing up. Even Princess Sara, like some twentieth-century Cinderella, reluctantly turned back into a humble scullery maid about to go to work. I proffered my present and a clumsy embrace while incoher-ently muttering something or other about why I was hurrying off. She wasn't buying it, and her big blue eyes seemed to be asking what was wrong. Ignoring their question, I stumbled out the door.

For hours I walked the Oakland/Shadyside section of Pittsburgh along tree-lined streets, past fashionable boutiques and old Victorian mansions, vainly trying to get my head together. It didn't take long to get a handle on why Sara's coming of age and the song she sang hit me so hard. It was indeed later than I thought. Compliments did not come easily from Rose, and the highest compliment he could bestow on another human being was an understated, "He's serious." My life was passing "as quickly as a wink," and it would never pass Rosean muster as serious. Sara was now 21. I would be 21 in a few months. Was I serious about her? Was I serious about spirituality? Was I serious about anything? Or was I, as Rose liked to derisively put it, merely a "pusillanimous piddler" instead?

I now knew at least one damn good reason why I didn't tell Rose about *Isis Unveiled* and the man who gave it to me. I no longer saw the incident as a favorable omen. Instead I now saw it as a ghostly admonition, something like Jacob Marley back from the grave on Christmas Eve to warn Ebeneezer Scrooge. A warning about how I would end up if I didn't quit toying with life and finally commit body and soul to something worth doing. I recalled a quote from the great ninth-century Chinese Zen Master, Huang Po, and now it seemed like a perfect fit for me and my half-stepping ambivalence. "Oh, you students of Zen! You must work hard and never slacken in your efforts. Because if you do, if you do, you will end up a common ordinary man."

My God, I thought, as fine, wind-whipped shards of icy drizzle stung my cheeks. *Huang Po wanted to light a bonfire under the asses of his students. But he didn't threaten them with hellfire or reincarnation as a lowly June bug. No, he threatened them with the worst thing he could possibly imagine: ending up a common, ordinary man.*

Every time I looked into one of the storefront windows lining Walnut Street, Shadyside's main drag, I saw a common ordinary man with one foot on the gas and the other on the brake peering back. I was ostensibly seeking the Truth while constantly hedging, keeping secrets, dealing in half-truths, and occasionally indulging in a common ordinary man's common ordinary lies.

I was keeping Sara in the dark about my true relationship with Rose for fear I would scare her off. I couldn't share my feelings for Sara with Rose because I was afraid he would scare *me* off. I didn't dare tell Sara how I felt about her because I was terrified she would reject me, or maybe even worse: accept me. I scrupulously hid Rose and the Zen Studies Society from Orysia and the Russian History Department because I was afraid their disdainful disappointment would tarnish my hard-earned golden boy status. Meanwhile, I continued to feed my professors and parents the convenient fiction that graduate school and my eventual career were still my top priorities because I was determined to keep all my options open. When conflicts among all these balls I was frantically juggling inevitably arose, I wasn't adverse to trafficking in lies (especially with myself) to cover my tracks. Finally, I shared none of these Byzantine palace intrigues with Rose, of course, because I was afraid if I asked for his advice I just might have to take it.

The common denominator was fear, and all this torturous backing and filling, hedging and double talk was only exacerbating the disappointment in life and myself that sent me to Rose in the first place. But I felt powerless to do anything about it. I was spiritually, psychologically, and emotionally stymied: trapped, just like at Hotchkiss, in some woebegotten no man's land. Stuck between the heroic, all-in, Rosean "100 percenter" I desperately wanted to be and the pathetic, poor man's excuse for a hesitant Hamlet I painfully was. If, like Demian, all I ever wanted was to live in accordance with my own true self, the task now seemed to have metastasized from merely difficult to utterly overwhelming.

I retraced my steps down a deserted Walnut Street, the trendy shops now long since shuttered for the night. I lived on the corner of Copeland Street and Walnut, but when, from force of habit, I wheeled onto Copeland I blew right by our five-bedroom house until I ran out of street. I turned left onto a slippery sidewalk strewn with mold-blackened leftover leaves.

From somewhere off in the distance, I could hear the faint sound of a solitary church bell apparently up late and tolling to itself for company on such a dank and lonesome night.

My epiphany at Sara's party made my situation as stark as the occasional brace of headlights shimmering off an icy Ellsworth Avenue and into my eyes. I wasn't committed to *anything*, and I was unwilling to commit because I was a coward too terrified to make the personal sacrifices that "living the life" required. I still longed for that clean, clear, decisive "single point of white-hot intensity called *life*" that the Vietnam veteran so movingly described and Rose so heroically represented, but now it only seemed farther away than ever. To put it even more starkly than those shimmering headlights: Rose was a *man*, and I was not.

> To put it even more starkly than those shimmering headlights: Rose was a *man*, and I was not.

The black night turned bitterly cold, but I barely noticed, and as I continued my winding pilgrimage through Pittsburgh's windswept East End all these realizations, along with their concurrent anguish, coalesced into a dark, ominous cloud hovering over my head. Ironically, my frantic attempts to have everything were producing nothing but the sinking, sickening sense of a doomed man about to lose everything.

Something had to give. But whether it was merely going to bring down my tenuous house of phony cardboard bullshit, or me along with it, I couldn't tell. And that's what scared me most.

* * *

A week or so after all this midnight maundering, the phone rang. Amazingly, since like most of his generation he would rather gargle with ground glass than pay for a long distance call, it was Rose. He was coming up early for our meeting to do some research on his family tree at the Carnegie library across the street from the university. He invited me to tag along and added with a chuckle, "Don't get any ideas. I'm not going soft. I just want to see my cousin's face when he finds out we come from a long line of Kallikaks."

When I met him in the student union, Rose was drinking a cup of coffee with a faraway look in his eyes. Try as I might, I couldn't draw him out, and we just sat silently for a while before starting for the library. When we got to the small park between the university and the library he abruptly sat down on a park bench and motioned for me to do the same. A man walked by and Rose asked, "What can you tell me about that guy?"

His question caught me off guard, and all I could do was mumble, "Not much. He's in a hurry, I guess."

"He's not in a hurry," Rose said. "He always walks that way. He walks that way because his father walks that way, and that man's entire life is just one long, painful effort to be the man his father wants him to be."

Over the next ten minutes or so we repeated this exercise. Each time I drew a blank and Rose gave his analysis. His stories were so varied and full of detail that if it was anyone but Rose, or maybe Sherlock Holmes, I would've dismissed the entire project out of hand. Then, just as abruptly as it started, the exercise was over, and much to my relief, we continued to the library.

For several hours Rose worked diligently while I lounged around. As we were leaving the large, gloomy research room, Rose whispered, "There's someone here with a wonderful spiritual potential. Who is it?"

Again I was caught flat-footed, and more to comply than from any hope of success, I anxiously scanned the room. There were fifteen or twenty people sprinkled around, but I was so rattled that even if I'd seen a sign hanging from someone's neck, I doubt it would've helped. Sensing this, Rose jerked his head toward the far corner of the room.

"It's that woman over there."

Following his glance, I saw an attractive woman of about 25 sitting at a table, hard at work. To this day that's all I can say about her.

We left the library about 4, and since our meeting didn't start until 7:30 we had several hours to kill. Rose wanted to eat, so recrossing Forbes Avenue we headed for the fast-food joint near the student union. Rose ordered two regular hamburgers and a cup of coffee, and then, as he always did, conspiratorially whispered that regular hamburgers were the best deal on the menu.

The place was practically deserted, and we took a table at the very front with my back to the window facing the street and Rose sitting directly across from me. Something in the hamburgers lifted Rose out of his spooky mood, and he was again his old self. He said he'd been testing my intuition in the park and library, and he told me, almost urgently, that a well-developed intuition was essential to a spiritual path.

Spiritual intuition, he said, is a form of "direct thinking" that transcends ordinary thinking and feeling. Intuition is an "instantaneous computerization of all data to date," and Enlightenment is the ultimate intuitive insight, an explosive jump that "leaps the gap between life and death itself." According to Rose, a flash of intuition was the way all important problems were solved, and these intuitive leaps were the marks of all creative genius, spiritual or otherwise. Since I knew without asking I failed his intuitive tests, I asked how I could develop my intuition.

"Spiritual intuition is a state of betweenness," he continued as he lifted his faithful fedora off the table and placed it out of harm's way on an empty chair. "It lies halfway between the intellect and the emotions and uses them both. There are two ways of goin' about developing your intuition, things you do and things you don't. First, pick out a problem and make up your mind to solve it or bust. I suggest the problem of finding out who you really are. Next, you apply both the intellect and the emotions to the problem. The intellect represents knowledge and the emotions sensitivity. Use the intellect to learn everything you can and develop emotional sensitivity through compassion. Then use your intellect to check your feelings and your sensitivity to check your intellect. A group and a teacher can act as a check on your intuition as well.

"Make predictions about yourself and other people and pay attention to how these hunches play out," he said as he worked his second hamburger. "When you're wrong, figure out why, and try again. The more data you absorb, and the more you crunch it, the better your predictions will be. Hell, it's the same formula for pickin' stocks, horses, or pickin' up girls. It all comes down to what you want in life. If you want something bad enough and concentrate long enough, your nose gets pretty damn good at sniffin' it out."

"So, what are things you don't do, Mr. Rose?"

"A spiritual intuition is a finely tuned mechanism," he continued while holding up his palms and flexing his fingers to illustrate his point. "Every scientist shields a carefully calibrated instrument from interference and background noise. Spiritually speaking, this means you live the life by screening out distractions. That don't mean a cave or monastery, but it does mean drastically simplifying your life. Most folks have so much nonsense going on that background noise overwhelms their intuition. They got so many conflicting priorities that the only intuition they ever develop is a sixth sense for when supper's on the table."

I winced. Once again Rose seemed to be speaking generally while nailing me personally. For a moment, my mind reeled. How much did Rose actually know about my own "conflicting priorities"? I tried, apparently successfully, to not let it show, and he went on.

"Avoid traumas that damage the intuition. Traumas are mice that chew the wires and distort the signal. Distorted signals lead to bad decisions. Bad decisions lead to more trauma and even worse decisions until your life descends into a death spiral of ever-increasing confusion. Stick to the Ten Commandments and you'll be OK. Be careful with sex. Some of the most traumatized people are folks who think the sexual morality that humanity spent a few million years of trial and error figurin' out no longer applies. Jesus said we must become little children, and that means maintaining your innocence or regaining it through celibacy or a healthy monogamous relationship. You'll never get valid intuitive readings if you're all tore up with shame and guilt."

Again Rose struck home: I knew what it felt like to walk for hours "all tore up with shame and guilt."

Again Rose didn't notice or, if he did, didn't let on. Instead, he launched into a more "esoteric" aspect of intuition. Once more, Rose the alchemist began talking of "quantum energy." He said the highest form of intuition came from redirecting this "voltage" away from its strictly "somatic" or biological functions and "sublimating" it "upwards." Like the Yogic doctrine of Kundalini, Rose believed that physical, sexual, emotional, and intellectual energy could be "transmuted" into spiritual energy.

In order to transmute quantum energy, he said, it must first be *created* through a sensibly healthy lifestyle of diet and exercise. Next it has to be *conserved* before it is "dissipated" through licentious living or trivial distractions. Third, this energy must be *controlled* as it struggles for release, a struggle the student experiences as *frustration*. Finally, it must be *focused*. Psychic energy created, conserved, controlled, and focused was the state Rose called *attention* or being "at-tension."

"That's why in that old Zen story the Master defines Zen as 'Attention! Attention! Attention!'" Rose said so emphatically he almost knocked over his coffee cup. "And that's what makes Zen so unique. Most folks gravitate to spirituality as a way to relax, blow off steam, relieve tension, and go with the flow. That's hogwash. Spirituality means coming to attention or at-tension and remaining at attention until the riddle of life and death is solved. Building an iron-clad attention span is like building muscles. It's hard damn work, but the longer you can remain at attention the better your intuition gets, and if you have the guts and determination to stay at it, you'll find—"

"So, old-timer, where'd you come from?" came a voice from behind Rose.

Startled, I looked up and saw six apparitions in gaudy, silver lamé costumes strung out loosely behind Rose. There were four college-age young men and two young women. Their faces were covered in heavy, glitter-spackled makeup, but it was their eyes, acid-bedazzled and shining like klieg lights, that really made their costumes. The speaker, obviously their leader, was a big, good-looking kid with a shock of dark, curly, shoulder-length hair sprinkled with glitter. He was standing directly behind Rose's left shoulder, and his sarcastic question and giggling entourage left no doubt he was goofing on Rose for their collective, acid-enhanced amusement.

These observations took less than a second, but before I had time to wonder how they managed to sneak up on us, connect their costumes with Ziggy Stardust and the David Bowie concert later that evening, or wonder why, of all the dinnertime diners now packing the restaurant, these kids zeroed in on Rose, he was already in motion.

Without betraying the slightest surprise at being interrupted or by the spectacle that greeted his eyes as he swiveled his chair, Rose smiled affably into the leader's face.

"Where'd I come from? I just came from jail."

The leader's smirk froze and his eyes darted around. He was not expecting this answer, or Rose's utter nonchalance, and it rattled him, but he was in too deep and lurched forward.

"Uh . . . um . . . why were ya' in jail?" he sneered. "Were ya' drunk or somethin'?"

"Why? Hmm . . . let's see . . . the why never occurred to me," Rose replied dreamily before the leader's words entirely left his mouth. "The what was more interesting than the why. Did I say jail? I meant a hotel. A dream about a hotel, or more exactly a hotel made of dreams. I thought it was the Waldorf Astoria of my dreams, but it was really the Waldorf Astoria of dreams. I was the indentured night clerk. You know, I kinda' kept the key to each keep. A hotel jailer—in jail but not really in jail. Anyway, I had a key to each room, and each room was a dream and in each dream was a dreamer. You know: dreamers, dreaming in a dream. And I recognized each dreamer dreaming in each room or dream, and you know who they were? They were you, you, you . . . " Rose went on, jabbing his finger at each of the six as he spoke.

"I knew you were all dreaming of me, but I didn't have the key to your dreams, so it became a bad dream of dreamers never waking up, and this nightmare was costing me sleep, so I had to check out. And that's how I ended up here."

The effect of this spontaneous speech, seamlessly delivered without pause or punctuation, was electric. Rose's would-be tormentors froze, and their acid-dilated pupils rolled up in their heads. Seconds slowly ticked by before one young man finally managed to break the spell.

"H-h-hey, m-m-man, you're freakin' us out!"

But even as he did, the leader waved him off, and without taking his eyes off Rose, said, "Cool it, man. This guy knows something."

Then, without introduction or invitation, he sat down in the chair next to Rose and asked, "What happens when we die?"

It was instant intimacy. It was as if the leader was rejoining a serious conversation he and his best friend had been pursuing for the better part of a lifetime, and Rose responded in exactly the same way. With that, the others crammed into chairs and began firing questions at Rose as fast as he could answer them.

I could scarcely believe my eyes, but what was stranger still was the way I found myself utterly marginalized. Only minutes earlier, six ghosts materialized out of the ether and now, through some bizarre displacement in space and time, I was the ghost. No one, including Rose, seemed to realize I was there, and I had the distinct feeling that if I did manage to say something they would all just look at me with barely concealed annoyance as if to say, "Who the hell are you?"

For the next couple of hours I became an observer eavesdropping on a very intimate conversation. There wasn't anything trippy about their questions or Rose's answers, but the utter rapport between Rose and these kids created a psychic barrier that, just like at Sara's party, left me feeling like the poor, crippled boy who can't keep up as the Pied Piper leads the rest of Hamelin's children into Paradise.

Then, without warning, one of the girls jumped to her feet. She was sitting at the opposite end of the table from Rose, and until then hadn't said a word.

"You're trying to manipulate them!" she spat out, quivering with rage. "Who the hell are you that you should tell them how to live their lives? What do you know?"

"What do I know?" Rose said softly while meeting her eyes. "Why, I know you. I know you inside out, like your veins were on top of your skin. That's what I know."

Rose turned away, satisfied to let it go. Stung, the girl hesitated, but she decided it was too late to back down.

"OK, so what do you know about me?" she hissed with a toss of her head.

"I know this," Rose replied evenly. "You are well on your way to becoming a dish rag. You were blessed with a spiritual potential that you are dissipating as fast as you can in a cloud of drugs and through your gonads. You've given up on yourself, and now you're determined to deprive these others of their chance by discrediting me."

The girl froze. After a few moments, the leader said, "Missy, do you have your ticket?" She nodded.

"Cool. Why don't you meet us there?"

Without another word she put on her coat and left, and the session picked up exactly where it left off.

Eventually, it was time for their concert and our meeting. Rose and his newly acquired devotees raucously poured out onto the sidewalk and headed up Forbes Avenue. I was straggling just out of earshot as Rose repeatedly said things that produced roars of laughter and mutual back-slapping. We came to a halt at the student union, and one by one the kids solemnly thanked him and shook his hand. Everyone, including Rose, seemed moved and sorry to part, but as Rose turned to go he suddenly whirled back.

"Wait a second, I almost forgot—"

Instantly all heads dipped conspiratorially, eagerly anticipating a parting dollop of darshan from the guru.

"Higamous hogamous woman's monogamous; hogamous higamous man is polygamous."

For a second there was stunned silence, and then the whole acid-soaked sangha erupted into laughter. This called for one more round of handshakes and hugs and then, just as mysteriously as they appeared, Ziggy Stardust and his Spiders from Mars melted into the misty darkness.

As Rose and I headed into the student union, all the suppressed emotion of this crazy day and my crazy life bubbled to the surface. Was the magical appearance of this ersatz Ziggy and his spidery Martian backup band yet another example of that damn necromancer Rose conjuring events to hammer home his points?

"Wow, Mr. Rose, I can't believe what just happened. Why didn't you ask them to come to the meeting?"

"What?" Rose replied, arching his eyebrows. "They're blasted on acid. By this time tomorrow they'll be wonderin' if I exist. Acid opened up their intuitions, and they could feel me. I guess that's a good thing, but we can only pray that now that they got the message, they remember to hang up the phone."

"But here's what I don't get," I said with rising excitement, ignoring his reply. "It's like . . . well . . . it's like all day you been trying to tell me something or show me something about intuition. I don't know . . . it's just . . . well, like that acid rap you laid on those guys. I mean, it was like you were telling them that life is all a dream they're dreaming, and since they're also on acid, which really, if you think about it, is just another kind of a dream within a dream . . . is that what the Yogis mean by Maya?" I paused as I tried to maintain my verbal footing. "And since you were inside their heads . . . I mean on rapport with them . . . it was like you were intuitively dreaming their dream along with them, but you could wake up any time you wanted, but they couldn't. So is that what you meant when you said you didn't have the key . . . "

"It was some of that and none of that and bullshit besides," Rose interrupted, stopping me dead in my tracks.

"Listen," he continued brusquely. "You got a pretty good head on your shoulders, and you think you're going to figure it all out. You might as well sort all the grains of sand on the banks of the Ganges one by one. I got a better idea. Why not make the trip? Why not go there? Just go there. Then you'll stop pestering me with all these foolish questions."

I walked right into another Rosean sucker punch, but despite his stinging critique, I spent the next several days frenetically sorting sand, searching among the finely ground grains for what Rose was really trying to say. On the surface it was clear: cosmic consciousness was not an intellectual puzzle to be figured out incrementally step by step. It was something right out of Hunter S. Thompson: a gonzo, fear-and-loathing, madcap, full-tilt boogie, open-air convertible, head rush to an ethereal Las Vegas, an otherworldly netherworld way out in the desert and a million miles from nowhere. A mystical modality outside space and beyond time that might accept an occasional guest but could never be comprehended.

But it was the enigma wrapped in the message that really kept me up late sifting silica along the Ganges of my gyrating ganglia. Rose also seemed to be saying I would never resolve my personal dilemma intellectually either. Commitment was not something I could intellectually do, it was something, like an acid trip or an orgasm, that must happen to me.

There also seemed to be something new and newly unsettling in the sandy subtext of Rose's parting shot. After failing all his tests I felt left out and left behind by Rose and his acid-drenched disciples. Was this intentional? Was Rose on to me? Was he disgusted, running out of patience, pushing me away?

Ken Kesey told his fellow Merry Pranksters, "You're either on the bus or off the bus." You're either all in or all out. Maybe Rose's metaphysical version of Further, the Pranksters' garishly painted, psychedelic bus, was pulling away without me. But Kesey and his Pranksters had a catalyst. They used LSD and The Electric Kool-Aid Acid Test to help them get "on the bus" and take the trip.

That's what I needed: a spiritual catalyst, a cosmic shove, a noetic nudge to show me the way. But what form of catalyst? And how would I find it before it was too late?

Chapter Ten

THE SUMMER RETREAT

And so each venture
Is a new beginning, a raid on the inarticulate,
With shabby equipment always deteriorating
In the general mess of imprecision of feeling,
Undisciplined squads of emotion. And what there is to conquer
By strength and submission, has already been discovered
Once or twice, or several times, by men whom one cannot hope
To emulate – but there is no competition –
There is only the fight to recover what has been lost
And found and lost again and again: and now, under conditions
That seem unpropitious. But perhaps neither gain nor loss.
For us, there is only the trying.
The rest is not our business.
—T.S. Eliot[26]

In the spring of 1973 Rose announced a summer "intensive" at his farm. While it would mean forgoing the money I would earn working, I instantly signed on. From the safe distance of Pittsburgh, I thought

171

this opportunity might just produce the catalyst I was looking for. Since Rose needed the rent from the farmhouse we would have to camp out. So in late May, Ray and I arrived in my iridescent-green 1963 Ford van that I decided would make a perfect summer hermitage on wheels. We also arrived with a full-grown German shepherd I picked up at the pound and named Dharma. Through some reasoning that now escapes me, I got it into my head that a dog named Dharma, like a Day-Glo green van, was essential to a successful Rosean retreat.

Everyone had to fend for themselves, so Ray and I brought food, sleeping bags, a Coleman stove, and a portable toilet consisting of little more than a seat with aluminum legs. There was no refrigeration, we would be carrying water from the spring, and even the outhouse by the trailer mysteriously sprouted a "Women Only" sign. The trailer was occupied by Frank and Jeanne, 26-year-old married schoolteachers from Pittsburgh who initially showed up at my house after the abortive Kung Fu revolution. Rob, having temporarily left his phalanx of half-frozen frogs to their own devices, was participating, and there were also four students from Kent State University where the son of an old friend of Rose started another group called The Pyramid Zen Society.

Ray and I parked the van on a more or less level, grassy piece of land under a gnarled box elder about fifty yards from the unpaved road and joined the others in the open space behind the trailer. Rose was telling a story about a friend who recently remarried after a painful divorce.

"I love my wife so much," the man told Rose with tears in his eyes, "and I'm so afraid I'm going to screw it up again. What do I have to do?"

"Everything, and I mean *everything*, has to change," Rose replied.

"What do you mean?" the newlywed said with alarm. "I'm a good person; I don't drink or run around."

"That's not what I'm talkin' about. Your first marriage failed because you are a businessman who happened to have a wife. To make this new marriage work, you must become a husband who happens to own a business."

"You're right," the man said after thinking it over. "What do I have to do?"

"You don't *become* a husband by sayin' 'I do.' Stay awake and put your wife first. When your wife and your most important client are on the phone, put the client on hold and take the call from your wife. It's like a diet. You don't *become* a thin person on good intentions; it's one decision, one resisted potato chip, at a time. You *become* a husband the same way. And here's where faith comes in. While you may not be able to see it now, as a good husband you'll be a better businessman as well."

Rose told us spirituality works on the same principles. It's not what we say, think, or feel that defines a spiritual path, it is what we *do*. He reiterated that we could never *learn* the Truth, we could only *become* the Truth. Over time, and by habitually putting our spiritual goals first, we gradually *become* a spiritual "vector," and the momentum behind this vector would carry us safely through the inevitable spiritual trials that lie ahead.

As he spoke, I recalled Rose's own great spiritual trial when he hit rock bottom only to find he had become a vector irretrievably committed to the Truth whether he liked it or not, a vector he described as a "runaway train with eighteen years of steam behind it." Like an exhausted, demoralized, but well-trained soldier whose legs keep moving from pure habit long after his mind and heart have given up, Rose's vector kept him staggering forward against all odds and ultimately pulled him through.

While I enjoyed Rose's story, I was anxious for him to settle in and begin his orientation for our summer intensive. I expected an overview, maybe a handout on our daily routine, and then, perhaps, a chance to talk about our own objectives for the summer.

I knew what my goal was: I wanted to get to the bottom of all those energy jolts between me and Rose. The best description for these experiences I've ever heard came from a woman describing PMS. It was this *tension* that seemed to well up from nowhere with an ever-increasing intensity until . . . well, that was it: until what? Then just as quickly, it would be gone, leaving me relieved and wondering if anything happened at all. After my first experience on the street outside the Theosophical Society I decided to ask Rose about this phenomenon, but even now, almost a year later, I was still putting it off. While I wanted Rose to confirm that these experiences were spiritually significant—maybe even the germ of that magical catalyst I was looking for?—what I really wanted was to find out they were merely the result of too much caffeine, post-adolescent jitters, and an overactive imagination.

What I might've said if Rose asked remains a mystery because he suddenly yawned, stretched, looked at his watch, mumbled something about the time, fired up the Oldsmobile, and roared off in a cloud of dust toward town. We were all taken aback by his abrupt departure, but we just assumed he would return in the morning and take it from there.

Rose didn't show up the next day. Or the next. Or the next.

At first we were busy unpacking, getting used to ice-cold baths at the spring and, for the men, using the sandy racetrack as an open-air toilet. Then we tried meditating, reading, hiking, and anything else we could think of. But as one hot, sticky, fly-infested day piled wearily into the next, we became increasingly antsy. Something had to be done. Hell, maybe Rose had a heart attack, and we'd end up like those fanatical Japanese soldiers who held out for twenty-five years in the Philippine jungle patiently awaiting orders while unaware that World War II was long over. Since we didn't have a telephone and no one wanted to face Rose alone, we all squeezed into my van and headed for Benwood.

When we knocked on his door Rose greeted us affably and, without inviting us in, said, "So, what's on your mind?"

This innocent question and his relaxed manner was the last thing we expected. "Well, Mr. Rose," I finally said, "we haven't heard from you and, well, the truth is, we're kinda, I mean . . . we're kinda wondering . . . well . . . "

"You mean you're bored to bejesus!" Rose roared. "Is that what you're tryin' to say?" We nodded sheepishly.

"Good. Now that I have your attention, maybe we can get some work done."

Rose owned an abandoned house in Benwood, and he set us to tearing it down for lumber in order to build a bunkhouse at the farm for future retreats. Everything was to be salvaged, including the nails, and since Frank was the only one with some carpentry to his credit, he was put in charge. He was also put in charge because, though it never occurred to us, Rose had a family to feed and wasn't getting rich hosting free retreats. He picked up a number of painting and roofing contracts that summer and would be available only intermittently on an "as needed" basis.

Rose was right. Like no lecture ever could, idling for days dramatically illustrated why every monastic tradition emphasizes manual labor. We were eager for our first day, but when we arrived at the site, Frank asked to speak to me privately.

"Mr. Rose says you're not allowed on the roof."

"Why?" I sputtered. Even I knew a house was torn down top to bottom.

"He says your head's up your ass. He says you're so busy laughing and teasing other people you'll fall and break your neck. Then he'll have to drive to Pittsburgh to tell your mother."

I was speechless. I started this damn group. I was Rose's first student, the apple of his eye. Clearly there was a mistake. But Frank, not without sympathy, said there was no mistake, and made an end to the conversation.

I wasn't even allowed to pull nails from the lumber cascading from the roof but was set to work *straightening* the bent ones. By the end of the day my effort wouldn't have garnered 35 cents if the nails were new, and mine sported the square heads of the previous century and were half rusted away. When quitting time finally rolled around, I jumped into the van and made a beeline for Rose. He met me at the door.

"You're not going to believe this, Mr. Rose," I said as if setting him up for a bad joke. "Frank said you don't want me on the roof. I figured he misunderstood you."

"He didn't misunderstand anything," Rose said flatly. "I told him your head is so far up your ass I'd need a team of mules and a day and a night to extricate it. You're so busy amusing yourself at other people's expense you'll fall and break your neck. Then I'll have to drive to Pittsburgh and tell your mother." After neatly echoing Frank's "you'll shoot your eye out" response to my request for a BB gun, he shut the door in my face.

As usual, Rose knew his mark. I continued to seethe but was so determined to prove him wrong that I went back to straightening nails with a vengeance. My determination paid off, and I was eventually given more valuable work. But I never did reach the roof that summer. I only metaphorically managed that many years later, when, with the benefit of hindsight, I was ready to admit that some of the most valuable work I ever did was banging away on those worthless nails.

* * *

Soon we settled into a routine of work, meals, freezing baths, group meditations, and sleep. The work progressed, and gradually the center of gravity shifted to the farm, where we began erecting the bunkhouse. Rose stopped by to check on our work, and a couple of times a week we drove into Benwood to spend a few hours sitting around his kitchen table. These sessions were often merely social; we would just chat and listen to Rose tell stories. Sometimes the conversation turned serious, but it seemed to depend on Rose's mood or our eagerness to ask questions.

As to reading, diet, fasting, and specific contemplative practices, much to my surprise, these were left to our discretion. At the time I felt this absence of "canned" spiritual techniques, liturgies, and drill sergeant supervision keenly. Like most people, I hated blank sheets of paper. But Rose loved the opportunity blank paper provides. He insisted that people's penchant for one-size-fits-all "practices" was an egotistical desire for the same safety, security, control, passivity, predictability, and predefined outcomes that authentic teaching labors so hard to undermine. My later business experience bore this out. Everyone is for getting outside the box in theory, but if someone actually touches the damn box, wholesale panic ensues.

> Rose loved the opportunity blank paper provides. He insisted that people's penchant for one-size-fits-all "practices" was an egotistical desire.

Rose relied instead on psychological shocks designed to "knock the head off dead center" just long enough for "direct realization" or epiphany to slip through the intellectual defenses of the logical mind. He defined Zen as "a series of leaps and shocks." Of course, none of this prevented him from ranting generally about people who asked for, but seldom heeded, his advice. Inspired by one of these tirades, I went to him and said I was willing to do anything he recommended without reservation.

"You'll do anything?" he said, arching his eyebrows skeptically.

"Yes," I whispered, no longer so sure.

"Anything?"

This time I barely nodded.

"Good," he said. "Learn to think for yourself."

Talk about a blank sheet of paper! This command was so far outside the box it stunned me, but it might very well be the best single piece of advice I ever received.

None of this means Rose was a New Age advocate of "anything goes." He had his own meditation system, and he was frequently rejected for being too rigorous, inflexible, even dogmatic. But Rosean rigor was at the level of principle, and at the level of practice he allowed plenty of room for individual differences. Rose was like a master of spiritual music: he insisted we learn the principles of melody and harmony, play with passion and in unison, and come in on cue and on key. But he was indifferent as to whether we played the violin or piano, preferred chamber music or rock, or played with our left hand or right.

As the summer progressed, I couldn't see much of anything that might be termed "spiritual" going on, but I was enjoying myself too much to really care. That summer I experienced for the first time the incredible sense of well-being that accompanies hard work, simple food, good fellowship, restful sleep, and the absence of worry, dissipation, and trivial distractions. I lost some baby fat, learned how to drive a nail, got a tan, forgot my worries, and found myself happier than I'd been in a very long time. I forgot all about telephones, running water, refrigerators, flush toilets, and everything else so painfully missing when I first arrived. I even began looking forward to cold baths in the moss-encrusted bathtub fed by the spring.

I also made a new friend.

Al was a student from Kent State. He was a stocky, blue-eyed Canadian of English/Irish extraction. The golden-brown ringlets bouncing off his shoulders along with a dashing mustache to match made him look, for all the world, like that swashbuckling movie star he apparently believed he was. Al invariably wore khaki shirts and shorts, high leather boots, a wide belt, and a broad-brimmed felt hat that made him look like he was either on safari or an Aussie Light Horse cavalryman fresh from the Boer War. If that wasn't romantically swashbuckling enough, he had painstakingly hand embroidered his shirts with the turquoise-beaded talismans of some obscure Canadian-Indian tribe that only he had heard of.

Self-supporting and living on his own, Al loved to regale us around the campfire with tales of how he bested incipient poverty and a ferocious Ohio winter by heroically living out of the tiny tent he clandestinely pitched each night somewhere on Kent State's campus because he couldn't afford to live in the dorms. Affable, witty, big-hearted, high-spirited, Al was perhaps the only human being I ever met who was even more hopelessly romantic than me. And we quickly formed a fast friendship over our mutual interest in military history, military hardware (especially tanks!), and derring-do deeds of mythic proportion in general. As usual, Rose, with his West Virginia penchant for turning a short "I" into a long "E," came up with the five-word description that most perfectly captured the chivalrous character of noble Sir Alan: "Al is dedeecated to dedeecation." (Rose always defaulted to a long E pronunciation of words like *dedicate* or *indicate*. Even fish often became *feesh*.)

Of course, no battle is won so easily that there aren't casualties, and as the summer wore on, the battle of the bunkhouse was no different. The only difference was it was Rose's possessions and tools that were taking the losses, and by extension his patience. One of Rose's antique chairs, worth hundreds of dollars, chopped a hole in its seat and transformed itself into a portable toilet. Rose's saws developed an uncanny knack for finding the nails the nail pullers missed, and several foolishly ruined themselves in this way. Then Rose's cast-iron tack hammer, which had no business trying to drive a ten-penny nail, tried to do just that, and its head broke off midstroke, nearly taking off a human head in the process.

One day Rose noticed his wooden ladder had built itself into the bunkhouse right under our noses. At first he merely shook his head and chuckled, but when someone suggested we teach the ladder a lesson by chopping it out rather than redo a day of our precious work, he rolled his eyes heavenward, muttered "Oh, Jesus Christ," and insisted on mercy for the obstinate ladder instead.

Hiding behind the passive voice aside, these things and many more actually happened. What's more embarrassing is we were so rude, insensitive, and self-absorbed we assumed all this collateral damage was an acceptable price to pay for free labor on a 20-foot-by-20-foot, make-work shanty of a bunkhouse. We were so blind we were blissfully unaware of the storm clouds gathering around our heads until it was too late to seek shelter.

One day Rose arrived unexpectedly at the site with his son James. He'd stepped on a nail at one of his own jobs, and he was walking with difficulty, running a fever, and looking, as he would say, peaked. We just finished installing the triangular trusses for the roof, and Rose climbed painfully up the ladder to have a look. He gazed along the peak for a minute or so and, without saying a word, climbed heavily back down. Then he called us over.

"Let me tell you guys something," he said, his blue eyes blazing from fever or something else. "I taught myself carpentry by building a house from oak because I wanted it to last forever. I cut trees off this farm and hauled them to the mill for lumber all by myself. Then I held the nails with vise grips as I drove them because oak is so hard, they'll bend if you don't.

"And I did this after working all day to feed a family. Hell, I nearly fell off the ladder a dozen times—I was that damn tired. But I still built that house to quarter-inch tolerance all the way around.

"It took three years and I barely finished," he continued, his voice rising, "when the politicians decided to put a bypass through the dining room. They took my house in the interest of the public and their Mafia friends in the construction trade and offered me ten cents on the dollar for my trouble. So I spent the next three months in a sandwich board picketing the courthouse at my family's expense. It was hopeless, but when the bulldozer rammed that house, I got the satisfaction of watching it slide off the foundation all in one piece. And you know what? I'd do it all again."

Then he turned and again gazed at the roof. When he turned back I didn't recognize him. His pallid cheeks were flecked with red, and there was so much cold fury in his eyes my own eyes widened as my heart sank.

"What the fuck do you guys think this is?" he screamed as spit flew out of his mouth. "Do you think this is some kind of fuckin' game we're playin'? Well, you may be playin', but this is my *life's work* you're fuckin' with. I told you guys to cut those trusses *square* and install them *true*, and what do I find? The fucking ocean. You fuck up everything you touch. Hell, you've lost, busted, and abused tools I've had a lifetime and my father and his father before me. That chair you turned into firewood so the weeds wouldn't tickle your asses was my great-grandmother's—and it's all because you're a bunch of Peter Pans on a lark and just don't give a fuck."

For a moment or two he just stood there out of breath, seething, but his face was so contorted I knew he wasn't finished.

"You're going to tear this down and do it again. And if it still ain't right, you'll do it again, and again, and again," he screamed, pounding his palm with his fist. "If you got to take this fuckin' box of sticks back to the rubble it came from and start over, you'll do it. If you intend to half-ass your way through life, go right ahead, but do it with someone else. I've waited thirty-five years for a group, and I'll wait thirty-five more, but whatever we do we'll do *right* even if I have to do it myself and drop dead doin' it."

Without another word, he limped away.

As soon as he left we set about feverishly correcting our work, fixing tools that weren't hopeless, and cleaning and oiling the rest. But we were so stunned and ashamed we scarcely spoke to each other.

The next day Rose returned for another inspection. As he painfully hauled himself up the ladder once again, I felt like the architect for the dome of St. Peter's Basilica watching the scaffolding come down in front of the Pope and praying the dome didn't follow suit.

Rose climbed down and grunted, "Now you're talkin.'" Nothing more was said about the incident.

Rose's outburst reduced me to a jumble of emotion. I'd never seen Rose like that, and I never heard him use that kind of language. I felt that in light of our youth, inexperience, the rotten lumber, and our nonexistent wages, our job was "good enough" and he completely overreacted. Worse, in giving in to rage, he utterly lost control, and this didn't fit my conception of a spiritual teacher. I felt utterly let down.

A few days later, I went into town to see him on a routine errand. He greeted me affably, and I was impressed by the absence of any stiffness in his manner. We conducted our business, and I was leaving when he said, "Wait a second." He looked at me intently for a moment.

"First things first. I meant everything I said out there, but we'll leave it at that. The whole time I was also inside your heads. Frank was so mad he could've killed me, but he'll get over it. You, you didn't get angry. You were completely let down. You still are. You thought you knew me, invited me over for tea, and then I busted up all the furniture.

"But that ain't the half of it. You're let down because it's dawning on you that daddy don't have all the answers, that daddy might be human, and that daddy can't do this work for you. That's good, because I ain't your daddy, and the best thing I can do is rid you of that notion any way I can."

As I drove back to the farm, I was amazed at how neatly Rose read my mind and put words to my emotions. He was absolutely right, but I was more confused than ever.

What I couldn't see was Rose had a completely different perspective. To him, our labor was a form of prayer, and the kind of relativistic comparisons and "good enough" compromises that might be adequate to a merely human undertaking were utterly unacceptable when God was involved. To him it was ridiculous to speak of Truth if you couldn't install trusses true.

Spirituality for Rose was a habit, a way of life, a spirit of excellence. There was no compartmentalization. A seeker was never off duty, and everyday life supplied the opportunities for paying attention or living "at-tension."

Rose's reaction to our slipshod work was a broadside against that "mutually modulated conspiracy of mediocrity" he warned tempts all communities. Although I always agreed with him in principle, when he applied his philosophy to me, I felt hurt, unappreciated, and disappointed in him.

My reaction was also another example of my desire for control. Deep down, I was desperately counting on spirituality to take me beyond human emotions like rage and, especially, depression. Rose was supposed to provide a bulwark against all the chaotic emotion and irrationality of my life, and seeing my hero behaving like a mere mortal threatened all this.

But as bad as all this was, things were about to get far worse. Like a Russian doll within a doll, while all these Rosean storm clouds were gathering around us, others were gathering at a much lower altitude— around my own head.

Chapter Eleven

THE COMING OF THE LORD

The inner freedom from the practical desire,
The release from action and suffering, release from the inner
And the outer compulsion, yet surrounded
By a grace of sense, a white light still and moving,
Erhebung without motion, concentration
Without elimination, both a new world
And the old made explicit, understood
In the completion of its partial ecstasy,
The resolution of its partial horror.
—T.S. ELIOT[27]

Phil was a student from the Kent State contingent who got on my
nerves. He was a thin, old-school hippie with a bad complexion and
an ostentatious leather headband I think he slept in. He seemed to
think he was God's chosen because he was mild-mannered, ate organic chickpeas with chopsticks, drank decaffeinated green tea, and
reeked of sandalwood incense. He also was one of those elitists who

flaunt their elite status by disdaining elitism—as if he'd already won the game by refusing to play.

In retrospect this analysis was only partly true, but I needed a victim to help pass the time, and these putative traits put Phil at the top of the list. As we were tearing down Rose's house in Benwood to salvage the lumber, I started needling him for the amusement of one and all, and as the summer wore on, I became very good at it. My favorite tack was to engage Ray in a conversation about turning Rose's farm into an amusement park and dirt motorcycle haven. I would go on at length, designing in all the environmental travesties I could think of until, right on schedule, Phil would drop his chopsticks into his organic gruel and storm off in a rage.

One day, just after we started assembling the bunkhouse, Rose took me aside. "Phil was in to see me," he said.

Uh-oh, I thought. Gathering my composure, I said, "What about, Mr. Rose?"

"He says you cap on people. You pretend you're teasing, but you're really establishing a pecking order with you as head rooster."

I didn't know what to say, so I stammered, "What did you tell him?"

"I told him to work harder, get smarter, and learn to cap on you. I told him I wasn't running a spiritual convoy that only moves as fast as the slowest ship."

As he walked away, I thought, *That's telling him, Mr. Rose. The damn snitch! Phil's such a wimp he can't even face me himself.*

Of course, now that I felt I had Rose's blessing, I went back to giving Phil the business with renewed relish.

A couple weeks later Rose again took me aside. "Phil was in to see me again," he said blandly.

"What about, Mr. Rose?" I asked, feigning curiosity.

"He said Dharma barks all the time, and he can't meditate."

"Do you agree with him? I mean, Dharma only—"

"No, no," Rose said, waving me off. "I told him to learn to focus his mind regardless of distractions." He walked away, leaving me muttering to Dharma, "Good dog. *Good* dog."

* * *

Nothing more was said until a couple weeks after Rose's blowup over our wobbly trusses. Frank announced that Rose would be commuting to the farm to personally oversee the final stages of work on the bunkhouse. He arrived early the next morning, and the first thing he did was start in on me. No matter what I said or did, Rose delivered a putdown. All morning this continued, and Rose added to my humiliation by making no attempt to temper his insults with the cleverness and humor I knew came so effortlessly to him. It was just one crude, sarcastic hammer blow after another.

At first I was shocked, but I quickly caught on. I'd been dishing it out, I'd ignored his warnings, and now Rose was stepping in to even the score. As the shock wore off, I decided I had it coming, and resolved to just bear up under the onslaught until Rose was satisfied I'd learned my lesson. I figured I was in for a few hours of hell. But the torture outlasted the day—and the next one, and the next. The atmosphere at the job site became oppressive. I dreaded each day. Little by little I was driven back onto myself. I became so absorbed by my inner dialogue and chaotic emotions I was oblivious to everything else. I began bumping into things and making mistakes, and this played right into Rose's hands.

Desperately, I tried to decide what to do. One minute I was halfway to my van headed home. Then I changed my mind: I wasn't going to give the bastard the satisfaction. Then I reacted to this reaction.

187

My God, am I here to learn, or win battles with the teacher? Next, I wondered if it was all a test: Rose always said he wanted fighters, so maybe I was supposed to take a swing at him. But if I was wrong, that would finish things between us. Perhaps Rose had his reasons even if I couldn't see them. Maybe surrender—submissive endurance—was the answer to this nightmare of a paradox, this mother of a Zen koan. I instantly caught this thought halfway and cut it off. *What the hell are you thinking?* a panicky voice interrupted. *Are you so snowed by the bastard that no matter what cruel, unfair, unjust thing he pulls you'll write it off as Zen? That's not surrender, that's insanity. Where will it end, surrendering your firstborn son?*

Seconds later, I changed my mind again. Had I no faith? After all the things I saw Rose do, why was I forever doubting when things got sticky? Besides, what did I know about justice and fairness? When Phil wanted justice, he was just whining. Maybe everything Rose was saying was true, and I just couldn't face it. *That's not it,* another voice would cut in. *What you can't face is being wrong about the guy. Admit it. Cut your losses. You knew he was a nut when he lost it over the damn trusses. Instead, you wrote it off to fever, and now you're making excuses again. You're just too damn proud and in too deep to admit you made a mistake.*

Around and around these competing voices swirled with increasing velocity, creating an emotional vortex of ever-tightening spirals sucking me down. I soon stopped taking any of these arguments seriously; they were all so perfectly reasonable and so perfectly contradictory they canceled each other out. Instead, I just watched in dumb disbelief as they rushed through my head, rising and falling like overlapping bits of half overheard conversation leaking from a passing train. Paralyzed and afraid, I lost confidence in thinking itself. Which, of course, only gave me that much more to think about.

My life degenerated into long days and even longer nights as I wandered around in a daze like a decapitated man carrying his own head. I ate little and slept less.

I felt like a newly unemployed member of a snooty country club suddenly reduced to a social pariah. Things with my fellow Rose students were so awkward that, while I'm sure it's an exaggeration, my memory of mealtimes is me sitting on one side of the campfire and everyone else on the other. I didn't have a soul to turn to. I felt absolutely alone—except for Dharma.

Only Dharma was on my side, and after supper we would walk my overheated mind around the farm until everyone else went to sleep. One evening I sat on a sandy mound by the racetrack and immediately lost track of everything, including Dharma. I must've stewed for an hour or more because when I came back to the world, it was pitch dark. Dharma, rooting around nearby, had apparently created the noise that broke the spell.

I needed a friend in the worst way, so I whistled and gratefully heard him bounding through the underbrush in my direction. He was a black dog, and I didn't see him until he was already clambering all over me. Suddenly the smell was overpowering, and I realized with a shock he had been to the portion of the sandy racetrack the men used as a toilet. Dharma was covered with human feces.

My disgust turned to dismay when I realized that, to clean him up at the spring, I would have to return to the campsite for a flashlight and face the others with this latest example of how far the mighty had fallen. But there was nothing else to do, so grabbing him by the collar with one hand and my nose with the other, I started back. When I arrived, the terrible stench I brought with me created the grand entrance I imagined. Everyone started grimacing, moaning, and clutching their noses. As I stepped into the firelight looking for a flashlight, suddenly their complaints turned to laughter. I didn't get the joke for a second or two, but I finally realized I was smeared head to foot with human excrement. Dharma even carefully anointed my face with his soiled muzzle.

My only friend had turned on me as well.

Grabbing the flashlight, the dog, and a change of clothes, I headed for the spring. As we cleaned up, all I could think of was what Rose would make of this latest misadventure when someone told him about it. And I knew someone would.

For whatever reason, Rose didn't join us the next day, but sure enough news arrived from town that he wanted us to come to Benwood that evening. I went like a man to his own execution.

As we gathered around his kitchen table, the tension was oppressive. Rose added to it by just sitting quietly for a few minutes, seemingly engrossed with his fingernails.

"Well, well," he finally said in a voice dripping with sarcasm. "I am deeply embarrassed. I owe you guys an apology." He paused to let us wonder where he was going with this ironic opening.

"You see, I invited you down here under false pretenses, and though I didn't intentionally mislead you, you've been misled nonetheless. You came under the impression I'm some kind of Zen master. Well, I think we just found out who the real master around here is.

"Now, whatever you may think of me, I do have sense enough to know when I been outgunned, outclassed, and just plain licked. But at least I ain't the only one been licked, eh Augie? Heh, heh, heh."

His laughter was intentionally forced and humorless, and though the others laughed along, they were clearly straining at it.

"Think about it," Rose continued, folding his arms and leaning back in his chair until the front legs hovered a few inches off the floor. "Zen says, 'Those who know don't say, and those who say don't know' and 'expect the unexpected.' How much more unexpected can you get than a master in the form of a dog who not only don't say but can't? Here's a real Zen master right under our noses in more ways than one, and we didn't even know it until he revealed himself in such a spectacular fashion."

Rose was warming to his subject now, and successfully giving the impression that he was addressing everyone while obviously singling me out.

"Stay with me, and I'm sure you'll see what I'm drivin' at. Zen is all about wordless transmission. A real Zen master don't use words, he goes right to the heart with a sign, a gesture, a symbolic act. Zen's 'a direct pointing at the Mind of man.' So while I been spinnin' my wheels bustin' verbal hammers on Augie's ironclad head, Dharma gets fed up, steps in, and shows an amateur how it's done.

"You see, somehow Augie got it into his fat head he's Dharma's master, and if that ain't bad enough, he don't even treat Dharma like a student. No," Rose said, leaning forward again and tapping his index finger on the table for added emphasis, "he treats him like a dog whose sole purpose is to jump through hoops for Augie's amusement. I guess that ain't so surprising, come to think of it." He shook his head sadly.

"Augie treats a lot of folks that way. Anyway, Dharma decides something drastic got to be done if Augie is ever gonna' realize just how full of shit he really is. So, like a true Zen master, he neatly sidesteps all the hot air and smears him head to toe with the genuine article. Now that's direct communication for you! It's pure genius for them that's got eyes for it, or, maybe I should say, *noses* for it. Heh, heh, heh."

On and on and on he droned as I descended into blackness. I was utterly defeated. There wasn't a single thought in my head, just the unintelligible white noise of his singsong voice. The others gave up trying to laugh and just sat there squirming, but still he went on. Only Al seemed sympathetic. I could see anger in his eyes as he glared at Rose, and I was incredibly grateful for this tiny show of support.

The next thing I remember is driving back to the farm. I was finished. I couldn't take another second of this. I didn't know what I was going to do if the torture continued. I only knew I was at the end of my rope.

When I arrived at the job site the next morning, Rose was already there, and he greeted me so naturally I knew my ordeal was over. In fact, he reestablished a friendly relationship so easily I felt like it had all been some kind of bad dream. Perhaps it was merely by contrast, but over the next few weeks he seemed to treat me with a special kindness. When I became mildly ill with a stomach virus, for example, he insisted I take to bed in town so he could monitor my progress while personally dosing me every four hours with Pepto-Bismol. I don't think my sainted mother ever treated me more solicitously than Rose did over those few days.

* * *

The mood of our retreat reverted to the relaxed jocularity that preceded the crisis at the bunkhouse and my ordeal. The bunkhouse was finished, and before I knew it summer was winding down and it was almost time to return to school. With little to do out at the farm, we spent much of those waning days hanging around in Rose's kitchen in Benwood socializing, talking philosophy, and just enjoying ourselves.

One day the mood was particularly relaxed. There wasn't room for us all around the rectangular kitchen table, so I was sitting a little behind Rose's left shoulder as he sat at the head.

Rose was telling a story about a group of older women who, hearing he could hypnotize, asked for a demonstration at one of their teas.

"I don't know what I was drinkin', but I accepted the invite," Rose said, shaking his head. "First thing some old battle axe who already buried three husbands starts pullin' on my cheek and says, 'Oh, Richard, you look so young, you don't have a single wrinkle.'

"But I managed to parry that thrust. I told her well-stuffed sausage skins like me never have wrinkles."

Rose asked for volunteers to be hypnotized. As a trust experiment to determine the best subjects, he stood behind each volunteer and asked her to fall backward into his arms.

"Anyway, the last volunteer was built like a hogshead barrel and went 280 if an ounce.

Without thinkin' I told her to fall over backward. Over she came like a Redwood in a dead swoon, and before I knew it she's in my arms and the blood's rushin' to my head. My eyes were popping, and I almost had a stroke gettin' her back on her feet. I was so winded I staggered to the bathroom to take a blow. Believe you me," he finished gravely, "it was everything I could do to keep that old bloat off the floor and out of the basement."

While everyone was laughing, it occurred to me that this relaxed atmosphere, among witnesses, with Rose distracted, offered just the safe venue I needed to ask about those little jolts of energy. I hadn't experienced one all summer, but they were still nagging at me, and with the retreat almost over, I decided it was now or never.

I leaned in toward Rose, fully intending to come right to the point, but at the last second I lost my nerve and scaled my question back to something safer. "Mr. Rose," I said as nonchalantly as I could manage, "you know, sometimes I think if I just let go something might happen to me."

Before I finished Rose's eyes were already locked on mine.

"Yes," he said dreamily, as if he'd been waiting for eons for me to deliver my line so he could deliver his. "But you'd have to cry. And Augie doesn't cry now, does he?"

Instantly a shock wave of energy stunned me, knocking me off balance. This was my deepest secret, a secret so deep it was a secret even to me. At some point during my traumatic Hotchkiss ordeal, I'd unconsciously locked away all my chaotic emotions as a self-protective mechanism, and I hadn't been able to cry since. This dark secret rushing to the surface stunned me again, and with another surge of energy I realized Rose knew all along. He orchestrated everything to bring me to this point. No, it was more than that. It went back before our first meeting, before our births, before . . . Then I realized how crazy this was, and that stunned me again.

All this took less than a second, and before I could recover, my world dissolved into a series of stronger and stronger energy surges. Surges that left me amazed, then amazed at how amazed I was, and then amazed at how amazed at how amazed I was. Faster and faster these stunning, recursive shocks piled, one on top of another, until there wasn't an instant to figure out what was happening and regain my footing. Overwhelmed, I felt myself mentally falling over backward under the force of these repeated blows.

Rose's face, and then the room itself, receded at light speed until I was mentally racing through black, empty space with abject terror adding its own impetus to the process. All I desperately wanted was just one tiny split-second to catch my breath and take stock, but there wasn't even enough space between shocks to scream. Instead, my awareness, my sense of self, became detached from my thought processes altogether. I could only watch in dismay as thoughts flashed by my mind's eye as if on a screen, one replacing the next with such velocity I couldn't even take them in. With thinking left far behind, there were no longer words, just realizations. I was like a submarine at four times its maximum depth, and all around me alarms were going off as rivets popped out of the hull. Something even more fundamental than thought was giving way, and I fought with all my strength to hold on.

Then *something was there*. And this *something* wordlessly offered me a chance to see myself as I truly was. A whole new way of seeing was being offered, and all I had to do was tilt my mind's eye to take advantage of it. But instead, just as silently, I wordlessly screamed out in abject terror: "No, no, my God, NO!" What if what I was about to see wasn't *me*? What if I was an alien and not human? What if I was a monster? What if I didn't exist at all?

All these questions and millions like them were embedded in my instantaneous and negative reply. My horrified "no" echoed through empty darkness because, with my answer, whatever it was that invited me to see myself vanished, and the opportunity was gone.

With its departure, I finally felt I was gaining a grip. It was tenuous, like hanging onto sheer marble by my fingernails, but it was there nonetheless. I have no idea how long I hung there, but eventually I noticed that, like coming down off LSD, I was gradually revving down. By minute degrees the room came back into my field of vision. There was Rose, looking down at his hands folded in his lap, while the others seemed silently caught up in the mood.

There was still only one emotion, fear, and the first thought I had after what seemed like an eternity of thoughtlessness was, *Please, God, as long as Rose doesn't look at me, I think I'll make it, but if he looks at me I won't be able to take it and I'll fall.* He didn't look but continued to sit quietly. Then I thought: *Please, God, I'm closer now. As long as he doesn't speak to me, I'll make it.*

He didn't speak to me.

Finally my emotional feet touched the ground again, and I sat there breathing heavily. This went on for some minutes, and then, when all danger had passed, Rose turned to me. He had tears in his eyes, and his face was the face of the father welcoming home his prodigal son.

"Mine eyes have seen the glory of the coming of the Lord," he said. I broke down in tears.

* * *

The next thing I remember is being back at the farm. Remarkably, all the terror had been transformed into clarity of purpose, a clarity so pure it was accompanied by a profound exaltation. I tried my best to tell the others what happened. They told me I was "gone" for the better part of an hour, and that Jeanne cried out, "My God, look at his face!" only moments after the first shock wave hit me. Besides this initial outburst, the "spirit" so quickly and completely blanketed the room that everyone was plunged into a deep meditative silence, a silence broken only when Rose finally spoke of the coming of the Lord.

For the remaining few days of my stay at the farm, this sense of clarity and exaltation stayed with me. My one clear memory of this period is a profound sense of: *Of course. How could I have missed it before?* Life was so beautiful and such a gift, I wondered at how we all conspire to make it so hard. I remember going to the grocery store one day and being shocked by all the pain, confusion, and sorrow I saw on all the faces. I wanted to rush up and hug them all and tell them . . . But that was just it: tell them . . . *what?*

Finally, I drove into town to say goodbye to Rose before heading back to Pittsburgh. We had not seen each other since my experience in his kitchen. Rose greeted me warmly, and we spoke for a while about our plans for the university group. Then it was time to go, and suddenly there were tears streaming down my face.

"Mr. Rose," I blurted, "I don't want to go. I want to stay here with you . . . stay at the farm. I see everything so clearly now: a bag of rice, a jug of water, a sleeping bag, and this work. I don't need anything else. I don't want to go back."

"I know," Rose said, and the tears in his own eyes left little doubt that he really did. "But you don't understand. You can't stay here. You'll only fall asleep. You need the struggle, the friction of life to keep you growing. Your destiny is out there."

I knew he was right, but when I got to the door I turned back. "Mr. Rose," I said too loudly, startling myself. "What happened to me?"

Rose was already sorting through some mail. "What happened?" he said quietly, looking up at me over his glasses. "I thought I told you. 'Mine eyes have seen the glory of the coming of the Lord.'" And he went back to the mail.

Over the years, at various times and in various places, in good times and bad, I asked that same question, always hoping for an elaboration. Each time Rose would look at me with fresh surprise and say, "But I told you. 'Mine eyes have seen the glory of the coming of the Lord.' What else could you possibly want to know?"

Chapter Twelve

BACK TO THE FUTURE

What might have been is an abstraction
Remaining a perpetual possibility
Only in a world of speculation.
What might have been and what has been
Point to one end, which is always present.
—T.S. Eliot[28]

It was a hot, sunny, early September afternoon in Pittsburgh, and after wandering around a bit I found a brick building on Eighth Avenue sporting the sign I was looking for: LABORERS DISTRICT COUNCIL OF WESTERN PA LOCAL 1058. Facing me and the street was a busy, middle-aged receptionist snugly tucked behind the thickest glass window I'd ever seen. Glancing up from her paperwork, she leaned into the microphone on her desk, pressed a button, and with a faint whiff of annoyance, said, "What do you want?"

The outdoor speaker above my head amplified her voice as well as her annoyance, and it took a few flustered seconds to realize her bullet-proof ticket window offered a small, louvered vent for replies. Bending over slightly, I said, "I want to work for the union."

She shoved a 3-by-5 notecard through a small slit under the vent with curt instructions to fill in my name and phone number. I complied and she breezily said, "We'll call when there's work." Switching off her microphone, she returned to her papers.

Her blasé demeanor as well as the unprofessional card she perfunctorily proffered strongly suggested the next stop for my name and phone number was the circular file under her desk. But I was determined to work in heavy construction at union scale, so, ignoring her chilly brush-off, I pressed on.

"Excuse me, Ma'am. Would it be OK with you if I stopped by occasionally to see if there's work?"

"Sure," a disembodied voice from the speaker replied. "Knock yourself out. It's a free country after all."

I turned and ambled off down the street.

Even without elaboration from Rose, I knew terror and immaturity prematurely aborted my spiritual experience in his kitchen. I was obviously not ready, as Rose would say, "to take the trip." Several years later I found an apt description of my experience as well as my horrified reaction in the teachings of the famous ninth-century Chinese Zen master, Huang Po. "Oh, you silly students of Zen! You fear falling into the void with nothing to stay your fall. But that is ridiculous: there is no void and there is no ego to fall."[29] Obviously, there was still work to do.

However, that singular, white-hot clarity of purpose followed me back to Pittsburgh, and the first thing I did, much to the dismay of my parents, was drop out of the University of Pittsburgh. What college offered now seemed trivial, even absurd, but I later regretted not telling my mentors, like Orysia in the Russian History department, that I was dropping out. I probably didn't know how to explain an inexplicable decision with words I just didn't have, but in any case, I rudely failed to show up for the first day of class.

I then told my roommates I was moving out of our quarters in Shadyside in favor of a newly rented house I was turning into an urban "ashram," or spiritual community, by renting bedrooms to the more serious members of our Zen Studies Society. (Despite dropping out as a student, I would still be chairing our campus meetings.)

Next, I needed a job. I wanted a physically demanding occupation, something to keep me in shape while freeing my mind for sundry transcendental ruminations. It was these objectives that sent me on my hero's quest to the legendary Land of Local 1058 and its mythic Threshold Guardian, the baleful Lady Behind the Glass Wall.

These decisions, though consequential, were comparatively easy. Much more difficult was ending my relationship with Sara. So difficult, in fact, that despite my firm intentions, I was still putting it off.

I wandered around Pittsburgh for a while, and when I got to Horne's department store, I hesitated before braving the store's revolving glass door. When I was pushing 3, my mother and I shared one of these revolving compartments on our way into Horne's for some Christmas shopping. As we were making our exit, one of those dastardly doors grabbed my head and wedged it firmly between the rubber jacketed tip of its outstretched arm and the concave outer wall. The frantic efforts of my mother and an army of sales clerks responding to my screams proved ineffectual, and I remained tightly fixed until a maintenance crew finally pried my tiny head from the jaws of that fiendish door.

By 1973 I no longer attributed malicious intent to inanimate objects, but I still superstitiously debouched into Horne's with a quick little skip-step just in case that twirling dervish of a door once again took a fancy to my head.

Jousting with revolving doors, cruising around Horne's, and grabbing a cup of tea at the coffee shop killed an hour or so, and soon I was once again facing 1058's formidable Lady Behind the Glass Wall.

"What do you want now?" she said impatiently.

"Well, you said I could stop back to see if there's work."

"But I told you an hour ago there isn't any work!"

"Yes, Ma'am, I know. But a lot of things can change in an hour."

Luckily, I tempered my temerity with that same mischievous "good little bad boy" smile I often used to great effect in tight spots on the sainted Franciscan sisters at Saints Simon and Jude grade school.

Little by little the irritation drained from her face, and, despite herself, her lips began curling into a faint semblance of the same bemused smile that graced mine. But catching herself, again just like the nuns, she feigned some faux anger and gruffly said, "No! There's still no work!"

Rebuffed yet again, I resumed my urban odyssey. In light of my newfound commitment to Rose and spirituality there was no future for my relationship with Sara. Sara was the "marrying kind," and until I reached my spiritual objectives, marriage was not an option. The situation was further complicated by my decision to formalize our still non-physical relationship (as well as my own virginity) by becoming a celibate Brahmachari. But despite my firm intentions, I was still not able to broach the subject with Sara. She didn't even know I'd dropped out of school and moved out of my shared house. I was just making things harder by putting it off but . . .

"You again!" came the now-familiar voice from behind the impenetrable glass. It was five o'clock, and I was just in time to catch her rolling down the blinds on her street-level human aquarium before calling it a day.

"No," she started to say, "there's still *no* . . . " But she failed to finish because we were both too busy laughing while pointing at each other through the glass wall. Eventually, still laughing, she finished rolling down her blinds while teasingly bending over and waving bye-bye until her huge glass eye completely closed for the night.

At 8 AM the next morning I was standing at attention as those same blinds stubbornly blinked once or twice before reopening for another day. At first she was startled, and then: "*You!* I can't believe it! Listen . . . my goodness. I got to get someone to talk to you!"

Switching off her microphone and whirling around in her high-backed chair, she launched into a high-spirited debate with a dark-skinned older man with snow white hair. It was like watching a silent movie, but the acting was so good I quickly divined the plot. The beleaguered Old Sorcerer adamantly didn't want to see me while his now thoroughly beguiled Guardian was just as determined he would. Back and forth the agon raged, my fate in the balance, until the cranky old alchemist finally threw up his hands, shrugged his shoulders, and, making eye contact with me for the first time, wearily waved me inside. With a big, self-satisfied smile, my newly won rank-and-file guardian angel pressed a button, a buzzer sang out, and the gates to Local 1058 and my union job in heavy construction magically swung open.

The next morning I was formally invested with a bright orange hard hat on Interstate 79 just south of Pittsburgh in the brand-new work boots and gloves I proudly bought just for the occasion.

* * *

I spent the next several weeks playing that Old Sorcerer's sunburnt apprentice as I frantically heaved a continuously replenished mountain of heavy gravel into an endless series of spellbound wheelbarrows with an oversized coal shovel my Italian colleagues affectionately called an "Italian spoon." The relentless parade of wheelbarrows were "Italian Cadillacs," and I eventually shoveled so much gravel without making the slightest dent in that damn pile that I wearily decided Italian spoons and Cadillacs were collectively honeycombed with invisible holes.

Shoveling gravel all day did give me ample time to rehearse the noble breakup scene I was preparing for Sara. But though I saw her almost every night, I just couldn't pull it off.

Then one night I dropped into The Portfolio just as Sara was getting off work. I needed a noisy public place bustling with people to break the spell and bolster my resolve. We took a table in a corner and ordered hot tea. My well-rehearsed speech instantly turned to mush as I tried to tell Sara why I couldn't see her anymore. Sara didn't say much. She mostly just looked down at her tea, and I distinctly remember marveling at how beautiful she was. Listening to my incoherent prattle, I became increasingly frustrated by my inability to say what I wanted to say. Suddenly I blurted it out.

"Sara, I am not leaving you. This is not my idea. If it was up to me, I'd never leave you. Never."

Sara looked up and softly said, "I know." She did know, and I was deeply moved by this tiny sliver of understanding, a precious strand of understanding not a single soul in my wide circle of friends and family seemed to share.

But when I kissed her goodbye, she whispered through tears.

"Augie, it's not fair. If things don't work out for you with the buddhas, you can always come back to me. But if things don't work out for me, what am I supposed to do?"

I headed down the street, but I was so upset I strode right past my van and kept walking. I was heartbroken. I missed Sara already. But there was also an ominous warning floating among her parting words. What if things didn't work out for me? Then what? Since returning to Pittsburgh this hadn't even occurred to me. Stopping dead in my tracks, I shuddered as I brushed up against the third rail of spirituality for the first time, that lonely wasteland and special psychological hell lying halfway between Heaven and earth. What if I sacrificed Sara and everything earth has to offer only to find that the heaven I longed for was a fleeting will-o'-the-wisp, forever receding, always just beyond my grasp? What if all I managed to do was turn myself into some misbegotten, grotesque gargoyle, a misshapen, half caterpillar, half butterfly, mooncalf of a Caliban stuck and slowly suffocating in some cramped and lonely cocoon called the Main Hotel—unfit, unworthy, unwelcome in either Heaven or earth?

Sara's parting words gave me an unexpected and totally new insight, a fresh stomach-churning glimpse into just how deadly serious things were getting. Leaving Sara wasn't like giving up meat, dropping out of school, changing living arrangements, or even becoming celibate. All these sacrifices were retrievable, easily reversed. Sara represented an entirely new life, an earthly life with endless possibilities, and this opportunity, despite her promise, was closing and closing permanently. I suddenly felt like a family man with a huge mortgage trying to catch up with his stomach on the down elevator after quitting his secure, high-paying, "perfectly good" job in order to bootstrap some half-baked, back-of-the-envelope, entrepreneurial dream.

The thought of sacrificing Sara and still coming up spiritually short was so painful I began entertaining a "best of both worlds" scenario where I knocked out Enlightenment in a year or so and came running back to Sara. But this sent fresh chills up my spine. *No*, I thought, *that's cheating. That's hedging. That's hanging back. You're trying to game the system. Holding on to earth with one hand while reaching for Heaven with the other is exactly the kind of thinking that will lose you both Sara and Enlightenment.*

As I passed the Kunst bakery on Forbes Avenue (Sara's favorite, by the way), now shuttered for the night, I recalled an interview with an undefeated former prizefighter. The champ loved his chocolate cake, but throughout his long career he never ate a single slice. He was asked how often he fought.

"On average, once a year."

"Once a year? In fifteen years, you couldn't risk one lousy piece of chocolate cake?"

"Listen," the steely-eyed fighter replied. "I didn't want my final thought as the lights went out, maybe forever, to be, 'I wonder if it was that damn piece of chocolate cake!'"

Any thoughts of reaching Enlightenment and getting Sara as well was like trying to have my chocolate cake and eat it too. It was a one-way ticket to some desolate park bench in spiritual Palookaville feeding Carnegie's pigeons and bitterly wondering whether I failed because I always held something back "just in case." I didn't want to end up like some wannabe entrepreneur who keeps his day job as a hedge only to end up wondering if he failed because he hedged.

When I finally returned to my parked van, I realized Sara's heartfelt farewell added a new dimension to the sense of purpose I received in Rose's kitchen. Sacrificing Sara added desperation to inspiration, and I silently promised Sara I would not let our mutual sacrifice be in vain. I would reach Cosmic Consciousness or die trying.

> **Little did I know I was destined to spend the next twenty-five years in the spiritual desert wandering in ever-tightening circles until, little by little, I began to give up on God and, even more so, on myself.**

Over the next few months, as the pain of our breakup slowly ebbed away, the self-confident exhilaration I brought back from Rose's farm re-asserted itself. I'd successfully cut ties with my "old life," and now I eagerly anticipated what was to come. Despite Sara's warning, in my euphoria and naiveté I was utterly convinced that having heard His footsteps in Rose's kitchen, the Lord would be along any minute.

Little did I know I was destined to spend the next twenty-five years in the spiritual desert wandering in ever-tightening circles until, little by little, I began to give up on God and, even more so, on myself.

* * *

A *whoosh*, followed by a heavy *whop*, suddenly broke the windy silence as our parachute, struggling to open, jolted the creaking clockwork of space and time in 1996 back into gear. I was rudely snatched from my timeless, womblike reveries about my past, first by the noise and sudden deceleration, and then by my chute's safety strap slowly inching up my chest to my forty-four-year-old neck until it partially restricted my breathing. The tandem jumper floating on my back urged me to enjoy the scenery, and though I tried, that pesky strap across my Adam's apple rekindled all my prejump apprehension. All I wanted was to firmly plant my dangling feet back on familiar terra firma.

The pro shouted in my ear: "Get ready to land!" He flared our parachute and, just below, I watched Mother Earth gently wafting up to embrace me. But as I touched down, there was a loud *crack*. I watched in amazement as my right foot turned completely around—something I didn't know it could do.

Crumpling to the ground, I realized my ankle was broken. Then the pain hit. It took forever for the ambulance to arrive, but I put the delay to good use by roundly cursing skydiving, skydiving schools, the "expert" strapped to my back, and, for good measure, his mother as well. All at the top of my lungs. The Duke students stood round as the school's medic cut off my pant leg and bloody shoe and applied first aid. But as sometimes happens in high-stress situations, amidst the pain, confusion, and nonstop cursing, I became strangely detached. I remember Meredith, a student I never really noticed before, kneeling at my side and staring at me with so much wide-eyed compassion in her bright green eyes that I was moved.

While waiting for the orthopedic surgeon to arrive at the hospital, I became frightened. A broken ankle gushing a shoe full of blood couldn't be good. Like a little boy with a boo-boo, I plaintively asked my nurse if I was going to be OK. "You're conscious," she snorted as if I needed a shrink more than a surgeon. "That's more than I can say for most of the damn fools they bring in from that school."

The doctor said I compound fractured the tibia and fibula bones in my ankle, and the broken skin was producing all the blood: I would have to be operated on immediately.

I awoke on my back, my foot raised, and a morphine drip stuck in my arm. I couldn't urinate, so I was catheterized as well. When the surgeon came in, I was counting on some encouragement.

"You've taken quite a shock," he said. "You drove a hell of a lot of energy through that ankle. It took fifteen pins and four screws to knit it back together. You shattered the bones that broke the skin. All I could do was press the pieces back in place like piecing together a mosaic out of tiny pieces of glass. You'll walk again, but a stiff ankle, a limp, and chronic pain are all real possibilities."

I was devastated by his prognosis and the cold professional way he delivered it. After he left, I began weeping uncontrollably. Then I began to panic. I panicked because I would never walk again. I panicked because I would never urinate again. I panicked watching myself panic over irrational fears. Finally, I panicked just because I was panicking.

Then it hit me. My panic had nothing to do with my ankle. I was panicking over my mortality. I was looking death right in the face without any psychological buffer. *Sure*, I thought, *you'll go home this time, but if you're panicking now, what will you do when someday the doctor tells you you're a dead man?*

Horror filled me to bursting, and even as it did, I had to face the fact that after twenty-five years on a spiritual quest, when I desperately needed something to fall back on, there was nothing there. *Nothing.* I knew *nothing.* I believed in *nothing.* It was all a pretense, a crock of nonsense designed to get me out of bed in the morning and make me feel superior to other people.

Now I knew the truth. I was going to die someday. Someday soon. And there wasn't a damn thing I could do about it.

I told no one what was happening for fear that their panic for *me* would amplify the panic *in me* beyond my breaking point. Like a child trapped in a freezer, icy panic so utterly overwhelmed my physical voice that no one but me in my dark and tiny universe could hear my screams.

Chapter Thirteen

DARK NIGHT

Here is a place of disaffection
Time before and time after
In a dim light: neither daylight
Investing form with lucid stillness
Turning shadow into transient beauty
With slow rotation suggesting permanence
Nor darkness to purify the soul
Emptying the sensual with deprivation
Cleansing affection from the temporal.
Neither plentitude nor vacancy. Only a flicker
Over the strained time-ridden faces
Distracted from distraction by distraction
Filled with fancies and empty of meaning
Tumid apathy with no concentration
Men and bits of paper, whirled by the cold wind
That blows before and after time,
Wind in and out of unwholesome lungs
Time before and time after.
—T.S. Eliot[30]

"Good morning, Mr. Turak!" chirped a middle-aged nurse in a white, smartly starched uniform. "How are we today? Did you sleep well? Yes, I know, it's hard sleeping on your back with your leg in the air. But as we nurses like to say, doctor's orders! I hope the morphine helps. Speaking of which, how's that pain today?"

The hospital was a marvelous model of assembly line efficiency. The job description of each nurse or candy-striper was so finely delineated I decided the young pillow fluffer who expertly fluffed my pillows twice a day was recruited exclusively for her prodigious pillow fluffing expertise and nothing else. Whatever their unique tasks and talents, the one thing the entire staff shared was a sunny, optimistic disposition oozing oodles of analeptic good cheer.

"Shame on you! It's such a bright, sunny day, and here you are with your blinds closed. What say we brighten things up a bit, roll up these shades, and put some light on the subject? Or, in your case, the customer. Is that OK with you? Great! That's going to make you feel so much better! You'd be surprised at how many of our patients . . . "

* * *

Start with a thick base of traumatic injury. Add a heaping tablespoon of icy panic. Leaven with a big dollop of severe depression. Finish with massive amounts of morphine, and you end up with a surrealistic stew of altered states well beyond anything Owsley, The Grateful Dead's psychedelic acid chef, or even those hoary harridans from *Macbeth*, might cook up. After all, Shakespeare's witchy Scottish sisters had only the eye of a newt, toe of a frog, wool of a bat, and tongue of a dog to distill cauldrons of dour and dirgeful prophesies with.

My crushed ankle kept me in the hospital for a week, and while this witches' brew of pain, panic, depression, and morphine produced many sensory distortions, I felt its most egregious effect on my experience of time. Like Billy Pilgrim in Kurt Vonnegut's *Slaughterhouse*

Five, I was dreamily "unstuck in time," floating in and out of past, present, and future without any distinguishing markers to limn one from the other—a fantastical experience that only exacerbated my persistent panic attacks. Then at the oddest moments, time would just stop: smack dab in the middle of a sentence, I would slip into a momentary, morphine-induced reverie only to reemerge thirty seconds later right on cue without the slightest inkling my arrow of time had temporarily ground to a halt, much to the amusement of staff and visitors alike.

My stark private room was kept antiseptically clean almost to the vanishing point. The walls were alabaster, but whenever I floated into the future, they shimmered so brightly I wondered if some half mad, high-tech alchemist had invented a psychedelic version of impossibly pure, super-white paint. All my forays to this shiny future took me to the bottom of the same psychological cul-de-sac: my hospital bed morphed into a death bed, and I was forced to watch with morbid fascination as my breath quickened, then shallowed, until I hyperventilated into the certainty I was literally witnessing—while experiencing—my future death. The shimmering walls pulsated in time to my ragged breathing, egging me on, until they began shrinking into the white marble lid of my slowly closing sarcophagus. Eventually, this chest heaving, claustrophobic hallucination reached its panicky peak. I'd take a loud, noisy, death rattle of a deep breath, only to have this terrifying nightmare reset and begin again.

My surreal sojourns in the present were not much better. The TV in my room became an almost sentient being hell-bent on sadistically repeating the movie *Point Break* over and over.

This story was filled with hauntingly familiar skydiving scenes and a limping Johnny Utah, played by Keanu Reeves, who insists on jumping off walls and out of airplanes while painfully landing on his injured knee. Despite gobs of morphine, I was in so much pain the mere thought of ever putting weight on my crippled ankle again was psychologically excruciating. Yet despite my distress, I became so morbidly mesmerized I masochistically refrained from flipping the channel even though, every time Utah landed on his damnable, badly damaged knee, I silently screamed in sympathetic agony.

My gossamer present did contain many well-intentioned visitors, but they seemed to be on the other side of an enormous abyss, as if that Eternal Boatman, Charon, had marooned me on the far deserted shore of some cold, black, fathomlessly unfordable River Styx. Everyone seemed a million miles away, and I anxiously traced the genesis of this gaping gulf in space and time to the terrible secret I possessed that they could not share: *I knew I was going to die and they did not.*

This unbridgeable chasm was particularly painful since most of my visitors were spiritual students and fellow seekers I'd gathered since leaving the cable TV business and moving to Raleigh in 1985 to take a job as vice president for a software startup. By 1987 I felt my prospects for ever reaching my spiritual objectives were rapidly dwindling, and despite my worldly success—or, probably, because of it—recurring bouts with my old two-headed nemesis, depression and self-loathing, were becoming more frequent, severe, and long-lasting.

As a tonic for all this burgeoning anxiety, I gave a series of lectures about my Rosean adventures to several hundred college kids at North Carolina State University. Even if my own spiritual prospects had faded, maybe I could find some solace in helping others—despite my own life now representing more of a cautionary tale than a shining example. My Rose stories were enthusiastically received, and some NCSU students started a campus club, to follow up. They called their club The Self Knowledge Symposium (SKS) and I agreed to chair weekly meetings. The SKS quickly spread to the University of North Carolina and then Duke University, and about twenty-five adults who attended other public lectures began gathering at my house on Friday nights as well. Then, in 1993, I bootstrapped a garage startup software company with my brother Tom, a business colleague, and three members of the SKS including Dave Gold, an old friend from those heady early days with Rose and the Zen Studies Society.

These well-meaning friends, family, fellow seekers, and students eagerly tried to lift my spirits, but they all made the same cardinal error. They mistook the Augie in the hospital bed with his leg in the air for the same man who flew up in a small plane straining for the heavens a few days earlier rather than the shattered Humpty Dumpty excuse for a man who tumbled in pieces back to earth.

These wonderful well-wishers came loaded with spiritual books, flowers, and heartfelt get-well cards. They said all kinds of warm, uplifting, spiritual things. All of which I now found cloyingly irrelevant and sickeningly sweet to the point of half-maddening exasperation.

Dumbfounded by their inane, bovine, trance-like ignorance, I wanted to shake them by their collective lapels and scream, "What the hell kind of nonsense are you droning on about? The Titanic is going down under our feet, the icy water is over our knees, and you're wondering what's for supper! Can't you see we're all going to *die*? *Wake up!*" But that was just it . . . wake up to *what*? To the nightmare I was living? I bit down hard on my tongue and silently played along even as my ingratitude, misplaced anger, and secret deception threatened to smother me with shame, guilt, and remorse.

The toughest part of passing through what passed for my present was Jonathan. Jonathan was the good-looking, clean-cut, all-American son of a Methodist minister and the dedicated student leader of the University of North Carolina's SKS chapter. Every day he would smile boyishly, pull up a chair, and softly read to me from *The Bhagavad Gita*, the Gospels, or T.S. Eliot's *Four Quartets*. Unable to focus on what he was reading, I would just watch him through tears of anguish. In his high-minded innocence and steadfast devotion, Jonathan was me all those many years ago, and now I felt like a phony and utter fraud for successfully conning him and so many others with some half-assed heroic version of myself that I now knew was misleading, even false. But I didn't know how to make it right or what to

211

say, and so, as the incomprehensible words he read slowly swept over me, the gulf between us seemed to grow wider. His daily visits became such a painful source of self-accusation and recrimination I wanted to tell him to stop coming but didn't have the heart, so I suffered in silence instead.

With the future and present of my hospital stay inhospitably riddled with terror, anger, guilt, and shame, I dreamily wandered more and more into the past, looking for consolation and escape while trying to figure out how a spiritual adventure that started out with so much lofty promise back in Richard Rose's kitchen in the summer of 1973 could go so horribly wrong.

* * *

It was early fall 1974. Taking a deep breath, I began pounding on the rectory door of Holy Rosary church in Cleveland, Ohio's Little Italy neighborhood. I was about to give up when, with the loud squeal of a sliding bolt, the heavy oak door cracked open and an elderly, gray-haired, obviously Italian priest peaked out.

Introducing myself, I said, "I'm an old altar boy from Pittsburgh, Father. I don't know anybody, and I slept last night in the back of my truck. Do you know a place in the neighborhood that might be for rent?"

The old priest smiled benignly and, through a thick Italian accent well-suited to the task, said, "Introibo ad altare dei."

"Ad Deum qui laitificat juventutem meum," I automatically replied.

Passing this pop quiz from the old Latin Mass earned a former altar boy this priest's imprimatur, and this gentle man soon sent me in search of a parishioner, a certain Mrs. Maci, with directions on how to find her house.

Acting on a sudden impulse, I said, "Father, may I please have your blessing?"

Bowing my head, I was flattered when he once again trusted me with the Latin version. "In nominee Patris, et Filii, et Spiritus Sancti, Amen."

As I headed back toward Mayfield Avenue in search of Mrs. Maci, I was glad Father didn't ask me how I arrived at Holy Rosary, fresh from sleeping in my truck, bathed and freshly shaved. I had brazenly walked right by security and into nearby Case Western Reserve University's gym for a shower. Since I didn't think my initiative would add much in the way of luster to my character, I conveniently omitted that detail from my humble tale of the Pittsburgh-to-Cleveland pilgrimage of an errant "old altar boy."

Rose's vision was to create a hub-and-spoke system. Feeder groups on college campuses in various cities would funnel serious students to him and the farm for more advanced—or what he liked to call "esoteric"—work. After two years of hard labor, Pitt's Zen Studies Society, while not exactly thriving, was more than holding its own. So Rose suggested I go to Cleveland and start another group. That was it. No money, no handbook, no accommodations, no contacts, no job referrals, not even a flipping map. Just a solo, lone wolf, metaphorical parachute drop into the terra incognita of Cuyahoga County to start a group.

Luckily, someone from our Kent State Zen group hailed from Cleveland, and he suggested I anchor my efforts in the Little Italy neighborhood. Little Italy was directly across Euclid Avenue from Case Western Reserve University, and the no-nonsense truculence of the fiercely self-reliant Italians offered a safe port, eye-of-the-hurricane refuge from the raging storm of urban unrest, crime, and decay blighting the rest of Cleveland's East Side.

As I walked along Little Italy's Mayfield Avenue for the first time, my senses were overwhelmed by the sights, sounds, and smells of this Italian village far from the boot of Italy. An urban village I soon fondly considered home. There was not one or two, but several, fruit stand-fronted little Italian grocery stores, and the redolence from the capicola, prosciutto, mortadella, pancetta, an infinite variety of salamis, San Daniele smoked trout, and huge wheels of pungent mozzarella and parmigiana cheese wafted out open doors and into the street. There they met, mingled, and were ultimately perfected by the aroma of freshly baked Italian bread from Presti's bakery. Inspired by these fragrances and the rumblings they elicited from a grouchy and unbreakfasted stomach gone supperless the night before, I took a hiatus from my quest to find Mrs. Maci and wandered into one of the stores instead.

I felt like I was entering a whole new world. A world uprooted and transplanted straight from the old one eons ago. The well-worn tongue-and-groove oak plank floor was sprinkled with old-fashioned wooden barrels bursting with olives, pickles, briny Italian peppers, and a dazzling array of dates, figs, and other dried fruits. The groaning shelves suggested the imported olive oil from various Mediterranean sources were huge best-sellers, and for a young man schooled from infancy by Eastern European immigrants who knew a good, cured meat, smoked fish, or aged cheese when they tasted one, the deli choices were mind-boggling.

The burly man behind the counter in a full-length apron was about 50, and sans the chef's hat and mustache, he made for a pretty fair facsimile of Chef Boyardee. He hailed me with a jovial "Buongiorno!" and I could see by the way his smile lit up his face and highlighted his extra chins it wouldn't take much to turn it into laughter.

"Hi," I said. "I'd like some stuff for a sandwich. What do you recommend? I like just about anything as long as there's enough of it! What's your special?"

"Excusa," he replied. "I no speaka good English. Cosa vuoi? I mean, you get something?"

It took effort from me and patience from him, but five minutes of mutual finger pointing, head bobbing, and shoulder shrugging later, we managed to narrow my choices and fill my order of very reasonably priced meat, cheese, and olives. Then we hit a snag.

I have never been a coffee drinker, and by 1974 I was already addicted to caffeine straight from a cola bottle but, in deference to my ascetic lifestyle, or more probably my vanity, I only drank diet versions. But every time I tried to add a diet cola to my order, my nuovo amico behind the counter, Adolfo, offered a sugar-laden Coke or Pepsi instead. It soon became abundantly clear he didn't know what the word "diet" meant, so I fell back on that universal, time-tested, semantical technique for making incomprehensible words magically comprehensible in any language: *volume.*

"*Diet* cola," I repeated, this time more slowly and a bit louder. Adolfo still seemed perplexed, so I further simplified the problem.

"DI-*ET,*" I said, this time emphasizing each syllable while upping the decibels considerably. When this proved fruitless, I gave it one more shot, enunciating *"DI-ET"* so loudly I startled us both.

Frustrated and fresh out of ideas, I spread my palms out over my midsection and began massaging my stomach to suggest I was watching my weight even though I was pretty thin at the time.

Instantly, the cloud of confusion cleared, and Adolfo's eyes lit up with a huge smile of recognition. Reaching down with both hands for his own ample belly, he avidly began working it while roaring with laughter like a jolly Italian Saint Nick merrily jostling his bowl full of jelly. I have no idea what he thought I was trying to say with my initial gesture, but before I knew it I was in tears laughing while jiggling my own stomach in *tenuto* time with his.

I never did get my diet cola, but from then on Adolfo and I were on the best of terms. I saw him almost every day behind his counter or loitering in front of his store chatting amiably in Italian with the locals. Whenever he saw me, even from half a block away, he would drop everything, grab his belly, shake it vigorously, and roar with laughter. And since he clearly expected me to reciprocate his heartfelt greeting in kind, I always did.

Reluctantly leaving Adolfo and my dreams of a diet cola behind, I crossed Mayfield Avenue, went into Presti's, and bought a couple of freshly baked rolls. I lived on Italian cold cuts and olives for the first month or two that I lived in Little Italy, and I soon mastered the fine art of greeting Presti's baker by name while toting a pound of Adolfo's imported, sweet, unsalted butter just as he was wheeling out racks of Italian bread, piping hot, straight from the oven.

Returning to the street, I tore the rolls apart, loaded my culinary acquisitions and, after two or three ravenous bites and a half-dozen black olives, resumed my quest to find Mrs. Maci.

Mrs. Maci turned out to be a pious, respectable, bosomy, bespectacled woman of about sixty-five with her still jet-black hair worn up, a wide nose, no waist, and formidable hips. Feisty, loud, and voluble, she adumbrated, emphasized, and repeated everything she said with a vast assortment of gesticulations inextricably linked to a collateral collection of colorful facial expressions. Mrs. Maci was, in short, exactly what you might expect in an older Italian woman who loved to cook, made her own pasta, stewed sauce from scratch from vine ripe tomatoes, and still had one foot firmly ensconced in the old country. Her hand gestures and lively facial features came in handy because Mrs. Maci spoke very little English, and even when I did finally convince her I did not speak Italian, she still often loudly and insistently addressed me as if I did.

Mrs. Maci lived with her tiny, wizened, 95-year-old mother on the first floor of her red brick house amidst a small, immaculately kept yard with colorfully seeded cedar flower boxes in front and an obligatory vegetable garden in back. Her mother did not speak a word of English, and due to this collective language barrier, I never could ascertain whether Mrs. Maci had children or what happened to her husband.

Mrs. Maci led me to a private entrance and up a flight of stairs adjacent to her standalone one-car garage at the end of a concrete driveway that led to the street. (Mrs. Maci drove very infrequently, but when she did, she always trundled her miniature mother into the passenger seat, backed onto the street, and floored it, whiplashing her mother as if she were a limp rag doll fast asleep or dead as she did. Her mother reminded me of an ancient Italian astronaut as her wildly flopping head and torso were quickly plastered to the seatback by the punishing G forces of Mrs. Maci's getaway. I found these mother/daughter takeoffs so amusing I always made a special effort to be at ground zero any time I heard the rumbling ignition of her late model Buick starship firing up.) At the top of the steps was another door with about three locks that opened into the tidy kitchen of a furnished apartment.

Mrs. Maci was obviously very proud of her flat, and as she showed me around I managed to overcome the language barrier somewhat with some well-deserved compliments.

"Wow, Mrs. Maci, did you make these curtains?"

"Si," she said while beaming with a hint of girlish embarrassment.

"I knew it. They match the tablecloth and napkins too! Do those bedspreads come with the apartment? I hope so. They're like works of art. Did you make them too?"

"No, no," Mrs. Maci said, shaking her head before proudly adding, "mi mamma make them."

The rent was right, and I'd already taken a nonverbal shine to Mrs. Maci and, apparently, she to me, so I took the apartment on the spot with a month-to-month verbal lease.

I had very little money and even less time to lose, so the next day I walked to Case Western and made a beeline for the student affairs office. A friendly young administrator told me starting a campus Zen club meant filling out a form, writing a constitution in compliance with the university's guidelines, and getting fifteen students to sign up as members. Once my group was approved, I could book an auditorium for a Rose lecture at no charge and apply for funding to promote it. She, of course, assumed I was a Case Western student myself, but since she didn't ask for my student ID, I discretely decided it might prove counterproductive to disabuse her of this misconception.

I found an empty office with an unguarded typewriter and quickly typed up the forms and my Zen Studies Society constitution. It was now about noon, so I headed for the cafeteria. I found a crowded table, sat down, and proceeded to outline my scheme to about ten to twelve students.

"Excuse me, guys. I'm in a bit of a catch-22. I want to start a Zen group on campus. I am trying to book a lecture to find members for my club, but the administration says I need fifteen members to book my lecture."

I asked the students to sign up while reassuring them that if they were not actually interested in Zen, "I promise, you will never hear from me again."

They loved the idea and the mischievous temerity behind it, and my newly won campus co-conspirators fairly elbowed each other out of the way in their eagerness to sign on. After an encore at another table, I had twice the student ID numbers I needed. I returned the documents to the young lady in student affairs who was startled to see me again so soon. We chatted awhile and, after a cursory review of my paperwork, she let me book a venue provisionally for my Rose lecture while awaiting official approval. Thwing Hall held about 125 people, so I booked it four weeks out and headed back to Chez Maci with the satisfied sense I'd done pretty damn well for my first day on the job.

Arriving with a fresh loaf of bread from Presti's, I was amazed to see that Mrs. Maci anticipated me. My bed was made, the place tidied up, and I was delighted to find freshly baked lasagna with homemade sausage and a salad in the fridge! Rather than renting a modest apartment, I was apparently booked into a five-star, full-service resort on the Italian Riviera.

This VIP impression was only reinforced over the following days as Mrs. Maci treated me like the only son of a doting mother just home, miraculously unscathed, from a foreign war. She even hand signal-insisted I surrender my soiled laundry into her capable hands for washing and ironing.

I returned to Case Western the next day, and my patroness in student affairs let me use an idle typewriter. I typed up a press release for Rose's upcoming lecture and sent it out to all the media. A few days later I managed to borrow a phone as well and began hounding the outlets about my release. While I had a number of minor successes, I struck gold when I snared an interview on *Jabberwocky*, a one-hour show on WMMS, Cleveland's top rock station. Then I convinced the *Cleveland Plain Dealer*'s religion editor to interview me about the lecture as well.

The *Plain Dealer*'s editor kept me on tenterhooks for weeks as the interview failed to appear in the paper. Then, three days before the lecture, on my umpteenth follow-up phone call, he told me to "tune in tomorrow." The next morning I discovered a full column spread on page 2 of the paper with big black letters screaming: *Zen Leader to Speak at CWRU*. The piece was excellent publicity and, as Huck averred in *Huckleberry Finn* about Mark Twain's "other book," *Tom Sawyer,* the article was "mostly true except for a few stretchers." Most notably, a stretcher where the writer inexplicably failed to double-check his source and erroneously described me as "August Turak, a student at Case Western Reserve." But I was so thrilled by the article that when I called to thank him, I charitably chose to spare him the embarrassment of a rookie journalistic mistake and painful retraction by not calling it to his attention.

When I wasn't badgering the local media, I managed to get our nascent student organization officially approved and weasel a grant from the student activities board for posters and several quarter-page ads in the campus newspaper. I spent the intervening days before Rose arrived papering the CWRU campus with hundreds of posters: posters with the bad habit of disappearing almost as fast as I could hang them. Effective postering, as I learned from Pitt, is an uphill struggle requiring scads of staples, masking tape, and long hours of recursive trips to the same bulletin boards, telephone poles, storefronts, and bare walls. Especially if you adopt the intensive strategy of posting in verboten high traffic venues in hopes of temporarily garnering some higher visibility.

* * *

Rose made the two-and-one-half-hour trip from Wheeling to Cleveland, and I proudly met him at Thwing Hall with a standing room only crowd and some gas money also provided courtesy of the university. His talk was a hit. Lots of kids signed up for the Zen Studies Society, and by the time he started his return journey later that same night, I was confident we had the makings of a group.

On the surface everything was proceeding well, but behind the scenes there was trouble brewing at Manse Maci. The Greek goddess Calypso fell in love with the wandering Odysseus and kept her boy-toy captive on her island for seven years. I increasingly felt like a kept Augie, held captive in Mrs. Maci's mythical flat, slowly smothering under a heavy, handsewn quilt of motherly affection from this Italian incarnation of Ceres, the Roman goddess of Mother Earth.

I once rented an apartment from my immigrant, Slovak grandfather who lived across the street. I adored my grandfather, and we shared a first and last name, but he never seemed to get the hang of distinguishing between *his* building and *my* apartment. At all hours of the day and night I would hear his master keys jingling at the door as he announced yet another unannounced visit with cheerful iterations of "Hoop! Hoop! Hoop!" Sometimes he would sneak up on me in the kitchen, and more than once he tracked me to the flat's unlockable bathroom where, if I happened to be in the bathtub, he would offer to wash my back and wouldn't take no for an answer.

Like my grandfather, Mrs. Maci took the notion of *mi casa, su casa* far too literally. She was in and out constantly, whether I was home or not, and while she stopped short of bearding me in the bathroom, I am fairly certain that if I'd been so inclined and knew enough Italian to ask, she would've been more than happy to wash my back.

Of course, "mistakes were made" on my part as well. Al, my old friend from Rose's summer intensive, decided to join me in Cleveland. I was delighted to have his strong right arm at my side, and he soon proved his worth by sussing out that glazed donuts at Presti's bakery emerged hot from the oven precisely at midnight. (His donuts were exquisite, but the only word we ever managed to extract from Presti's ancient night baker was the interrogatory "Something?" he invariably used to elicit an order. Al began referring to him as "Something," as in "Let's go see Something and get donuts!" even though I am quite sure his parents christened Something something else.) Anyway, my rude mistake was not telling Mrs. Maci I was taking in a roommate, and though she didn't object in Italian or English, I could see by her sullen reaction she was put out. She never did warm to Al or even acknowledge his existence, let alone do his laundry.

Then I managed to inadvertently flip my toothbrush into the swirling toilet bowl only to helplessly watch as it instantly disappeared. Unfamiliar with the workings of toilets, I assumed that since the toilet was still flushing freely the toothbrush was long gone. However, the first time Al added toilet paper to the mix we ended up with a wet floor and a shrieking landlady madder than a wet hen. Somehow, I managed to interrupt Mrs. Maci's Italian tirade long enough to tell her we would mop the floor and fix her beloved toilet, and she reluctantly retreated to her own place.

As luck would have it, Rose arrived early the next day for one of our meetings. I had to work fast before he tried to use our clogged toilet. So, after some small talk, I worked up the gumption to say, "Mr.

Rose, we have a bit of a Zen koan on our hands. Since solving unsolvable koans is your specialty, I was wondering if you could help out."

Rose was on to me instantly. Raising one eyebrow, he said, "Who do you want killed? Hope it ain't the old lady downstairs. She seems nice enough, and she might have Mafia friends in the neighborhood. Anyways, I didn't bring a pistol."

I smiled and pressed on. "Well, you see . . . I flushed my toothbrush down the toilet and, well . . . now the toilet is backing up. Mrs. Maci is super ticked, and I don't have the money for a plu—"

"Oh, Jesus Christ! How in hell did you manage that? I brush my teeth in the sink. You oughta' give it a try. Besides, flushin' a toothbrush down a toilet takes finesse. A koan like that requires a Master, and you ain't even a novice. How many tries did it take you before the toothbrush finally went down?"

Rose spent the next several hours fishing my toothbrush from the trap under the floor with the plumber's snake he kept at the ready in the back seat of his Olds for just such emergencies. As he vigorously worked the snake, Al stood at his elbow and said, "Here you are, the most enlightened guru in America, maybe the world, and you're busy trying to exorcise some damn fool's toothbrush out of a demon-possessed toilet."

This set Rose giggling as he playfully beat Al around the head and shoulders with his faithful fedora until he ran him headlong out of the bathroom.

The dramatic denouement to the Mrs. Maci saga, however, was what Al and I came to call The Great Chicken Fiasco. Neither Al nor I knew a damn thing about cooking, but one night we decided to bake chicken thighs in the electric oven. Rather than put the meat in a pan or wrap it in foil, we simply spread a dozen fatty thighs out over the oven's baking rack and closed the door. Before long the drizzling drippings oozed onto the red-hot heating element at the bottom of the oven and caught fire. Black smoke billowed out, engulfing the kitchen, and though Al and I quickly doused the flames, the real damage was done. Moments later a coughing Mrs. Maci joined us in the smoke-filled kitchen, and this time there was no appeasing Mother Earth. On and on she ranted hysterically in incomprehensible Italian as her diminutive mother endlessly keened "Mamma mia! Mamma mia! Mamma mia!" from the bottom of the steps, dolorously wailing as if the pope himself had just expired in her withered arms.

"Please, Mrs. Maci," I said, "everything's going to be OK." Opening the oven, I added, "See, the fire's out, we'll open the windows, turn on the fan, and once all the smoke is out of here, we'll wipe—"

But when it became apparent my feeble efforts to placate Mrs. Maci and, by extension her moaning mother, were having no effect, Al took matters into his own capable hands and loudly said, "Goodnight, Mrs. Maci."

When this heartfelt farewell proved ineffectual, he pumped up the volume and reiterated, "*Goodnight*, Mrs. Maci!"

But this bon voyage too was ignored so he resorted to repeating over and over—at the top of his lungs.

"GOODNIGHT, MRS. MACI!"

Soon the entire Maci household degenerated into a smoky, coughing cacophony of my plaintive pleadings, Al's booming valedictions, Mrs. Maci's Italian hysterics, and her mother's lugubrious litany of shrieking "mamma mias."

Whether Al's thunderous efforts were instrumental or merely coincidental is hard to say, but after nine or ten of his eloquent goodnights, Mrs. Maci stopped screaming, muffled her mother, and both returned to their floor of the house.

* * *

Fed up and fully expecting to be evicted anyway, Al and I quickly unearthed an old, dilapidated, wood-sided, faded blue, ice cream parlor for rent on Random Road right off Mayfield Avenue. It was owned by identical twin brothers who ran their custom kitchen company next door. The place was divided into a large open space in front for customers and a smaller prep area in back. Anxious to see their shack start producing revenue, the brothers installed a fiberglass-enclosed, freestanding shower in the back room over the only available drain smack dab in the middle of the floor. The next day Al and I moved out of Mrs. Maci's and into our new "ashram," and though the accommodations were quite a come-down from the Italian Riviera, we felt like escaped prisoners who, having just safely crossed the Rio Grande, could finally take a deep breath.

As we were moving out, I was taken aback by Mrs. Maci's reaction. Rather than relief, she sat crestfallen at the kitchen table like she was helplessly watching her only son elope with a non-Italian, non-Catholic, chain-smoking divorcée who couldn't cook and she cordially despised. She even trotted out her best broken English in an attempt to change my mind. I was very fond of Mrs. Maci, felt sorry for her, and was deeply grateful for all her motherly kindnesses, but my mind was made up.

I never saw or spoke to her again.

Al and I quickly settled into new digs Rose always described as "like livin' in a piana' box." The front room was large, enclosed with glass windows, strewn with tables and chairs, and impossibly expensive to heat. So we closed it off and lived exclusively in the back. There was no air conditioning, and the only heat emanated from a single vent at the top of a standalone furnace with a dodgy pilot light that always seemed to doze off in the middle of the coldest nights. The vent's top-loaded location meant we were warm chest up and freezing cold chest down, and this made winter long johns de rigueur and turned showering into quite the adventure.

We picked up an old refrigerator and stove for next to nothing and installed them near the commercial sink that came with the place. While not exactly an outhouse, the bathroom, accessed by a short tunnel of corrugated fiberglass, was usually so chilly that bathroom reading was discouraged if not outright impossible. We slept in sleeping bags on wooden cargo pallets cushioned with foam carpet padding, and we stapled carpet scraps over cracks between the overlapping wooden siding of our uninsulated piana' box to keep cold drafts at bay.

By this time I was woefully short of money, and I decided to fall back on carpet installation. Unfortunately, we were in the middle of a severe economic recession and jobs of any type were hard to find. For five days I sat by the phone with the Yellow Pages on my knees calling every carpet store within fifty miles only to be turned down by them all. Undaunted, I went back to AAA Carpets and started over.

When I got to Kilgore Carpets, I got Mr. Kilgore on the line. After a moment or two he gruffly said, "Hey, didn't I talk to you last week?"

"Yes you did, sir."

"Didn't I tell you we had no work?"

"Yes you did, sir."

"Then why in hell are you bothering me again?"

"Well, a lot of things can change in a week, sir."

There was dead silence on the phone for a moment and then he said, "My God, I gotta' meet you. How soon can you get down here?"

Once again persistence paid off, and forty-five minutes later I was in Mr. Kilgore's office at the corner of East Fortieth and Chester on Cleveland's East Side. Mr. Kilgore offered me a job, but only as a helper for the two-dollar minimum wage. I gratefully accepted and started the next day.

Al got a job laying carpet with another company as well, and we settled into a routine of work, meetings, meditation, and postering. I honed my own lecturing skills at Cleveland State, Baldwin-Wallace, and John Carroll universities, and I occasionally drove down to Kent State University to chair a meeting there. On weekends I usually made the five-hour round trip to Benwood to discuss organizational issues with Rose while hoping I might catch some spiritual lightning in a bottle once again.

Case Western's Zen Studies Society slowly grew, and eventually there were six of us sprinkled around the floor of our Rosean piana' box evenly splitting the one-hundred-and-fifty-dollar monthly rent. We didn't have a radio, TV, stereo, or newspaper subscription. We didn't drink, smoke, do drugs, or date girls. We never went to the movies or registered to vote, and notwithstanding the occasional midnight donut run, we lived so simply I opened a savings account at Cleveland Trust and socked money away weekly while earning minimum wage. My only vices were reading constantly, eclectically, and voraciously, and the occasional trip to the mall with Al just to window shop and poke around.

I'd never worked harder, lived simpler, or been happier, but I didn't realize it until a temporary roommate caught me off guard. Gary was a high school friend of Dave Gold's from Pittsburgh. He was a first-year law student, and he needed a place to crash until a room opened up in the dorm. So we found him some unoccupied space on the floor of our ashram for his cot.

One day I came home from work at five o'clock as usual. I picked up the Zen Studies Society roster and began telephoning each member with a meeting reminder for the next night. Gary was eavesdropping.

"My God, don't you ever stop?" he blurted. "You're meditating before six, start work at seven, and bust your ass on your knees nine hours a day. Then you walk through the door and without eating or even bothering to take off your company uniform you start making calls. If you aren't at one of your damn meetings, you're putting up posters for the next one, and you keep at it day after day after day. I have no idea what the hell you guys are up to,

Until that moment I never noticed or gave it a thought. Groping for an answer, I finally just smiled and said, "It's the only game in town, man. It's the only game in town."

but I gotta' ask: where do you get your drive? You sure as hell aren't in it for the money."

I was startled by his question. Until that moment I never noticed or gave it a thought. Groping for an answer, I finally just smiled and said, "It's the only game in town, man. It's the only game in town."

* * *

I lived this way for four years: on my wits, audacity, and a fraying financial shoestring. I bought, hauled, installed, and finally learned to cook on a string of battered twenty-five-dollar stoves as me and my van parachuted onto college campuses in Akron, Columbus, Washington, D.C, Baltimore, and Boston. In Boston I lived in Cambridge, on Green Street, just off Harvard Square and gave lectures that kick-started Rose groups at Harvard, Tufts, Boston University, Boston College, and Northeastern. I also picked up my first job in sales in Boston, selling 3M copying machines when the carpet business was slow. I worked only intermittently but lived so frugally I was able to buy a new vehicle with cash: a Wimbledon white, one-ton Ford van I specifically ordered without a radio so I could spiritually ruminate for hours without distraction while driving from city to city.

Occasionally I'd spend a few weeks at Rose's farm for some spiritual R&R, but as the years wore on and the sizzling interest in spirituality on college campuses began to wane, Rose kept me on the hop distributing his books, organizing weekend retreats, promoting Zen intensives, bucking up sagging groups and, eventually, with Dave Gold, putting on a series of spiritual symposia in various cities. Events Rose called Chautauquas.

On the surface everything seemed to be moving ahead, but behind the scenes, just like at Chez Maci, trouble was brewing. This time between me and Rose. Trouble engendered by paternalistic smothering of an altogether different stripe. Once again there was a woman involved, but she was not a matronly, shapeless, Italian immigrant of a certain age. She was a vibrant, shapely, American girl in her mid-twenties.

Her name was Linda, and she also just happened to be married to one of my best friends in the Rose group.

* * *

I slowly realized the words buzzing around in my dope-addled brain were not Mrs. Maci's incomprehensible Italian after all. They were coming from my sunny, stiffly starched nurse in perfectly intelligible English as she finally finished fooling with the window blinds in my hospital room. Apparently I'd just emerged from one of my morphine trances dragging Little Italy and poor Mrs. Maci out of the past with me. Oblivious to my momentary, drug-induced absence, my nurse was well into the umpteenth verse of her paean to the recuperative power of unobstructed sunshine.

"I see it all the time," she said, leaning over to stick a thermometer in my mouth. "Now I'm not saying sunshine and fresh air is some kind of miracle cure, but I swear it's the next best thing!"

I dropped acid once and found myself watching *The Tonight Show with Johnny Carson*. Suddenly I was seeing through Johnny, his guests, and the show itself. No one wanted to be there, and they didn't really care about each other. The hilarity was forced, and they didn't really think the jokes were funny. It was all an act. A façade. Like kids playing make-believe, but with the added tragedy that Johnny and his guests didn't seem to realize how phony it was. It was just so . . . *sad*. *Is that it?* I wondered to myself. *Is that all life is, people playing silly games we don't even know we're playing? Is life all just a seeming with nothing real behind it?*

I remember how anxious this revelation made me feel, and that was exactly what I felt as I watched this highly trained, well-intentioned nurse expertly reading my thermometer. She had no idea what life was all about, and everything she was saying about blinds, sunshine, and the-devil-knows-what was just the idle prattle of a highly programmable automaton, prattling things some even more highly programmable automaton programmed her to say.

There was no *real* empathy or warmth. She would forget my name the moment she walked out of the room, and she was completely oblivious to the tragedy of it all. I wanted to hate her with all my might—but I couldn't. I couldn't because she was just like me, just like us all, doing the best we can with the pathetic hand we've all been dealt, and failing miserably at it.

I was left with just this terrible aching sadness for her, myself, and the whole world. But I said nothing. I just bit down hard again and said nothing because there was nothing to say.

Chapter Fourteen

BREAK WITH ROSE

There is no end, but addition: the trailing
Consequence of further days and hours,
While emotion takes to itself the emotionless
Years of living among the breakage
Of what was believed in as the most reliable—
And therefore the fittest for renunciation.
—T.S. ELIOT[31]

"Hi, Augie. How you doin' these days? We got a bet at the office about when you'll be back. I got the under, so I'm countin' on a speedy recovery."

Opening my eyes I saw Jay, one of my business partners, standing at the foot of my living room couch grinning at me over my blue orthopedic boot propped on a pile of pillows.

"I'm OK, I guess, Jaybird. Getting around on crutches. It's amazing how fast my leg is shrinking. Seems like every day I tighten this damn boot a little more. How's things at RGI?"

While not a member of the SKS or ostensibly interested in spirituality, Jay was one of the very few thoroughly decent human beings I'd ever known. We met in the late '80s when he was a novice sales rep and I was running sales for a company called Data Broadcasting Corporation (DBC) in Washington, D.C. Jay was a stocky, blond, blue-eyed cross between Elroy Jetson and Barney Rubble, hilariously funny and a brilliant born leader. In 1993 we started Raleigh Group International (RGI) on $2,500 and a nine-word business plan from another partner, Dave Gold: "We're smart guys; we'll figure out something to do." As CEO, Jay was my indispensable number two, or chief operating officer. Jay kept the trains running on time while I stayed on the road or on the phone trying to commandeer more trains.

When I finally got out of the hospital, Jay, on his own initiative, began showing up at my condo with armloads of charts, graphs, and progress reports on the business. Each time we reenacted the same charade: I pretended I was actually reading all his wonderful analysis and Jay pretended he didn't notice the stack of untouched previous reports on the coffee table beside the couch.

"Sales are up, and so are our margins," Jay said. "Not as much as I'd like, of course, but I got a few ideas, and if I'm right . . . "

* * *

After a week in the hospital, they still wouldn't let me go home until I could urinate on my own. Then, in order to put an end to my horrific deathbed hallucinations, I traded in my morphine for nothing stronger than ibuprofen. Not only did the hallucinations go away, but I began to urinate on my own. But they still wouldn't release me and kept catheterizing me, checking for infection.

When the urologist finally came in, I promptly humiliated myself by begging through tears, like a desperately homesick child, to go home.

"I think catheterizing me over and over is only going to end up introducing the infection they're looking for," I told him.

The urologist smiled, put his hand on my shoulder, and gently whispered, "I tend to agree with you."

This simple gesture of genuine sympathy hit me so hard I felt like my head would explode. Panic morphed into gratitude. A gratitude so intense I didn't think I could stand it. I wept convulsively while thinking, *My God, he understands! He's so kind, just so kind.* Over and over these words echoed, leaving fresh waves of ecstatic gratitude in their wake.

The urologist did send me home, and gradually the panic attacks went away as well. But as one dreary day on the living room couch oozed into another, I knew something was very wrong. I would lay there repeating to myself: "I've never felt this way before. I'm all hollowed out inside. I'm not just fragile, I'm all busted up."

The future seemed ominous, dark, and full of dread.

The best word for my emotional state is *somber*. While dark and exhausting, at times this mood could be almost comforting because it seemed strangely suited to the actual human condition. Stranger still, this melancholy mood heightened my sensitivity. I was deeply touched and wept profusely over the slightest kindness, like the sympathy of the urologist or Jay bringing reports he knew damn well I wasn't reading and saying nothing about it.

Overall, I was still spiraling downward. Ironically, the shock of being so deeply moved by these tiny gestures only seemed to exacerbate my slide. I felt like an artist whose inspirations so utterly overwhelm his talent that his art becomes a depressing exercise in frustrating futility. It was as if I was being torn apart by tiny God-glimpses into the way life *should* be, *could* be, was designed to be, but never *would* be—never would be because no one, primarily me, was living the right kind of life. No one was paying attention to what a miraculous gift life really is. I felt helpless amidst so much human darkness, and guilt for how selfishly and unconsciously I lived, and was still living, my life.

But the most terrifying thing about all this agony and ecstasy was I didn't have a single word or concept to help me navigate this disorienting jumble of exotic experiences. I was on a journey into the unknown without a guide, signpost, or familiar landmark, and like a long-suffering patient without a diagnosis, this meant my prognosis could be just about anything.

"Listen, I gotta' get back to the office," Jay was saying as, with an effort, I managed to tune back into the present. "We got a company full of 25-year-old kids. It's like tryin' to manage a litter of barely housebroken bear cubs. In any case, adult supervision is warranted. But your phone's in the kitchen and, now that you're hobbling around, feel free to call in once in a while. You're missed, buddy. You really are."

I added Jay's latest reports to the burgeoning stack and returned to a far more engrossing preoccupation: trying to unravel the mysteries encoded in the swirls of textured spackling dotting the ceiling of my condominium. Like a tongue to a sore tooth, I obsessively traced and retraced each pointy pattern until it seamlessly merged with an adjacent eddy of tangled putty. Each Gordian ganglia seemed to represent a node on Zen's interlocking Riddle of Life and Death.

But one plaster puzzle plastered just above my head was the most magnetically intractable of all: What went wrong between me and Rose?

* * *

In 1964 Bob Dylan presciently prophesied, "The times they are a changin'." By 1977 this was again true of the country as well as my work with Rose. The heady, optimistic mood of Woodstock had long since collapsed under the strain of the Vietnam War and Altamont, the abortive Rolling Stones concert where four people died. Echoing Altamont's dystopic devolution, the uplifting, life-affirming psychedelic music of the 1960s had, by 1977, contracted into the mind-numbing beat of that psychedelic soul killer: disco. The drugs of choice were a changin', too, as hallucinogenic mind-expanding "uppers" like LSD, mescaline, and magic mushrooms were being rapidly superseded by escapist "downers" like Seconal, quaaludes, and even scag, the street level *nom de guerre* for heroin.

The same soporific escapism was overtaking college campuses as well. In 1972, ten of Ray's crude Zen posters attracted a hundred students. By 1975, one hundred professionally produced posters barely brought in ten. A cartoon from *The New Yorker* summed up the changing mood perfectly: one well-dressed man at a swanky Manhattan cocktail party says to another: "I used to be into consciousness. Now I'm into money."[32] While the hard-partying, uber-materialistic yuppies, or "young urban professionals," had yet to make their appearance, MTV and the sybaritic excesses of the 1980s were in the offing—and closing fast.

In the face of this dismal law of diminishing spiritual returns, Rose despaired of reaching enough young people with his unvarnished mystical message to keep our precarious community viable. He decided to expand our outreach to older people and what he referred to as the "outer layers of the spiritual onion skin" in hopes that today's astrologist, spiritualist, or psychic healer might become tomorrow's hard-core seeker and mystic.

Moving away from our campus nomenclature like The Zen Studies Society and The Pyramid Zen Society, Rose rebranded our new, more eclectic efforts using the Truth and Transmission (TAT) name he chose as an umbrella for our activities, a name that also differentiated us from Zen and other established traditions.

At Rose's behest, we tried retreats called TAT Intensives, self-help called TAT Encounter Groups, and even the TAT Employment Cooperative (TEC), with results ranging from meager to nonexistent. Nothing seemed to reach critical mass, and the one thing all Rosean endeavors seemed to share was that dividends, such as they were, were only wrung from an obstinate universe by dint of hard, unremitting, uphill labor.

* * *

It was the spring of 1977. I was five years into my hitch with Rose and crashing in yet another ramshackle house, this time in the Maryland suburbs of Washington, D.C. The wall-mounted rotary phone in the kitchen was ringing insistently. With a sigh Dave Gold rose and carefully zig-zagged his way to the kitchen through mounds of precariously stacked mail pieces peppering the living room floor.

Dave and I were in Washington executing the fifth leg of Rose's latest "big tent" initiative, a series of weekend colloquiums he christened, as I mentioned previously, Chautauquas. These eclectic conferences were inspired by the immensely popular Chautauqua Movement of the early twentieth century. A movement that sponsored educational and cultural events featuring speakers, teachers, musicians, showmen, and preachers of the day.

Billed as a "confluence of minds," our four previous Chautauquas garnered sold-out crowds at twenty-five dollars a head in Pittsburgh, Cleveland, Akron, and Columbus. Dave and I were now determined to crack the big time by repeating the formula in Washington, D.C.

But at the moment my far more modest aspiration was just wishing Dave would pick up that infernal phone.

He finally did and sang out, "Augie, it's Rose!"

My heart sank. Penny-pinching Rose would never spring for a long-distance call unless it was bad news. And lately all the news from Benwood was bad. I retraced Dave's steps between piles of sorted mail like a prisoner heading to his own execution.

Before I could finish saying hello, Rose erupted. "What the hell's going on down there?" he screamed.

"Me and Dave are working on the D.C. Chautauqua. American University gave us their Kay Spiritual Life Center. It's a beautiful space, and we're sorting direct mail pieces by zip code so we can send them—"

"Don't give me that bullshit!" Rose interrupted. "You're hidin' under the bed. You don't call me, and you're hopin' the hell I don't call you! I told you the idea behind all these Chautauquas was usin' them to seed groups of more serious people. We had a big crowd in Cleveland, and now I hear the group you left behind already went belly up."

"But Mr. Rose . . . "

"Did I get the news from you? Hell no! You left Cleveland to die on the vine. When's the last time you attended one of their meetings?"

"Mr. Rose, I'm in Washington, D.C. I'm six and a half hours from Cleveland. I can't be in both places, and if I use the phone, you get all bent out of shape about long distance—"

"God damn it!" Rose roared. "I don't want any of your damn excuses. You think you're smarter than me, smarter than everybody, so you refuse to take direction and stick to policy. Every time I turn my back, you go off on your own and do whatever the hell that fat head of yours feels like doin'. I'm sick and tired of shouting myself hoarse and riskin' a stroke over you and your damn ego."

Then he hung up on me.

Looking around, I saw the thousands of direct mail pieces Dave and I just spent all night sorting in a whole new light. I didn't drink coffee, but I got so tired I'd washed down two heaping tablespoons of raw instant coffee with cold water just to keep going. I wrangled the venue at American University for free, as well as the speakers and mailing lists, and I somehow convinced the local post office to give us the nonprofit, radically reduced postage rate. I'd done all this while sleeping on the floor of a dilapidated house of a discomfited "friend of the group." A young man who was rapidly running out of patience with having his home turned into a direct mail clearinghouse.

"What did Rose have to say?" Dave asked gingerly.

"What do you think he said? He just screamed at me and hung up."

"Ah, the usual," Dave added with a grin.

Dave's father was a famous cantor in Pittsburgh, and his two older brothers were doctors. After graduating from law school Dave was about to give his proud Jewish mother her filial hat trick by passing the bar exam when a friend dragged him to a meeting with Rose. A complete skeptic, Dave started heckling Rose only to have Rose pull off a Pauline, road-to-Damascus conversion experience that knocked Dave clean off his high horse. He instantly became one of Rose's staunchest students, and Dave and I gradually became staunch friends.

Well-read and gifted with what my Irish mother described as a "yiddishe kop," Dave was also a great listener with a preternatural ability, born of compassion, to perfectly articulate in a few words what was troubling the soul of another human being.

"Dave, I'm at the end of my rope," I moaned. "Rose said I'm in hiding, and he's right. No matter what I do, I'm wrong. Every failure is my fault. We sold out four Chautauquas in a row with what? No money, just hustle and hard work, and Rose takes every miracle we pull off for granted. Hell, my big mistake was getting that minister in Cleveland to lend us his church for free. Now Rose expects every gig to be free."

Dave didn't say anything. Instead, he sympathetically offered me a seat by carefully repositioning several stacks of mail on a faded, threadbare sofa. As I sat down, my dejection morphed into anger. I told Dave I was losing confidence in Rose as a manager and as the leader of an organization.

"First it was campus Zen groups that cratered," I continued. "Then the TAT Intensives, the TAT Encounter Groups, and the TAT Employment Cooperative all fizzled. Now we're putting on low-budget, fly-by-night conferences for little old ladies who've been abducted by aliens to jump-start groups of alcoholic astrologists that fall apart the moment we leave town. Rose keeps saying if we boil enough psychics a few will bubble off into serious seekers. I'm still waiting to see it.

"Meanwhile, I'm five years in, dead broke, horny as hell, and we still don't have toilets or running water at the farm. Rose told me himself, 'Oogie, I know how you feel. Every time you leave one city for another, everything goes to hell, and you have to circle back to prop things up. It seems like me and you is doin' little more than runnin' in ever-decreasin' concentric circles until we clamber up our own backsides and disappear.'

"Then two minutes later he's back bitchin' and blaming me. And know what bugs me most about Rose? He's just like my old man. In five years, he's never admitted to being wrong, let alone apologized, for one damn thing."

I paused, chest heaving, for a few deep breaths. Dave headed for the kitchen, and from where I was sitting, I could see him putting a battered kettle on the stove for tea. "Keep talking. I'm listening," he said and, reassured by his thoughtful gesture, I upped the volume half a decibel and resumed my rant.

I told him there seemed to be something self-sabotaging about Rose that precluded success. One time the *East West Journal* agreed to interview Rose. I not only talked the editor into a splashy feature with a virtual unknown, but the interview was to be conducted by me. Landing a big spread, with editorial control, in the premier spiritual periodical was the perfect PR coup. Rose would finally take his seat among the other big shots in the burgeoning field of spirituality and personal growth, guys like Baba Ram Das, Ken Wilber, Werner Erhard, Chögyam Trungpa, Robert Pirsig, Alan Watts, Carlos Castaneda, Sri Chinmoy, and Thomas Merton. Super stoked, I made a beeline to Benwood to conduct my interview.

I arrived to find that Rose had already penned his interview, and when I read it my heart sank. It was a poorly written mishmash that needed a rewrite or at least some massive editing. But knowing how stubborn and sensitive to criticism Rose was, I downplayed my reaction. We began editing and he stiff-armed even the tiniest suggestions. As I continued to push, he lost his temper, so I gave up and submitted the article without any changes. A few days later the editor spiked the interview and quashed the deal. I was devastated, but Rose just brushed it off. There was not a word about my suggestions, let alone an apology.

"You know how I feel, Dave? I'm like one of those hapless sodbusters in a cowboy movie standing shellshocked in the middle of the street as some drunken gunslinger peppers his feet with bullets yelling, 'Dance! Dance! *Dance!*' No matter where I put my feet, Rose . . . "

As Dave proffered a piping hot cup of tea, I noticed it was all he could do to keep from laughing out loud. I gave him one of my best baleful stares only slightly distorted by the steam billowing off my tea and metaphorically out of my ears until he finally regained his composure.

"All that—or at least a big chunk of it—is true," he said as he pulled up a decrepit wooden chair with a cracked oval seat he'd fetched from the kitchen. "But on the other hand, it's all bull. Something else is bothering you, and it don't have a damn thing to do with whether Rose is incompetent, unfair, nuts, self-destructive, or all of the above."

I just kept staring.

"What's eating you is it's been four years since your big experience in Rose's kitchen. Four long years of sacrifice and hard work and, spiritually speaking, you don't have a damn thing to show for it. You're as far away from Enlightenment as ever and you want to blame Rose. But deep down you blame yourself, and that's why you're so bummed out."

Stunned by Dave's latest insight, my anger drained away and I told him about a recent incident that only hammered home his uncanny intuition. I was attending a community gathering at Rose's farm. By this time we'd taken over the farmhouse and built a wing on it for meetings. Rose was holding court as usual, seamlessly toggling between playing the guru and just playing around. Suddenly depressed, I left the meeting and retreated to the tiny living room. The shades were drawn, and I sat down on a rickety rocking chair next to a small table embossed with an old rotary phone. Through thin farmhouse walls I could hear rollicking laughter, and the louder it got the gloomier I felt.

"It's been four years since my experience," I said to myself, "and nothing spiritually has happened. Four years . . . " Over and over this dolorous dirge reverberated until I was rudely drawn from my dreary reverie by a throat being loudly and intentionally cleared. Rose was standing at the doorway with a coffee cup in his hand. He was apparently on his way to the kitchen for a refill when he chanced upon my mournful vigil.

"So," he said, "sittin' there thinkin' it's been four years and nothin's happened. Hah!" Breaking into loud peals of laughter, he resumed his quest for another jolt of home-brewed "gasoline."

Dave only nodded. He'd seen Rose at his preternatural best plenty of times and saw nothing remarkable in Rose telepathically reading my mind. Dave leaned forward, tipping his crippled chair precariously onto its front legs as he dug deeper into me instead.

"There's something else. You sound like a raw Marine recruit bitching about his crazy drill sergeant. Did it ever occur to you that all this hell is just a teacher doing his best to break your spiritual stalemate? You say you feel like some pathetic sodbuster helplessly dancing to the tune of random Rosean bullets. Well, hell, isn't that the way you're *supposed* to feel? Isn't that what we signed on for? Take any mystical story from any religion you want, and what's the active ingredient? Frustration. It's all about the teacher frustrating the student's ego. And what are his favorite tools? Irrationality, unfairness, paradox. Maybe it ain't you, but only your ego that Rose is forcing to dance.

'You say you feel like some pathetic sodbuster helplessly dancing to the tune of random Rosean bullets. Well, hell, isn't that the way you're *supposed* to feel?'

"You want Rose to play fair. He is. He's just playing ten-dimensional chess and you're only playing two. You want him to play your game by all those rules of polite society they drilled into you at Hotchkiss, and you're pissed because he won't. Rose is playing for much bigger stakes than whether these damn Chautauquas are a success or—"

"I know! My God, Dave, I know!" Oblivious to the hot tea I was spilling all over myself, I lurched to my feet and frantically began pacing, narrowly skirting our carefully stacked mail. "I been feeding myself that same damn speech for a year. I just read this super cool Tolstoy story. The teacher tells his student to walk mouthfuls of water from a brook and spit them on a dead, blackened tree stump until the stump comes back to life. The guy keeps at it for years. He finally reaches the end of himself. He surrenders, and lo and behold the stump blooms. A great story, but man, I just don't know how much longer I can keep spitting on all these Rosean stumps with nothing but lumps on my head to show for it. It's one thing to read cool stories like that—"

"And another when it's happening to you," Dave interrupted. We both laughed.

Dave's commentary exposed more issues than it settled, so I decided to make a mad dash to Benwood to surprise Rose and see if I could salvage the situation. With conference deadlines looming I had to make the ten-hour round trip in one day, but I was hoping that my willingness to make such a sacrifice would convince Rose of my sincerity.

As I raced up Interstate 270 toward the Pennsylvania Turnpike, I recalled Rose telling me years earlier I was the boy with the burning feet destined to just keep running until I got too tired to run any more. Maybe Dave was right: maybe madly whirling like a dervish to the tune of Rosean bullets was just his way of tiring me out faster. Perhaps I was letting my ego get in the way.

After years of celibately spitting on stumps, I'd built up quite a "head of steam," as Rose would put it. I was a dynamic, confident, charismatic young man, and the ironclad willpower and skill set I collected hustling for Rose had made me a match for just about any challenge.

While promoting Chautauquas, I discovered that interest in psychic phenomena and the paranormal was not merely the last bastion of lonely cranks sharing a bathroom in some old boarding house like Carnegie's Main Hotel. Many professional people considered practicing meditation, talking about Karma, eating brown rice, and investigating the paranormal a chic alternative to traditional religion. I enjoyed mingling in these upscale circles, and I was flattered to be treated like a boy wonder who would magically meld all their various interests into something resembling a movement.

I relished this approbation, especially from the ladies, and being lionized a bit was a welcome respite from the nonstop criticism I was getting from Rose. In other words, as my spiritual hopes faded, I was increasingly tempted by worldly compensation instead. So, in fairness to Rose, I could see that my ego as well as my vanity was becoming part of the problem.

Despite these admissions, as I exited the Pennsylvania Turnpike onto Interstate 70 toward Wheeling, what I was unable and unwilling to admit, especially to myself, was that for the better part of a year I'd been engaged in a massive deception behind Rose's back: an impossible romance which would ultimately prove fatal to my work with Rose . . .

. . . Linda was an attractive brunette in her mid-twenties with shoulder-length hair parted in the middle. Funny, bright, blue-eyed, and shapely, she was also married to Danny, a friend in the Rose group. Danny and Linda joined after attending some meetings in Pittsburgh, and Danny and I hit it off immediately. He was a square-jawed, blue-eyed, wise-cracking former football star and weightlifter. Most of the guys in our group were nerdy introverts, but Danny was definitely *cool*.

But Danny made two mistakes. The first was neglecting his beautiful wife. The second was trusting me. Despite being married, Danny became celibate and moved onto Rose's farm. Farm living was reserved for men, so Linda took one of the bedrooms in Rose's house in Benwood. Since I was constantly in and out of Benwood, Linda and I were thrown together quite a bit. Before I knew it, and long before I was willing to admit it, sparks were flying, and we were flirting big-time.

The plot thickened considerably when Linda volunteered to organize the preparation and sale of food and beverages at the Chautauquas Dave and I were promoting. This, of course, gave us reasons—and eventually pretexts—to meet alone.

At one tete-a-tete in Pittsburgh, Linda began shyly talking about how difficult it was to be married to man who was avidly practicing celibacy.

"I'm lonely," she said. "This is not what I had in mind when we got married. I'm sick and tired of hugging my pillow at night."

Rose often insisted that the biggest obstacle to finding the Truth is the insatiable human appetite for self-deception, compartmentalization, denial, and rationalization. When it came to Linda, I was frantically pulling all four levers. I knew I was intensely attracted to her while blithely maintaining the convenient fiction it was nothing to worry about. And definitely nothing that needed the guru's attention.

Then, just before Christmas of 1976, I got a card from Linda with veiled yet definite romantic overtones. I was so excited I carried her card in my coat pocket, reading it repeatedly until it became decidedly dog-eared. As Rose metaphorically wrote about his own Enlightenment experience, I was a charmed lover hopelessly fighting the spell while languishing into it . . .

. . . When I pulled into Benwood, the only surprise evinced by Rose was a couple of raised eyebrows.

"Mr. Rose," I said. "I only have a few minutes. The D.C. Chautauqua is coming up fast, so I have to get back. There's still a million things to do. But I wanted to talk to you. Things have been rough between us, so I was hoping we could clear the air."

Rose nodded.

"I know I've been screwing up and letting my ego get involved, but I just can't stand being wrong all the time anymore. It's tearing me up. So I got an idea. You just tell me exactly what you want me to do, and that's what I'll do. That way there won't be any misunderstandings, ambiguity, or incorrect interpretations. I'll just be another set of hands and feet for you, an extension—"

"Jesus Christ!" Rose erupted. "It ain't enough I'm workin' myself half to death, now you want me to do *all* the thinkin' too! Boys get told. Men think for themselves. It ain't enough that I'm losin' sleep wipin' everybody else's butt in this damn group. Now you want me to wipe your butt too!"

Rose ranted on for what seemed like forever, and when I eventually climbed back into my van, I was more depressed than ever.

* * *

Two weeks later Rose arrived in Washington for the Chautauqua with several group members in tow.

It was a fiasco.

The same formula Dave and I used to produce sellout crowds in Pittsburgh, Cleveland, Akron, and Columbus flopped in a far more discerning Washington, D.C. The no-name speakers I managed to book on a shoestring budget failed to sell even half the tickets we expected, and the people who did attend were far too sophisticated for those same speakers.

But the denouement of the two-day tragedy was the hypnosis demonstration. Our hypnotist was a thin, sharply featured, part-time instructor from some obscure college with a high-pitched voice and Van Dyke beard that made him look like some caped and top-hatted villain from a one-reel silent movie. I booked him sight unseen based on somebody's recommendation, and he arrived with an entourage of five or six of his students. After a short speech, he invited his students to the front of the auditorium and put them into a hypnotic trance. He then produced a pistol, handed it to a young man, and ordered him to shoot one of the young women.

Bang! Bang! Bang! The gun went off, acrid gunpowder smoke filled the air, and his victim collapsed on the floor. The screaming audience, cowering in fear, instantly went to ground as well. One well-dressed man in his late thirties came streaking up the center aisle, flew past Rose calmly sitting at the ticket table, and launched himself pell-mell out the front door.

Seconds later, the young lady popped back to her feet as our hypnotist blithely said the bullets were blanks and the whole scene a humorous hoax. Rose and I ran out the front door determined to head off the fleeing man before he could call the cops and report a murder.

From the top of the steps we could see him jogging across American University's campus quad several hundred yards away. Cupping both hands to my mouth, I shouted at the top of my lungs.

"Come back! It was all a joke! No one was hurt! *Come back!*"

Slowing down, he waved one arm limply in my direction and yelled over his shoulder, "You go to hell!" And kept going.

Apparently, the rest of the attendees didn't get the joke either. As I reentered the auditorium, I met the remnant of the shell-shocked audience silently filing out.

We eventually made our way back to the house. I was devastated, but by this time Rose, true to form, was relishing the disaster's more humorous elements.

"If I didn't see it with my own eyes, I wouldn't believe it. That guy came barrelin' up the aisle eyes bulgin', elbows churnin', fists pumpin', lips curled, and teeth clenched. I'll wager he wasn't two feet off the ground. Hell, when he came tearin' past the ticket table all I could make out was the top of his head. He was every bit of six foot and sprintin' full speed on what looked like his knees."

Leaving his chair, Rose went into a deep lunge and did such a spot-on imitation of the man he just described that everyone—but me—was rolling in laughter.

"Augie yelled after him to come back, but he told him to go straight to hell and kept on goin'. Can't say's I blame the poor fella'. He must be in the outskirts of Baltimore by now."

Utterly depressed, I staggered up the stairs, found an unoccupied bed, and curling up in a ball went to sleep on an empty stomach.

Linda had family in Maryland, and when Rose and his posse returned to West Virginia, she stayed behind for a visit. A few days later we met for lunch, ended up at a deserted public park, and spent the afternoon making out in the grass. While we never technically consummated the relationship, we got close enough to qualify as adultery.

Returning in Linda's car, we felt so guilty we barely said a word. We were like those apple-eaters, Adam and Eve, struck dumb with shame by the sudden realization they were naked.

A few days later I showed up in Benwood. At least Rose was still in the dark, and I planned to keep it that way. Rose was in the kitchen with a few visitors yukking it up. He greeted me warmly and even offered a cup of tea and a chair beside his. Relieved, I was just sinking back in my chair when Rose, taking advantage of the distraction provided by a particularly humorous story, leaned over and hissed in my ear, "So tell me. How was she?"

Over the next few chaotic days, as the scandal rippled through the group, I discovered that Rose was, of course, on to us all along. He even knew about Linda's dog-eared Christmas card. Showing more restraint than I frankly thought him capable, he had merely strung us along.

Those excruciating times are all a jumble, but I did see Linda one last time. She was too ashamed to even make eye contact with me. I saw Danny at the farm, apologized, and assured him I had not actually had sex with his wife. He nodded and walked away, a nonreaction which only made me feel worse.

Our deteriorating relationship, the failed D.C. Chautauqua, and now my fling with Linda made business as usual with Rose impossible. I went back to laying carpet in Pittsburgh with my brother Tom to make some money and let the heat die down.

One of our customers had a house trailer for sale, so I bought it and went to see Rose. "Mr. Rose, I know I screwed up. I know you no longer trust me. Frankly I don't trust myself. I want to move to the farm and live an isolated, contemplative life until I get my head back on straight. I bought this trailer. I want to haul it onto the farm and live in it."

Rose didn't evince any enthusiasm, but he didn't reject the idea out of hand.

One week later I got a four- or five-sentence letter from Rose. The gist was that rather than asking how I could be of service, I'd egotistically told *him* what *I* wanted to do instead. I do, however, vividly remember the letter's final sentence.

Leave me and the group alone!

* * *

Imagine you're tied to a long rope a giant is swinging in ever-widening circles above his head. As the earth recedes and the velocity increases, you are initially giddily exhilarated by your mild disorientation and the vistas revealed. But as more and more rope plays out the scenery blurs, vertigo sets in, and you are suddenly terrified and deathly sick to your stomach. When you reach escape velocity the giant lets go and your universe contracts into the endless tumbling, tumbling, tumbling of a tether-less astronaut lost in outer space.

This is what it felt like when I realized Richard Rose was no longer in my life.

Chapter Fifteen

A LEADERSHIP GURU AND TRAPPIST MONKS

Do not let me hear
Of the wisdom of old men, but rather of their folly,
Their fear of fear and frenzy, their fear of possession,
Of belonging to another, or to others, or to God.
The only wisdom we can hope to acquire
Is the wisdom of humility: humility is endless.
—T.S. ELIOT[33]

"Not feelin' too good, are you, Augie?" came a syrupy southern drawl, apparently straight from the ether.

By June of 1996 I was limping around without crutches and back at work. The rehab pros prescribed step climbing at my gym to loosen my stiff and still swollen ankle. Already an avid stepper, I threw myself into my workouts desperately trying to outdistance the deepening depression and incipient despair nipping at my heels. I was like a terminally ill cancer patient who, through tremendous effort, manages to resume his daily routine and even forget his fate once in a while, yet in the back of his mind the terrible truth is always looming, casting its dark shadow over everything.

Startled by this unbidden comment, I paused mid-stride long enough to see that the disembodied drawl belonged to Hugh, a man I knew strictly on a first-name basis and only from the gym. In his early forties, Hugh was a physically fit, blue-collar knockoff of rock legend David Crosby, with long brown hair parted in the middle and a thick handlebar mustache. Hugh worked in a furniture factory, and I pegged him for a good ol' country boy living for beer, NASCAR races, and not much more.

I was slightly offended by Hugh's intrusive observation, but I was too emotionally exhausted to give a damn, so I just wearily nodded instead.

"Feels like your heart's broken, don't it?"

A tingle rushed up my spine. That was *exactly* how I felt, though I'd never used those words before. Stunned, I nodded again.

"Yeah, we call it the soul hole. I'm here to tell you that you're in for two years of so much hell you'll be wishin' you was never born. But you *will* get through it. God'll be waitin', and you're gonna' love yourself a whole helluva' lot more than you do right now."

Without waiting for a reaction or reply, he turned on his heel and strolled out of the gym.

Hugh's prophecy set the universe spinning. My heart *was* broken, but what about all that hell he was talking about? Just how much worse could things really get?

By the time I got back to my office, Hugh's prognostications, coming from a virtual stranger, were even more disturbing. Part of me wanted to add this spooky incident to my long list of dramatic encounters with previous prophets: the Vietnam vet, Jay and his Near-Death Experience, the man who gave me *Isis Unveiled*, and even my first eerie encounter with Richard Rose.

However, I was more afraid I was beginning to superstitiously "see signs." Soon I'd be getting secret messages from television commer-

> I wanted a *rational* explanation. I was in no mood and far too fragile for angelic oracles in the guise of David Crosby doppelgangers.

cials, then meeting ghosts, until, as Rose would say, I melted into the florid wallpaper of madness all together. I was determined to get to the bottom of Hugh's newfound penchant for fortune telling. I wanted a *rational* explanation. I was in no mood and far too fragile for angelic oracles in the guise of David Crosby doppelgangers.

While I was accustomed to seeing Hugh daily at the gym, I never saw him again, and his sudden disappearance only deepened the mystery and rattled me even more.

* * *

Six weeks later I answered my office phone. Josh was a favorite of mine, a Duke University SKS student who recently graduated. I also envied him a bit because his rangy build, blue eyes, and long, wavy blond hair made him look so much like a rock star taking a break from the road to study civil engineering that the girls at Duke called him a chick magnet. I was thrilled to hear from him, but since I rarely heard from students after they graduated, I asked why he was calling.

"Well," he said, "I just wanted to let you know at least one of your students took you up on your challenge."

"What challenge?"

"You said we should do something meaningful with our summer vacation rather than just drink beer, get a tan, and chase girls."

"Did I? I don't remember, but I've given worse advice. So what are you up to?"

"I'm spending the summer at a Trappist monastery in South Carolina called Mepkin Abbey."

I shot bolt upright. Leaning forward, I began deluging poor Josh with dozens of questions.

Josh told me that Mepkin Abbey, unique among Trappist monasteries, offered a Monastic Guest Program. Open only to men, a monastic guest, or MG, wore a gray-hooded surplice while living and working "behind the cloister wall" as a temporary monk. Josh rose at 3 AM with the monks, attended seven services a day, called the Liturgy of the Hours, worked manually in the monastery's egg business, shared the community's simple vegetarian fare, and did it all while observing the legendary Trappist commitment to living predominately in silence.

As Josh patiently answered my questions, I noticed something else. I'd known Josh for four years, and there was something in his voice that suggested a newfound, quiet confidence, as if a struggling post-adolescent work in progress had finally found himself, or "settled into himself," in a meaningful way.

Suddenly I blurted, "I want to come!"

Startled, Josh said, "When?"

"Right now!" I fairly shouted. Then I realized I was at work and it was only Wednesday, so I added, "I mean Friday. This weekend."

"OK," Josh said. "Hold on while I go ask Brother John."

That was the first time I heard the name Brother John, the Trappist monk destined to play such a magical part in my life.

While sitting on hold, I tried to take stock of my spontaneous decision to seek refuge in a Trappist monastery . . .

At first glance it seemed like little more than a frightened, deeply depressed, and increasingly desperate man willing to try just about any damn thing that might pull him out of his tailspin. However, I was not completely unfamiliar with the Trappists. Thomas Merton, the New York intellectual who became a mystic and Trappist monk at the Abbey of Gethsemani in Kentucky in the 1940s, wrote quite a bit on Buddhism and especially Zen. He died in a freakish accident while attending a conference with Buddhist monks in Bangkok, Thailand. I read his books on Zen and Christian mysticism and was so impressed I almost became a Trappist monk myself.

Returning to Pittsburgh after my break with Rose in the summer of 1977, I reapplied to the University of Pittsburgh to get my degree, but then, on a whim, I called Merton's old Kentucky monastery, Gethsemani. I got the Guest Master and told him I wanted to come.

"Why?" he asked, taking me off guard.

"I want to learn how to pray," I blurted without thinking.

"Good answer!" he said with a laugh. "That's why we're all here."

I asked him what I needed to bring.

"Just a toothbrush, Brother, just a toothbrush."

My toothbrush and I were packed and ready to go to Gethsemani when the Guest Master called. There were several extraordinary conferences coming up on the monastic schedule, and the guest house was fully booked until after the first of the year. I was deeply disappointed, but then, on the very same day, a letter arrived readmitting me to the University of Pittsburgh. Taking this as a sign, I went back to Pitt in September and graduated in the spring of 1978. I still often wondered what might've been if I'd gone to Gethsemani and . . .

"Augie, great news!" Josh gushed as he came back on the line. "Brother John said come down Friday and ask for him. I got a surprise for you too!"

Two days later I set off on yet another quest, this time a pilgrimage to a Trappist monastery with one thousand years of spiritual mojo behind it. Mepkin Abbey was located near Moncks Corner, South Carolina, just outside Charleston, about 250 miles from my home in Raleigh, North Carolina. A bit of research revealed that the sprawling monastery rested on 3,132 acres nestled along the Cooper River as it meandered toward Charleston and eventually the Atlantic Ocean. Once a rice plantation owned by Henry Laurens, the president of the second Continental Congress in 1777, Mepkin later became the estate of Henry Luce, the founder of *Time Magazine* and *Sports Illustrated*, and his famous wife, the author, politician, and socialite Clare Boothe

Luce. In 1944 Clare Boothe's only daughter from a previous marriage was killed in an auto accident at 19. Two years later, still grief-stricken, Boothe became a fervent Catholic. In 1949 the Luces donated the land to Merton's Abbey of Gethsemani, and twenty-nine Trappist monks voluntarily left the blue grass of Kentucky for the swampy lowlands of coastal South Carolina to found Mepkin Abbey.

After about an hour on I-40 East out of Raleigh, I hit I-95 South and settled in for a few hours of monotonous highway driving punctuated only by an endless series of annoying billboards urging me to be sure to stop at the faux-Mexican-themed South of the Border tourist trap. I clicked on speed control, leaned back, and returned to the same task I'd been hammering away at since my skydiving accident: obsessively retracing my past trying to figure out how I got myself into such a dark and scary fix in the first damn place.

* * *

When I was traveling from city to city drumming for Rose, what passed for recreation was hanging out at bookstores, especially spiritual ones. One of my literary rituals was accosting the owners and asking, "Who are the coolest people in town? Who do you know who can teach me something about life?"

They would always happily oblige, and I met many fascinating seekers in this fashion. In fact, this is how I met many of the people Dave and I later booked as speakers for the Chautauquas.

During one of several sojourns in Washington, D.C., I went looking for the YES! bookshop just off M Street in the trendy Georgetown section of the district. Founded in 1972, YES! was famous for its eclectic collection of spiritual titles. After browsing for a while, I introduced myself to the owner and, as usual, pumped her for referrals.

She bustled around and came up with an old-fashioned rolodex bursting with index cards. Rifling through her sundry collection, she pulled one out. Written in pencil were the words "Louis Mobley" followed by a phone number with a 301 Maryland area code.

"Thanks so much," I said while jotting down the number. "But you got a million cards there. Why this guy? What makes Mobley so special?"

"I'll leave that to you," the affable owner said with a grin. "It's all about the Quest, ain't it? Let's just say this particular pilgrimage won't disappoint and leave it at that."

Thoroughly intrigued, I called the very next day. Lou answered and I related my conversation with the owner of YES!

"C'mon out!" Mobley practically shouted in a soft southern accent, as if he'd been eagerly expecting my call. "Stay the night if you want."

Mobley lived on five acres in a sprawling stone ranch house perched on the highest point of a 450-acre cattle farm in the rolling Maryland countryside. His driveway was a two-lane, tree-lined, straight arrow access road a mile long leading up to a circle in front of the hilltop house enclosing a well-maintained flower garden. On one side of the driveway was a private airfield with a dozen or so single engine airplanes snugly tied down along the runway. When I pulled up, Mobley and his family poured out to greet me as if I was a long-lost son given up for dead. It was amazing, even touching.

Mobley's son Ricky and his daughter, Karen, were in their early twenties, and his younger son, Chris, still in high school, was seventeen. Mobley's wife, Dorothy, better known as Dot, as well as the family dog, a yapping wire-haired terrier named Tuggles, rounded out the welcoming committee. Mobley soon whisked me away and took me on a tour of the acreage surrounding the house.

Mobley was 62, about five-foot-ten, trim, and radiating good health and good cheer. He was bald with a fringe of gray hair and beard to match, and it was hard to say whether the face behind the glasses with its prominent nose was handsome or if his clear blue eyes and perpetual smile just made it seem so.

Mobley was from Georgia and a Georgia Tech engineer, and despite his apparent affluence, he harnessed the thriftiness of a humble heritage to his mechanical proclivities through a number of living-off-the-land projects. He kept a large garden and a variety of fruit trees that kept Dot busy canning for winter. There was a back-up diesel generator for electrical outages, plans to move up to wind power, and an underground tank and fuel pump for the gasoline he bought wholesale.

In the backyard was a huge telescope with a highly polished lens that Lou, an amateur astronomer, hand-ground himself. The property boasted a Mobley-designed solar-heated water system for the house and the extra deep, oversized, spring-fed swimming pool made entirely from steel. Lou solar-heated the water as it came out of the ground, and this made the unheated pool usable six weeks earlier than it would otherwise.

While showing me around, Mobley kept up a patter of scientific instruction with so much boyish enthusiasm I was soon completely smitten. As we slowly wandered back toward the house, he pointed to his freshly tilled garden.

"Just look at that rich black soil!" he said reverentially. "Makes you want to spray whipped cream on it and go at it with a spoon. You know the secret?"

I shook my head.

"Woims," he said, using his Georgian pronunciation for worms. "Thousands of woims. We've been feeding the family for twenty years without a drop of fertilizer. The woims do it all," he concluded with a sigh of deep satisfaction.

We retreated to Mobley's magnificent oak-paneled, booklined study, and settling in with a couple of glasses of Dot's old-fashioned iced tea, Mobley told me he was a former IBM executive. He retired early, at 55, and was now devoting his life to his consulting business (in deference to Dot's sanity, as he put it) and his passion for spirituality and personal transformation.

"When I was a kid," he continued, "I used to lay on my back on the roof of our barn and spend hours staring at the stars. I started asking all the deep questions about life, truth, God, and got so fascinated I even wrote a book on it. But I made the mistake of showing it to my family. They told me I was nuts, so I put the book in the bottom of my sock drawer and tried to forget all about it."

Mobley rose from his mahogany desk and walked over to the large sliding-glass doors that opened onto the pool and the magnificent vista of rolling pastures beyond. I knew he was somewhere in the past, so I just waited for him to continue.

"I went to Georgia Tech, and then did engineering work in optics for the army during World War II. I joined IBM, initially repairing typewriters, but discovered I had a passion for education. After creating two successful training programs for supervisors and middle managers, Tom Watson Jr., IBM's CEO, called me in. IBM was growing far too fast to hire the talent we needed. He gave me a blank check and carte blanche to create the perfect setting for human growth. Can you imagine? I was still in my thirties. It was a dream come true."

Mobley bought the Guggenheim estate at Sands Point, Long Island in 1956, renamed it The IBM Executive School, and went to work.

Throughout the day and long into the night I sat stone mesmerized as Mobley led me on a labyrinthian journey through dozens of subjects like Systems Theory, Process Theology, Teleocratic Management, the Efficient Market Hypothesis, Eschatology, Operations Research, Management by Objectives (MBO), PERT charts, Game Theory, Organization Development (OD), moral hazard, Chaos Theory, Noam Chomsky's Transformational-Generative Grammar, the Hawthorne Effect, nested hierarchies, Occam's razor, supply side economics, String Theory, the Laffer curve, discounted cash flow analysis, astral projection, Number Theory, the Random Walk Hypothesis, Quantum Entanglement, Reductionism, Jungian personality types, Peter Drucker, and Targ and Puthoff's psychic phenomena experiments at Stanford Research Institute. None of this reflected the idle interest of the dilettante or the aesthetic inclinations of a late modern Renaissance man; Mobley seamlessly connected it all to his all-consuming, completely practical devotion to spirituality and human development.

I did end up spending the night, and when I finally staggered out the door I felt as top heavy as Melville's proverbial "supperless college student with all of Aristotle in his head." I was dazzled by the sheer candlepower of Mobley's omnivorous intellect. I couldn't imagine how any one person could have done so much thinking and amassed so much knowledge.

As a lifelong reader and incurable talker, I was always drawn to conceptual thinking. My roles as facilitator, lecturer, manager, and advance man under Rose exacerbated this tendency to the point that Rose often needled me about it. One day I was loudly expounding on the writings of the nineteenth-century German philosopher Arthur Schopenhauer when Rose interrupted. "Oogie," he said, laughing and shaking his head, "I'm absolutely convinced your head can only hold so much crap. I just hope I'm still around to watch it finally explode." Despite his teasing, I continued to read voraciously and lecture on what I read to anyone who'd sit still for it. Deep down, I didn't feel like I really understood anything until I could convey it to someone else.

So I wasn't just dazzled by Mobley's intellect and knowledge. I sensed he was someone who could help satisfy my own intellectual hunger. I was also intrigued by the fact that much of Mobley's work on human growth had been driven by IBM's organizational challenges. His insights seemed applicable to the challenges of the spiritual community Rose and I were then facing. But what excited me most about Mobley was a sense that he and Rose were largely in agreement on the rules and laws governing human development and spirituality. The difference was that Rose puzzled it out bottom-up while chopping wood and used personal experience and intuition to support his findings, while Mobley relied on a top-down approach gleaned from decades of hard-core scientific research funded by IBM. As I drove back to Washington, Mobley's table-pounding voice was still ringing in my ears.

"Children learn. Adults grow. Authentic leadership takes a revolution in consciousness, a becoming process, a kick-ass, bottom-up, inside-out, in-your-face transformation of being. You can't train a man into a leader any more than you can train a caterpillar into a butterfly. Somehow you have to concoct a transformational cocoon and coax him into it.

"The IBM Executive School," Mobley continued, "was a twelve-week residential program with only one goal: *to blow minds*. We didn't teach a damn thing. There were no teachers, no books, no tests. Rather than didactic lecturing, we created a curriculum of controlled chaos designed to generate mind-bending realizations, epiphanies, eurekas, ahas, wows, and gotchas. We used experiential exercises to show all those hotshot IBMers that everything you think you know is wrong. It was an *unlearning* process, an apophatic *via negativa*, and the goal was humility. It's not what you think but how you think that makes all the difference, and you never open up to new ways of thinking without tons and tons of raw humility."

This sounded a lot like the mysticism of Saint John of the Cross or Zen 101, and I could easily imagine Rose nodding his head vigorously while exclaiming, "Now you're talkin'!"

Mobley stayed with the IBM Executive School until 1966, and he modestly pointed out that his school churned out the leaders who made IBM the fastest growing and most admired corporation in the world in the 1960s and '70s.

* * *

After our initial meeting I planned to stay in contact, but Rose kept me so busy we lost touch. But after graduating from Pitt and spending another nine months laying carpet, I called Mobley once again.

"Lou, I have a proposition for you," I said on an early January morning in 1979. "You started a consulting business when you retired. I'm a pretty good salesman, and I'll bring in clients. I don't want to be paid. All I want is for you to teach me everything you know."

"I'll go you one better," Mobley replied. "You can move into our guest wing and share meals with our family. In the morning we'll meet in my study for one-on-one sessions. In the afternoon you can rustle up clients. But I do have one condition."

"What's that?"

"I insist on paying you for your work."

The very next day I left for Clarksville, Maryland, in the exurbs of Washington, D.C. eagerly anticipating my latest spiritual adventure as the live-in protégé of Louis R. Mobley. I arrived just in time to be snowed in for three days with the family. Undaunted by the prospect of several days at close quarters, we passed the time playing games, singing songs, eating Dot's amazing cooking, and enjoying each other's company. By the time the roads were passable, I was converted: there really are happy, loving, close-knit families, and nothing I saw subsequently while living with the Mobleys ever changed my opinion.

True to his word, when the skies cleared, Lou and I began meeting each morning in his study, and true to mine, I made hundreds of cold calls to local corporations and government agencies setting up appointments for his Mobley and Associates consulting business. As I became more adept at selling his services, Lou and I made dozens of trips to Washington, D. C., and some of our best conversations took place during our lengthy two-way commute.

While these rides revealed many philosophical affinities, as I got to know Mobley better I discovered that, as men, Rose and Mobley couldn't have been more different.

Rose was an earthy bull who relished a good heart-to-heart or in-your-face confrontation. Mobley was a southern gentleman who went out of his way to avoid interpersonal tension. Rose was so personally transparent that if he was wrestling with a bout of irregularity you were going to hear all about it; Lou was reticent about his private thoughts and feelings. Where Rose could be caustic and quick-tempered, Mobley was kind, even-tempered to the point of detached, always respectful. He could get riled up on occasion, but these episodes always seemed a trifle forced, as if a basically shy person had managed to overcome his shyness through great effort and still had to prove it every once in a while.

While Rose and Mobley shared a passionate interest in the mysteries of human nature, for Mobley this was primarily an academic exercise. Fascinated by the generic riddles of the human heart, he showed little interest in the deeper motives of the people he met. As a result he was a poor salesman incapable of the breathtaking, intuitive insights that were Rose's stock in trade. Mobley accepted everyone at face value, which made him seem innocently naïve, like an absentminded professor, touchingly out of touch.

While all this might be called the formal part of our relationship, I was finding my way informally through the controlled chaos of the Mobley household—and loving it.

Fascinating people of every description dropped in, wandered through, or stayed a week, providing an unending stream of thought-provoking conversation. I also found that Mobley, Dot, and the kids represented three completely different spheres of influence, and while I traveled freely among them, it sometimes meant divided loyalties and humorous contradictions.

Mobley was a hard-news junkie while Dot loved gossip. Sharing both proclivities, I was soon splitting my time between watching *Meet the Press* with Lou and hanging out in the kitchen with Dot as we married off, divorced, and generally straightened out the lives of everyone we knew. Soon I was calling her Mom, and she was baking her carrot cake more often because she knew how much I liked it.

Dot relied on intuition to instantly take the measure of people, and when Mobley demanded objective proof for her quick studies, an exasperated Dot would retort, "For God's sake, Lou, stop thinking so

261

much and open your damn eyes!" None of this was serious, but when Mobley shared his frustration with Dot's overactive intuition, I would find myself in the awkward position of diplomatically nodding at Dad while secretly siding with Mom.

My divided loyalties came to a head in the spring of 1979 when it was time to put in the garden. Mobley, Dot, and I were all avid gardeners, and I eagerly volunteered to turn over their huge garden with the family rototiller. As I was churning away, Mobley watched with obvious satisfaction as thick, black, heavy earth spewed up between the blades. Sighing deeply, he finally managed to tear himself away and drive off.

A few minutes later Dot appeared. Furtively looking around she asked, "Where's Lou?" I told her he drove off someplace.

"Good," she grunted.

She quickly bustled me into the passenger seat of her yellow station wagon, and a few minutes later I was furiously cramming 50-pound bags of 10-10-10 fertilizer from the local feed store into the cargo bay.

"I'm sure you heard about the damn worms," she said on our way home in her now overloaded and tail-dragging wagon. "Well, he's been raising worms and I've been adding fertilizer—for twenty years. What he doesn't know won't hurt him, and it's easier than fighting. But we have to work fast because I don't know where he went."

I was soon rapidly spreading fertilizer and turning it in to hide the granular evidence, and while I felt a little guilty about it—especially when Mobley waxed on about his beloved "woims" to anyone who'd listen—I also came to consider the whole cloak-and-dagger operation an amusing rite of passage. Everybody but Mobley knew about the fertilizer, and I felt my initiation into this secret society meant I was no longer just a houseguest but a full-fledged member of the family.

A year passed in this way, and then, in the late spring of 1980, Mobley took me on a long walk around the farm. He had a serious heart issue that would require surgery at nearby Johns Hopkins Hospital in Baltimore. In 1980 open heart surgery was still in its infancy, and

Lou would be out of commission for a long time: he might even be forced to abandon his consulting business. He suggested I move to New York City and join forces with another disciple starting her own consulting business based on Mobley's ideas.

While I was initially shocked to discover that Lou was so ill, I eventually agreed to his plan. Soon I was tying up loose ends and planning to hit the road once again. This time to a city so self-consciously full of itself that even its own denizens reverentially refer to it as simply "The City." There I tumbled headlong into one of

I became one of the original members of that madcap company of merry pranksters who conjured into existence that magic lantern of video music that defined the 1980s: MTV: Music Television.

gonzo Gotham's gyroscopic wormholes only to be spat out as one of the original members of that madcap company of merry pranksters who conjured into existence that magic lantern of video music that defined the 1980s: MTV: Music Television.

* * *

I'd fallen so deeply into my reverie about my stint with the Mobleys that I was soon seeing signs for Maynard, South Carolina, my exit off I-95 for Mepkin Abbey. From here, my pilgrimage took me over swampy back roads and through the pungent pine of the Francis Marion National Forest named for the legendary "Swamp Fox" of the American Revolution.

Speeding up, I continued toward U.S. Route 52 South, my last leg to Mepkin. As I resumed my ruminations, I was still, almost twenty years later, only dimly aware, if at all, that there were other, darker reasons for why I chose Mobley for a teacher. Reasons much deeper than innocent intellectual curiosity or his affinity with Rose.

Mobley also provided the intellectual ammunition I needed for my ongoing argument with a world that seemed so hostile to the kind of life I was trying to live, an argument I was having mostly with myself. As the years without a spiritual breakthrough dragged on, it was this argument that continually tested my resolve as I struggled to maintain my spiritual momentum.

For example, "the world" argued that I should face facts, give up this crazy quest, get married, settle down, and spend the rest of my life peacefully resting in the bosom of my family. After all, if it was good enough for everyone else, what made me so damn special? I, on the other hand, retorted that this was only the rationalization of a tired, horny, and disillusioned man desperately trying to get off the spiritual hook. Hell, did I actually know anyone just peacefully resting in the bosom of his family?

But when you play chess with yourself, it's impossible to outdistance your opponent. During my years with Rose I sensed, through a glass darkly, that while I might be beating back these worldly arguments, I wasn't decisively winning any of them. My spiritual grip always felt tenuous and in need of the bolstering of even better arguments. This bottomless demand for psychological reinforcement was the real reason I thought, read, and argued with myself and others so often and so intensely.

I was terrified that if I lost even a single argument, my fragile hold on spirituality would begin to crack. If I relaxed my white-knuckle grip for even an instant, I would surrender all right, but to all the wrong things. Despite these fears and all my vigilance, at the end of my tenure with Rose, I did lose an argument. I spiritually dozed off, surrendered to lust, and woke up rolling around in the grass with the wife of a close friend.

There is an issue with the concept of surrender: an issue most seekers either ignore or don't understand. What is the difference between spiritual surrender and merely giving up, giving in, or just plain quitting? What is the difference between *letting go* and finding Enlightenment and just *letting yourself go* and betraying a friend with his wife? The movement feels the same. Only the result is different.

The energy it took to battle fatigue, frustration, forgetfulness, self-doubt, and worldly seduction was itself fatiguing, and during my last years with Rose I experienced bouts of deep depression. These episodes often followed my biggest successes like a well-received lecture or a sold-out conference. What I wanted from success was the feeling I'd arrived, that I could finally relax, exhale, let down my guard. I wanted to know that whatever I achieved wouldn't immediately begin evaporating like a weightlifter's muscles the moment he stops working out.

Of course, the only vista success ever revealed was an endless series of larger and steeper hills yet to be climbed. No matter how hard I tried, enough never seemed to be enough, and this depressed me even more. Worldly success was just like Mick Jagger wearing my Uncle Sam hat: a shiny, fraudulent bauble garishly promising something it could never deliver. My prophetic fear after the Rolling Stones Concert back in 1972 that "eager anticipation followed by inevitable disappointment might very well become the pattern of my life" was coming to pass—with a vengeance.

However, there was something even deeper than disappointment, fatigue, self-contempt, and guilt behind my depressions: it was the unconscious feeling that I was fighting a hopeless rear-guard battle against some terrible truth that was stronger than me and gaining on me. It was this sense of hopelessness in the face of inevitable defeat that darkened my life and deepened my depressions.

I read a story, for example, from World War II about German prisoners from the battle of Stalingrad driven to cannibalism by starvation during a ghastly Russian winter. Two young brothers were among the captives, and when one of them died, the other sat on the chest of his frozen corpse to protect it from the savagery of his fellow prisoners.

For three days and two nights he fought to stay awake as the cannibals sat in a circle patiently waiting. When it became obvious the boy was cracking under the strain, the oldest of the cannibals began softly, monotonously, soporifically whispering.

"Son, why are you doing this to yourself? Do you want to end up like your brother? You see, it's no use, you must sleep eventually, and it will all come to the same thing in the end. Let me take you to your bunk so you can relax and get some sleep."

On and on he droned until the boy began weeping uncontrollably. Sensing his opening, the older man took the boy by the hand, tugged him to his feet, and gently led him from the room. Then the others leapt onto his brother's corpse.

The horror of this story went far beyond the fact that I had six younger brothers I loved very much. I felt like the brother desperately trying to stay awake while worldly voices, like cannibals, monotonously, tirelessly, remorselessly droned that someday, no matter how hard I tried, I must finally surrender, fall asleep, and lose my way. And since my fate was so clearly sealed, this Greek chorus relentlessly sang, why not spare the time, effort, and agony and sleep now?

During my time with Mobley I was already running a low-grade fever of incipient panic, and it was only by using Mobley's intellect as a defense mechanism that I managed to keep this panic safely at bay. The man who gave me *Isis Unveiled* tapped into this hidden horror, and that is why I reacted so viscerally to his warning about falling asleep as well as his cautionary tale from a man who had.

So while I was dazzled by Mobley's intellect, his organizational in-sights, his similarities to Rose, I only realized many years later why I really chose him as a teacher: Mobley held a fount of fresh argu-ments—the fresh arguments I needed for the ongoing battle between my longing for surrender and my terror at losing control.

I was terrified that letting go would only mean letting myself go, and that surrender would surely lead to the raving madness of some nameless nightmare: a nightmare as horrific as selling one of my own brothers to cannibals in exchange for a few hours of dreamless sleep.

*　*　*

When I reached Monck's Corner, South Carolina, I took a left at a stop light and traversed the last few winding miles to Mepkin Abbey on picturesque country roads pockmarked by small, whitewashed, African Methodist Episcopal churches. I was wondering whether I made a wrong turn when a sign for Mepkin Abbey appeared. I followed a two-lane road for several miles, passing a huge stand of renewable timber that a road marker said belonged to the monks. I finally came to a black-on-white sign on my right that said "Mepkin Abbey."

The gate was open, and I suddenly found myself on a long, straight, deserted road, dappled by gently rippling shadows cast by two apparently endless rows of ancient live oaks heavily laden with gray Spanish moss. This vista was so inviting I involuntarily hit the brakes, killed the engine, and sat there in the shadowy stillness breathing it all in.

The overarching oaks created a living tunnel of swirling branches that seemed to stretch off into eternity, and with a bemused half-smile I wondered if Jay's White Light might be patiently waiting at the other end for a world-weary wayfarer like me. It felt like I was straddling a magical threshold with one foot still earthbound by earthly cares while the other had left the world behind.

Just then two gray squirrels darted from the trees and started chasing each other in circles in front of my car. This broke the spell and I slowly continued on my way. At the other end of Mepkin's shadow-strewn driveway I was greeted by a sign in the free-form shape of a featureless Trappist monk pointing the way toward the guest center.

The center was a log style building with a full-length elevated porch. It was closed for the day, but a note taped to the door instructed me to ring the tall free-standing bell at the foot of the steps. I gave the woven lanyard a couple of yanks and was startled by the pealing of the bell as it rudely interrupted the pervasive monastic silence.

Several minutes later I heard rustling in the gardens to the left of the guest center as a Trappist monk emerged from a narrow, almost invisible path I hadn't noticed before. He was about sixty, slightly stooped, with gray thinning hair, kindly blue eyes, and a huge smile that couldn't be anything but Irish.

"You must be Augie," he said gently.

"Yes," I replied, nodding.

"I'm Brother John. Welcome to Mepkin. We're so glad to have you."

Chapter Sixteen

MEPKIN AND MEREDITH

The detail of the pattern is movement,
As in the figure of the ten stairs.
Desire itself is movement
Not in itself desirable;
Love is itself unmoving,
Only the cause and end of movement,
Timeless, and undesiring
Except in the aspect of time
Caught in the form of limitation
Between un-being and being.
—T.S. Eliot[34]

Brother John climbed into my car, and we retraced my tracks back to Mepkin's oak-lined main road. Turning left, we slowed for a round-about with a statue of Jesus in the center. The circle's first exit veered right to the monastic farm, the second led to the Luce Gardens directly ahead, and the third toward the monastery proper on our left. We took the farm road for a half mile or so until we came to Saint

Benedicts, one of several retreat houses tucked into the monastery grounds. Saint Benedicts was a tidy brick ranch with a grassy front yard and shaded veranda sprinkled with wooden rocking chairs.

"We inherited this house from the Luce family," Brother John told me while opening the unlocked door as I tagged along with my luggage. "It housed some of the staff who kept up the grounds, especially the garden. The Luce family cemetery is in the garden, so we do our best to keep it up for them."

"Wow, Brother John, these are magnificent accommodations. Is it all for me?"

"Josh insisted we give you the VIP treatment," Brother John said with a laugh. "He's a wonderful young man, and we're so blessed to have him."

Brother John handed me a trifold outlining the monastic schedule, told me the main meal of the day, dinner, would be served right after noonday prayer, and then humbly apologized for having to hurry off. I walked him as far as my car and offered a lift, which he politely declined. Then, by way of goodbye, he said, "You know, businessmen often come here on retreat. Sometimes they are so exhausted we never see them. They just sleep the entire time. We don't mind. If that is what they need, we're happy to provide it."

As I watched his slightly stooped shoulders stride briskly back toward the monastery, I couldn't help but wonder whether my haggard face was the inspiration behind his offhand comment.

Stowing my gear in one of the bedrooms, I took a seat on a rocking chair and began sifting through my first impressions. Most palpable was the monastic silence heavily seasoned by the piquant salt air wafting up the

Trappist silence was not just absence of sound: it was an almost animate presence peacefully enshrouding the entire monastery in a soothing mist of tranquil serenity.

Cooper River from Charleston. Trappist silence was not just absence of sound: it was an almost animate presence peacefully enshrouding the entire monastery in a soothing mist of tranquil serenity.

As I sat basking in Mepkin's glow, I recalled a hot summer evening long ago when all ten Turaks were gathered around the supper table waiting for my father to begin grace. Suddenly my mother jumped up and turned off the oven fan. I didn't even realize the fan was on, but instantly my shoulders relaxed as my pent-up tension drained away. In a similar fashion, it seemed as if Our Lady of Mepkin had just switched off some existential oven fan that had been anxiously churning away in the pit of my stomach for as long as I could remember. Mepkin, I decided, was like some numinous nexus or naval of the cosmos, that mythical place where Heaven and earth meet.

I was still dreamily preoccupied when a series of echoing bells reminded me that noonday prayer, or Sext, was starting, and dinner would soon be served. Leaping to my feet, I hurried off on foot toward the bells.

The monastery proper was laid out in a horseshoe shape. The black metal-roofed buildings, frescoed with a sandy shade of cement stucco, gave the Abbey a Spanish flavor. A flavor perfectly suited to a South Carolina landscape strewn with majestic live oaks dripping with gray Spanish moss amid frond-laden Palmetto trees. The main entrance was a covered breezeway with the monastic offices and adjacent library on the right and the refectory or dining hall on the left. Attached to the refectory at right angles was the senior wing and infirmary for the monastery's aged and infirm. In the right center of the open end of the horseshoe, seventy yards from the breezeway, stood the church. Its steps were shaded by a towering live oak with one massive limb resting comfortably on a red brick wall like some ancient, arboreal Methuselah, with his hoary head and beard, grizzled with Spanish moss, propped up on an elbow lost in thought. About four feet tall, this "cloister wall" bracketed the steps leading to the main entrance of the church. Behind this brick facade, on a bluff overlooking the Cooper River, were the single-story, stucco-clad dormitories for the monks. As a retreatant, I was free to roam the monastery and use the main entrance of the church but was not otherwise permitted behind this cloister wall.

There was barely time to take this in from the breezeway before the bells on the tall, free-standing belfry beside the church began tolling again, and a single file of monks slowly emerged from a side entrance. Leading this measured "cloister walk" of about thirty monks to the refectory was a tall, handsome, dark-haired, vigorous-looking man in his late forties I later learned was Father Francis Kline, the abbot. Unlike their youthful leader, most of the monks were bearded and gray, but right in the middle of this solemn procession was Josh in his gray monastic surplice shorn of most of his wavy blond hair!

After a delicious vegetarian meal eaten in silence as one of the monks read aloud from a book chosen by the abbot, I met with Josh for a few minutes before he hurried off to his afternoon work assignment. It was great to see him, and he seemed to radiate that serenity I heard so profoundly over the phone back in Raleigh.

"Hey, what happened to your hair? You look like Delilah caught you napping and clipped you into a clean-cut businessman," I said. "That must be the surprise you promised me."

Josh told me that Mepkin's barber, Brother Boniface, a German-born monk of almost 90, was so determined to test his skills on a full head of golden hair—a unicorn-like rarity in a monastery with an average age of 65—that Josh finally took pity on him.

"Brother Boniface is hilarious," Josh said. "He is so bent over with spinal arthritis he can barely shuffle let alone walk. But he never stops smiling and cracking jokes. He's not only the barber, he bakes the bread too. That's what's so amazing about all these guys. They're so positive no matter what. Anyway, Boniface sits behind me in church, and he kept teasing me about my hair, so I finally let him cut it."

I spent the afternoon wandering the monastery grounds and sitting on a high grassy bluff overlooking the Cooper River as it lazily made its way toward the ocean. After a light supper at five, I arrived at the church for Vespers well before six. Rather than the Gothic architecture I expected, it was a bright airy building modeled on a French village church with huge beams buttressing a high wood-paneled ceiling surrounded by circular pane glass windows. As I entered the sanctuary through glass-paneled doors from the vestibule, I came to a dark gray, almost black granite altar slightly elevated on a platform of the same material. On the other side of the altar, in the middle of the aisle, was a stone, freestanding, holy water font murmuring softly in watery prayer as it was continually refreshed. Instead of pews, beyond the font, on either side, were two elevated tiers of square oaken stalls facing each other across the aisle, the back tier one step higher than the front. After the stalls was a lectern, and beyond it a celebrant's chair under a massive crucifix facing the granite altar near the entrance.

Even though I was fifteen minutes early, many of the monks were already in their places deep in prayer. As I blessed myself with holy water, a monk motioned me toward one of the stalls, reserved for retreatants, slightly separated from the monks. As I took my seat, he quickly prepared my place with a marked Psalter and hymnal so I could participate in the service. Then, as he was about to return to his stall, he suddenly hissed in my ear, "The chapel is open all night!" Completely taken off guard, all I could do was nod knowingly as if this was the answer to my most fervent prayer.

At the stroke of six, the bells pealed. The monks stood, bowed to the altar, and the prayer leader sang out, "Oh God, come to my assistance!" The entire community took up the refrain, "Lord, make haste to help me!" A tingle ran up my spine. It was my first service at Mepkin, my very first prayer, and these supplications made me think of Hugh's prophecy at the gym: If the hell he foretold was going to be anything like the nightmare I went through in the hospital after my skydiving disaster, I wanted all of God's help I could get.

The rest of Vespers was magical. The brothers recited psalms set to Gregorian chant back and forth across the aisle while occasionally singing a hymn or reciting a standardized prayer. Twenty minutes later I was so caught up in the mood I didn't notice that one of the monks was at the lectern reading from Scripture until he was well into it.

" . . . and the Lord God came to him and said, 'What are you doing here, Elijah?' And Elijah replied, 'I have been very zealous for the Lord God. The Israelites have rejected your covenant, broken down your altars, and put your prophets to death with the sword. I am the only one left, and they are trying to kill me too.' And the Lord said, 'Go out and stand on the mountain and wait; for the Lord God is about to pass by.' And a great and powerful wind tore the mountains apart and shattered the rocks before the Lord. But the Lord was not in the wind. After the wind, there was an earthquake, but the Lord was not in the earthquake. After the earthquake came fire, but the Lord was not in the fire. And after the fire came a still small whisper. And when Elijah heard this, he pulled his cloak over his face and went out and stood at the mouth of the cave as God passed by."

Without warning, I completely broke down. Overcome, frightened, and deeply embarrassed by my inability to control myself, I rushed from the church. The next thing I knew I was wandering around in the parking lot in front of the monastery desperately trying to regain my composure. Looking up, I saw a hooded, slightly bent monk 50 yards away walking briskly down the road from the traffic circle toward the monastery. Apparently mesmerized by a spot on the ground just beyond his feet, he didn't glance left or right, but when he came abreast of me, he suddenly pivoted on his heel and strode straight for me. Before I had time to wonder why he wasn't at Vespers with his brothers, his wide unblinking eyes were only inches away, staring effortlessly into my own. His black cowl barely concealed a full head of tangled gray hair and his smooth, wrinkle-free face was as white as snow. His feverish eyes glittered with a wild manic light that seemed to insistently be asking me a deeply personal question.

Stunned, it was all I could do to mumble, "Uh, uh, my name is Augie Turak. I'm a retreatant. A friend of Josh's."

My cloistered grand inquisitor wasn't satisfied. He just kept silently staring as if—not interested in merely my name, rank, and serial number—he was minutely scanning my soul. Thoroughly flustered, I reidentified myself again and again, to no avail, as his ice blue eyes burned right through me.

Then, without saying a word, he turned on his heel and briskly strode away leaving me shuddering. I felt naked, completely exposed, and even when I later found out that this mysterious monk was Father Benjamin, an aphasic Alzheimer's patient on one of his last unsupervised strolls, it did nothing to allay the prophetic sense that, when asked to answer for my life, I was unable to do so.

I recall only one other incident from my first visit to Mepkin. I was in line at dinner behind a slowly shuffling monk with a bent back and long gray beard who was clearly well into his eighties. As he painfully and painstakingly stooped for a tray stacked knee high below the serving counter, I noticed a trace of foot-tapping impatience welling up inside me until he suddenly turned and handed me his hard-won tray with an impish air of childlike delight. This tiny act of selflessness seemed to encapsulate everything right about Mepkin and everything wrong with me.

* * *

Despite these unsettling experiences, or more probably because of them, I returned to Mepkin several times over the next few months. Then I wrote to Brother John, who headed the Abbey's Monastic Guest Program, about spending several weeks over Christmas as a guest. I was accepted, and as an MG I would live and work alongside the monks as a temporary member of the community wearing the same gray-hooded surplice I saw Josh wearing.

When I applied to Mepkin to visit at Christmas, I was still working at RGI and running the SKS even as my depression and feelings of foreboding continued to deepen. There were two upticks in my down market, however. Dave Gold was now facilitating the SKS meetings at North Carolina State and the University of North Carolina, leaving me with only Duke and the adult SKS meetings to worry about. And at Duke, I had Meredith.

Meredith—the same Meredith who looked at me with so much compassion in her bright green eyes after my skydiving accident—was now president of the Duke SKS. One brisk October evening during the fall of 1996, she was walking me to my car after our weekly SKS meeting as she often did to discuss organizational matters. As we were passing the tall Gothic spires of the Duke Chapel and noisily scrunching our way across a campus quad choked with dry leaves, Meredith told me that Duke offered "house courses" for credit. If a faculty member agreed to sponsor the course, and the syllabus was approved, anyone could teach one. She asked me to teach a house course in the upcoming winter semester.

My initial reaction was utter fatigue. It was taking all the energy I had just to keep up appearances—and not very well at that. I was sleeping twelve hours a night and waking up dead tired and deeply depressed. Despite my guilt over smothering Meredith's initiative— the very initiative I was always complaining the SKS membership lacked—I decided to beg off without hurting her feelings.

"Sounds like a great idea, Mere," I said. "But what about our regular SKS meetings?"

"We'll have the house course on a different night, and if you don't want to lead the regular meetings, I will."

"Getting approval sounds like a lot of paperwork, and I don't have time—"

"I've already submitted the paperwork," she said without blinking.

"But I still have to find an advisor and do a syllabus. I don't know whether—"

"I already have a faculty advisor," she breezily replied. "And I sketched out a syllabus. All you have to do is fill in the blanks. We'll knock it out in no time."

"But to make it worthwhile," I doggedly continued, "we'll need fifteen students who—"

"That's what I thought you'd say," she interrupted. "Any more than that and we lose the intimacy. I've already got fifteen and a few alternates in case somebody backs out. It's seven boys, eight girls, and I told them they still have to attend the regular meetings so we don't lose our momentum there."

Suddenly she was grinning in triumph at the gobsmacked expression apparently glued to my face. Game, set, match. Once again, I'd been completely outmaneuvered by this 20-year-old sophomore the other kids worshipped and affectionately called The Boss.

"Well, looks like I'm teaching a house course," I finally said. "And I appreciate the fact that for once you went to all the bother of making it seem like I ever had a damn thing to say about it." Then we were laughing so hard tears ran down our faces. It had been so long since I really laughed my face hurt.

* * *

Within the space of six months, Meredith became indispensable to me. She was not only the go-getter I always dreamed about for the SKS, she was my right-hand man and confidant. I didn't dare make the slightest decision at Duke without consulting her, and when I did, she was always two steps ahead of me. She was a straight-A student, spoke fluent Spanish, played the acoustic bass, and when she decided it was time to trade in my decrepit old car on a new one, she showed up at my condo unannounced and dragged me by the ear to the dealer. There she astutely asked so many technical questions and knew so much about prices that she ran the sales rep in circles until he finally turned to me and said, "Christ, where'd you find this girl?"

Meredith was so quietly charismatic that the other kids competed to do her bidding just for the pure fun of it. She never raised her voice, wasted words, or chewed anyone out. Instead, she relied on a tiny trace of disappointment in her bright green eyes or the slightest whiff of chilly aloofness to send shivers of shame down the spines of feckless slackers—including my own. Meredith was so popular and gifted at promotion that a typical SKS meeting of fifteen or so was now regularly attracting forty students.

One time, as Meredith was walking me to my car, I happened to mention my mother, who passed away twelve years earlier, in 1984. Suddenly she burst into tears. Flustered, I asked her why she was crying and, flustered herself, she blurted, "But it's all about your mom! Everything is! Don't you see? I mean, oh . . . I don't know what I mean." Turning beet red, she burst into tears again. Baffled and embarrassed by her outburst, I told her she must be thinking about her own mother, but as I drove from Durham back to Raleigh, I couldn't shake the eerie feeling that Meredith was trying to tell me something important she couldn't quite articulate. It was as if there was a disconnect between her heart and her head, and what her heart made her say, her head couldn't comprehend.

This happened so often and was so disconcerting that one time, probably to dispel my own anxiety, I teased her about it. I told her she was my Pythian Oracle of Delphi incoherently blurting out, under the influence of sacred fumes, arcane prophecies that made no sense and too much sense all at the same time.

"You know, Mere," I laughingly told her, "one of these days I'm going to sit you down in a chair and force you to tell me in the Queen's plain English everything you know about me and my destiny."

She just stared and said nothing, but my joke so obviously hurt her that I immediately regretted it, and yet it was as if her anguish was further evidence for all I was intimating.

Of course, the one thing I was too terrified to share with Meredith or anyone else was the deepening depression inexorably dragging me down. I was afraid to tell anyone because, just like with Rose and those "little jolts of energy," I was afraid that sharing my terrible secret would trigger some tidal wave of despair I could no longer resist.

* * *

My first Christmas at Mepkin was initially uneventful, which was exactly the tonic I needed, at least temporarily, to stabilize me. Brother John walked me to my room behind the cloister wall and I was touched to see "August Turak MG" on my door. My quarters looked like a small room in an inexpensive but squeaky clean motel. There was a single bed, a rocker for reading, a desk and chair, a free-standing lamp, and a small, recessed closet with a cloth curtain for a door. The floor was carpeted, I could control the room temperature, and it came with a private bathroom, a couple spare blankets, and a Bible on the bookshelf. It was perfect.

At 3 AM two alternating chimes sounded in my room to wake me for the 3:20 service of Vigils. Vigils were followed by thirty minutes of meditation in the church and then the discipline of Lectio Divina (divine reading) in our rooms until Lauds at 5:30. At 6 AM breakfast was served, then more silent contemplation until Mass at 7:30, followed shortly afterward by Terce at 8:20. All services except Mass followed the general pattern of chanting psalms, singing hymns, and scriptural readings. After Terce, it was time for work, and the monks lined up in the small "chapter room" inside the church as Brother John assigned the day's work. Besides noonday prayer and Vespers, there was also a short service called None conducted in situ at our places in the refectory right after lunch. Finally, there was Compline at 7:35 in the evening. At the end of Compline we sang the Salve Regina followed by the Angelus. The entire community was then sprinkled one by one with holy water by Dom Francis, and we went off to bed just in time, or so it seemed, for the chimes to go off at 3 o'clock so we could do it all over again.

Except for Sundays and holy days when there was no work, this was the unvarying pattern. Once the romance of wearing a habit wore off, I found the rigorous schedule demanding, but the challenging routine was more than offset by the rewards. Little by little the psalms and prayers worked their way into my brain, driving out the more mundane concerns I brought to Mepkin with me. After a week or so the monotonous rhythm actually seemed to pick me up and carry me along like a spiritual surfer riding a 1,500-year-old wave. Like Eliot's "still point of the turning world," Trappist time also seemed to simultaneously speed up, slow down, and stand still, and try as I might, I could never seem to recall whether some biblical text I found myself pondering came from Lauds that morning or Vespers three days before.

On my first day, I lined up after Terce with the other monks for my work assignment. When I got to Brother John he lit up, lightly touched me on the arm, and gently whispered "Eggery." Then he thanked me so warmly it felt as if I must be doing him a personal favor. It was moving . . . and humbling.

The Trappists are officially the Order of Cistercians of the Strict Observance (OCSO). Trappist is actually a nickname that traces its roots back to the Cistercian monastery of La Trappe in France. Founded in 1098, the Cistercians in turn are an offshoot of the Benedictines (OSB), and they still adhere to the arduous sixth-century Rule of Saint Benedict. The Rule is founded on the twin principles of *ora et labora*—prayer and work—and the work aspect of the monastic charism requires each monastery be self-supporting.

In 1996 Our Lady of Mepkin (all Trappist monasteries are officially named for the Virgin Mary) was supporting herself by selling the eggs from forty thousand chickens, and Brother John had just assigned me to work in the eggery, or grading house, where all those eggs were processed.

Borrowing a bicycle from the monastery's fleet, I set off in the cool salt air for the eggery. The grading house was a long concrete block building located just beyond Saint Benedicts, the house where I spent my first retreat. Inside was an interwoven series of serpentine conveyor belts and suction cups that washed, checked, graded, and packaged the eggs as they made their way to local restaurants and grocery stores. Brother John soon arrived and told me with a smile that the machinery was so antiquated that spare parts were now as rare as, well . . . hen's teeth. He then flipped a switch and the antediluvian machinery huffed and puffed itself to life with a metallic roar. Brother John put me to work as "the loader," and I was soon feeding cardboard trays of twenty-four freshly harvested eggs onto the conveyor one after another while scanning each egg for the occasional crack. I had just decided that the noisy contraption reminded me of the Wizard of Oz describing the Tin Man as a "clinking, clanking, clattering, collection of caliginous . . . " when I felt a tap on my shoulder.

"Hi, I'm Brother Nicholas," boomed a lanky monk with a gray beard, fierce blue eyes, and a Cleveland Indians baseball cap with half the brim sliced off. "You know, all I want for Christmas is a hatchet I can bury in Father Malachy's head! Welcome!" Then he burst into throaty peals of laughter at the stunned look on my face before taking his place on the line. Father Malachy turned out to be a kind and gentle monk in his eighties with a beaming, beatific brow more deserving of obeisance than the sharp head of a hatchet, and as I came to know and love both monks, I eventually realized that even godly Trappists must have their pranksters like Brother Nick, who couldn't resist a little humorous hazing at the expense of a monastic rookie.

Monotonously loading trays of eggs onto a conveyor belt day after day gave me plenty of time to think, and as one week, then two, slipped away, I eventually got around to thinking about why I was at Mepkin in the first place. It was almost a year since my skydiving accident, and it was stone cold clear that nothing I was doing on my own was helping. My accident shattered me as well as my ankle, and ever since I'd been reduced to a shell-shocked observer helplessly watching life's meaning ooze through the cracks in my soul like the yolk from one of Mepkin's mortally wounded eggs I occasionally plucked from a tray and discarded. I was way over my head and needed help.

So, screwing up my courage, I asked Mepkin's charismatic young abbot, Father Francis, if I could speak to him privately. Several days later I arrived at his office anxiously hoping I could tell him my story without humiliating myself in the process by going to pieces.

Despite the fact that Father Francis lived, prayed, and worked in the closest possible proximity with his brothers at Mepkin, they held their vigorous, youthful-looking abbot in such high regard it bordered on awe. Though he was kind, affable, always polite, there was something so lofty and refined about him that he seemed unapproachable even though he was not. Father Francis had been a childhood prodigy on the organ, and by the time he graduated from the prestigious Julliard School of Music in New York, several of his Bach recitals had been simulcast nationwide, and he was already sitting on a recording contract with a major label.

Then, still in his early twenties, he shocked everyone by "throwing it all away" by entering the Trappist monastery of Gethsemani in Kentucky.

In the early 1990s Francis was elected Abbott of Mepkin, and besides playing the organ at services, he spoke several languages, wrote music and books, and was passionate about art, architecture, and environmental issues. He was also a gourmet chef who was as comfortable cooking a meal for the community or helping with the chickens as he was raising the money he used to rebuild the monastery.

Dom Francis studied theology and philosophy in Rome, and I eagerly looked forward to his homilies for their depth, but best of all, as Brother Stephen, Mepkin's lovable prior (or second in command), whispered almost conspiratorially to me one day, "Francis is a mystic, you know." The word *holy* is woefully out of fashion and, in any case, not one I would lightly use, but for Father Francis it is the only word that will do.

Despite my stint in New York working around celebrities with MTV, I was a little starstruck by Francis, and when I showed up for our first private meeting, I felt a little guilty for taking up his time. While not lavish, his office was roomy and brightly lit with a desk facing two chairs on one end and a sofa, coffee table, and two easy chairs at the other. Francis motioned me toward the sofa, and as he settled into one of the chairs, I took a big gulp and, by way of an icebreaker, said, "You're not going to holler at me, are you?"

Dom Francis laughed out loud.

"Listen, if I was going to holler at you," he said, "I'd be sitting on one side of the desk and you'd be on the other. The sofa is reserved for good people and friendly conversations."

I spent hours anxiously preparing my speech, but when Francis implied I was "good people" worthy of his time, I instantly became emotional, forgot it all, and just blurted, "Father Francis, I don't know what's happening to me. I feel like I'm falling down a deep, dark shaft in an elevator that's broken loose from its cables. Every once in a while the elevator seems to catch on something and comes to a screeching stop. For a minute or two I just huddle in the corner with my chest heaving. Then I take a deep breath and try to psychologically get to my feet, but as soon as I get to one knee, the elevator breaks loose, and I plunge again."

Backing and filling in a disjointed way, I eventually managed to fill Francis in on my skydiving accident, my experiences in the hospital, my spooky encounter with Hugh at the gym, my inexplicable reactions to the prophet Elijah during Vespers and, afterward, Father Benjamin in the parking lot.

"I know it sounds crazy because it sounds crazy to me, but it's like none of this stuff is an accident. I mean, it's like there's something behind it all that's trying to swallow me up. There's even this girl, one of my students, and she keeps knocking me off balance with crazy stuff too. I can't stop thinking that, maybe Elijah sent Father Benjamin, or maybe Hugh was trying . . .

"Father, I don't know what I'm saying. Maybe I'm just cracking up."

I took a deep breath, wiped my nose, and waited for Francis to say something. But he just continued to sit quietly with a serene look on his face that clearly said: Go on, I'm listening. So I continued to gush.

"I used to joke with my SKS adult group that if I was not careful, I'd soon be getting cryptic messages from the television. Then about four weeks ago that's exactly what happened. I was flicking through the channels and landed in the middle of this old movie from the '40s called *David and Bathsheba.* I only caught this one scene, maybe five minutes, but it hit me so hard I cried for a week.

"Father Francis, I went thirty years without crying at all. I couldn't even cry at my mother's funeral. Now I cry all the time and at the slightest things, and I end up utterly exhausted, ashamed, and more depressed than ever. Worst of all, I don't even know why I'm crying. I'm crying right now, and I don't know why."

Eventually what sounded to me like a long, self-indulgent jeremiad just petered out. Dom Francis got up, pulled me to my feet, and gave me a hug. Then he smiled and said, "My God, are you ripe!"

He told me that in the monastic tradition my depression was called *acedia*—a period of spiritual dryness where we feel listless and abandoned by God.

"The incessant weeping is not unusual either: it's called the Gift of Tears. Mystics like Saint Theresa associated the Gift of Tears with 'compunction'—the feelings of guilt, shame, and remorse we experience as we face the truth about ourselves. It seems to me that is what your encounter with Father Benjamin triggered. It was like looking in a mirror.

"But you must hold your ground and never lose heart. I know what you're going through right now feels like anything but a blessing, but if you hang in there and never lose faith, I know God will eventually answer your prayers.

"On a practical level, I notice you've been volunteering for extra work. That's good spiritual therapy. Stick with it. But above all, Augie, trust the process. The monastic tradition is a 1,500-year-old process that has helped thousands of people like me and you. Trust that process."

Just being in Francis's presence made me feel much better. I asked for his blessing, and as I was leaving he told me he would ask Mepkin's former abbot, Father Christian, to "work with" me. He said Father Christian was "a good man" and said it with so much feeling I was moved.

Two days later I arrived at my choir stall for Mass and found a note from Father Christian. He asked me to meet him in his office during the hour after Vespers and before Compline when the general rule of silence was relaxed so private conversations could take place.

While I'd never spoken to Father Christian, he was so remarkable I'd been watching him closely for some time. He was a small, lean, slightly bent man in his late eighties with a shaved head and a long white beard who seemed to burn with an unquenchable intensity like a human version of the biblical burning bush. Despite his years and spare frame, there was nothing feeble about his stride; no matter where he was heading, he seemed on a mission to get there and nowhere else. Christian had PhDs in philosophy, theology, and canon law, and when he was the celebrant at Mass, I always enjoyed his homilies for their no-nonsense tone and keen intellectual insights. If Father Francis epitomized holiness, Father Christian personified piety. He ate almost nothing, was always the first to arrive for a monastic service, and he never slipped into idle conversation. Even his quick, purposeful walk seemed to be the "Do Not Disturb" sign of a man utterly absorbed in prayer and the contemplation of matters too weighty to share.

Every night after Compline, instead of retiring, I noticed Christian retreating all alone to the small chapel off the main sanctuary. One night, from curiosity, I followed and found him kneeling on the hard ceramic floor in front of the tabernacle with his forehead touching the floor and his arms outstretched. Kneeling in the rear pew, I watched him through a dancing halo of flickering candlelight, almost hoping for the slightest movement. But when fatigue and sore knees finally overcame fascination and forced me off to bed, he was still prostrate and utterly motionless, more like a timeless vision of ceaseless prayer than a flesh-and-blood human being.

* * *

I arrived for my meeting with Father Christian downright intimidated. Francis only seemed unapproachable, but from what I could tell, Christian, with his gruff severity, actually was. He greeted me politely but formally, motioning me into a plain wooden chair while pulling up another for himself. "You like poetry, don't you?" he asked. Startled by this opening, I hesitated for a moment and then nodded.

"Thought so," he said through a tight smile. "You been watching me, but you didn't know I've been watching you, did you?" Without waiting for my answer, he reached for a plain sheet of paper on his desk and handed it to me. On it was a poem by Gerard Manley Hopkins, a nineteenth-century poet whose work I was unfamiliar with. Father Christian asked me to read it aloud.

My own heart let me more have pity on; let
Me live to my sad self hereafter kind,
Charitable; not live this tormented mind
With this tormented mind tormenting yet.
I cast for comfort I can no more get
By groping round my comfortless, than blind
Eyes in their dark can day or thirst can find
Thirst's all-in-all in all a world of wet.

Soul, self; come, poor Jackself, I do advise
You, jaded, let be; call off thoughts awhile
Elsewhere; leave comfort root-room; let joy size

286

At God knows when to God knows what; whose smile
's not wrung, see you; unforeseen times rather – as skies
Between pie mountains – lights a lovely mile.[35]

When I finished, Father Christian nodded and growled, "What's your exegesis?"

"This poem is me!" I stammered without thinking. "I just keep hammering and hammering at myself, and I'm so exhausted."

"I know," Father Christian said softly, and with so much warmth, that I instantly realized I'd just met one of the wisest, kindest, most compassionate people I would ever know.

Chapter Seventeen

PROPHETS AND MTV

Men's curiosity searches past and future
And clings to that dimension.
But to apprehend
The point of intersection of the timeless
With time, is an occupation for the saint—
No occupation either, but something given
And taken, in a lifetime's death in love,
Ardour and selflessness and self-surrender.
—T.S. ELIOT[36]

Eventually I managed to reiterate for Father Christian the same strange disjointed story I offered Father Francis a few days earlier. From behind steepled fingers, Christian listened patiently while nodding occasionally or absently stroking his long gray beard.

When I finished, he smiled grimly, gave both armrests a sharp rap with the heels of his palms, and exclaimed, *"Deus Absconditus!* You're being purified through suffering."

In answer to my obvious bewilderment, he reached for a heavy, well-worn, Oxford dictionary, which, perfectly in keeping with a man of his erudition, he kept cheek by jowl with his ancient Underwood manual typewriter. Licking his fingertips, he riffled through the pages until he found the entry he was looking for.

"*Deus Absconditus.* The apparent absence of God from those who seek him, or from dire circumstances where the godly are in extreme trouble."

Closing the battered tome almost reverentially, Christian returned the volume to its place on his plain vanilla, yellow pine desk and, swiftly switching gears, asked me to elaborate on the movie I briefly mentioned to him and Father Francis, *David and Bathsheba.*

"I saw that movie," he said. "It's from the late '40s or early '50s if memory serves. Gregory Peck plays David, and Susan Hayward, Bathsheba. Back then I was a Franciscan teaching seminary and still slothfully taking in a show now and again," he added through a half smile. "Tell me about it."

I was momentarily taken aback by what seemed like a strange take-away from a long story, but gathering my thoughts, I haltingly began.

"It was . . . it was, I don't know, about six months ago, Father. I was aimlessly flipping through TV channels when I stumbled on a scene near the end."

David and Bathsheba are alone and amorous, I continued, when Bathsheba playfully hands David his lyre and asks him to sing her a few of his psalms. A cloud passes over David's face, and he tells Bathsheba he no longer plays or sings because God abandoned him long ago, and without God his psalms lost all their beauty and meaning. Instead, his hymns became a torturous reminder of all he'd lost.

Hearing a commotion, David descends the palace stairs only to be confronted by his abandoned wife Micah, their young son Absalom, and an angry mob led by the prophet Nathan. Nathan denounces David for murdering Uriah because of his unnatural lust for Uriah's wife, Bathsheba. The famine wasting Israel and killing his people, Nathan proclaims, is God's retribution for David's sin.

Ashen-faced and overcome with guilt, David rushes from the palace and into the tent where the Ark of the Covenant is kept. Falling to his knees, he tells God he knows his sin is far too great to be forgiven. He asks God to spare the people by taking his own life instead. David, however, has one final request: he asks God to let him relive, for one dying moment, what it felt like when he was a boy and walked with God. Then he reaches for the Ark of the Covenant knowing full well that no man can touch the Ark and live.

Just as his hands touch the Ark a pyrotechnic explosion fills the screen, and a beautiful boy appears. He is walking alone through the mountains tending his sheep when a supernaturally tender masculine voice calls, "David . . . David . . . David . . . "[37]

My voice caught in my throat, but Christian merely leaned forward sympathetically and, with a nod, urged me to continue.

"All at once, Father, tears were streaming down my face. It was so agonizingly beautiful it was almost more than I could stand. Then the scene changes and Nathan is anointing the kneeling David by name as he pours sacred oil over his head and lets it roll down over David's ecstatic face. I began crying harder. Frightened, I turned off the TV, clenched my eyes and fists and tried to stop crying. But effort had the opposite effect: my crying became convulsive, and suddenly I was floating above my body, utterly detached, calmly watching myself cry with morbid fascination. It was like . . . I don't know, it was like watching myself speaking in tongues or something."

When I finally stopped crying, I told Christian, I was utterly hollowed out. I was exhausted and the room seemed alive and shimmering. Like a dazed soldier knocked forty feet in the air by a shell blast, I anxiously began checking myself. I seemed all right, but beyond feeling so drained and frightened, I felt incredibly vulnerable. It was like some invisible hand effortlessly slipped through all my defenses, grabbed me by the scruff of the neck, and shook me half senseless.

"But then, over the next week or so, Father, at the oddest of times, I would hear 'David . . . David . . . David' coming from everywhere and nowhere, and I would go to pieces all over again. I had to pull my car over to the side of the road one time until I could get control of myself. When these experiences finally subsided, all I remember is a profound sense of relief."

I became emotional in the retelling, and Father Christian waited until I regained my composure. Then he calmly said, "I thought so. The last piece of the puzzle. It ties everything together."

Baffled by this opaque comment, I waited for an explanation.

"Let's look at each event in turn," he said. "First, we have your story about King David. Then your emotional reaction to the story about Elijah and God passing by, followed by your encounter with Father Benjamin in the parking lot.

"David is a prophet. Like him you are experiencing *Deus Absconditus,* the loss of God. And again, like him, you are nostalgically longing for a time in your own youth when, like our second prophet, Elijah, you experienced your own version of God passing by. Father Benjamin completes our prophetic triptych: he's Nathan prophetically confronting you for whatever you did or didn't do. The grave sin, so to speak, that you blame for your divine abandonment and spiritual desolation. Finally, also like David, you're convinced that your sin is unforgivable and irredeemable. It's too late for you, and that's why you incessantly torture yourself.

"But I don't want to assume too much. First of all, does any of this make sense? If I'm not too far off, can you recall a specific incident or period of your life that fits the profile?"

I was so dazzled by Christian's concise speech and breathtaking analysis that for a full minute I was unable to respond. Not only did his observations make sense, they were so obvious I couldn't imagine how I missed them. Yet what terrible sin could I have possibly committed that sent not one or even two but *three* weapons-grade prophets on a mission to kick my ass? Once again, my stomach churned with the sickening sense that the walls were closing in, and Stephen King's time-munching Langoliers were greedily nipping at my heels.

I eventually managed to tell Father Christian about my experience in Rose's kitchen in the summer of 1973 and how Rose described it as "the coming of the Lord."

"Father Christian, God passed by so closely I could practically feel his breath on my cheek. It was so intimate it was almost like—yeah, it was almost like—He was calling *me* by name. This revelation left me with such an overwhelming spiritual hunger I dropped out of college, broke up with my girlfriend, and spent years like some late-modern Israelite wandering around in the American desert looking for more. But then . . . I don't know, Father. Then . . . "

"Something went wrong," Christian interrupted with a wry smile, "and now the bottom is out of the tub."

"Yes, Father, and I've been driving myself half-crazy since my skydiving accident trying to figure out what it was."

Christian glanced at his watch, and I realized those infernal Langoliers had chewed through our precious time together. Compline was looming, so I asked for his blessing. Before he graciously complied, however, he gave me an assignment.

One reason why so much of Trappist prayer life takes place before dawn is because, in those wee hours, the mind is not completely awake, and the ever-vigilant ego is still half-asleep. It's in this twilight state, Christian said, that the ego leaves its psychological defenses lightly manned. He told me to slowly reread the story of Elijah in the spirit of *Lectio Divina*, passively inviting the story to "read me" rather than actively trying to "grasp" the text.

"Let the story wash over you until you slip into something akin to a waking dream," he said. "Then, just let the Holy Spirit take you wherever you need to go."

This predawn suggestion made abundant sense. It also came with a healthy pinch of guilty salt, one too embarrassing to share with Christian. So far, all my efforts at early morning contemplation had come to grief. I kept nodding off to sleep and, for the first few days after meeting with Father Christian, much to my chagrin, this pattern continued. I would slowly begin reading the story, but a few seconds later, or so it seemed, I would awake to the sound of chimes summoning me back to church for Lauds or to the refectory for breakfast.

Eventually I did manage to hold onto this twilight state of Rosean "betweenness" for a few minutes at a time, but all I earned for my efforts was a frustrating blizzard of trivial thoughts and shadowy images. Then one morning, just after Vigils, I decided to switch things up by retreating to the chapel rather than my room. There, alone among flickering candles and the vestigial vibrations of a prostrate Father Christian perpetually absorbed in prayer, I slowly began repeating a text that by now I knew by heart.

"*. . . Then the word of the LORD came to him, saying, 'What are you doing here, Elijah?'*"[38]

For some reason, almost like a Yogic mantra, I began repeating, "What are you doing here, Elijah?" As I sank deeper into reverie, the reverberating words took on a life of their own.

"What are you doing here, Elijah?"
"What are you doing here, Elijah?"
"What are you doing here?"
"What are you doing?"

* * *

I awoke with a start with my head throbbing and the fluorescent lights over my head blazing away like klieg lamps searing my eyes. I was momentarily disoriented, but then I recalled that I was lying on my back on the carpeted floor of my spacious, well-appointed office on the 28th floor of 1133 6th Avenue in tony midtown Manhattan. Reaching under my head I felt for the balled-up jacket of my bespoke, custom-tailored, Paul Stuart suit which, according to the wall clock, I'd unceremoniously wadded into a pillow only a few minutes earlier. My untimely awakening was apparently occasioned by my office phone buzzing incessantly.

Dragging myself to my unsteady feet, I picked up the phone and growled, "What is it, Sheri? I thought I asked you to keep everybody out of my office and hold my calls."

"Yeah," she coolly replied through her heavy Brooklyn accent, "but there's a woman on the phone. She's from Sammons Communications, so I thought you might want to take it."

Jeannie did work for Sammons but, unbeknownst to Sheri, it was not a business call. This shapely young woman was flying in to spend the weekend with me. We met at a cable TV trade show and, after subsequently spending four splendid days with her in sunny southern California, I reciprocated by inviting her to New York.

Jeannie was boarding her connecting flight and would be landing at LaGuardia in a couple of hours. I breezily told her to take a taxi to my apartment on East 77th Street between York Avenue and the East River, and I would leave money with the doorman to cover the fare. I knew damn well that any guy with even a modicum of propriety would be at the airport to meet a terrific girl like Jeannie, especially on her first trip to the City, and that tiny tinge of timid disappointment I heard in her voice suggested we were of like mind on the subject. But lovely Jeannie was far too sweet to say more, and I was just too tired and, by now, probably too spoiled to really give a tinker's damn.

I collapsed in my chair and tried to sweep the mental cobwebs away long enough to take stock of my situation. I was in one of those classic man-about-town fixes that eventually made being an "upscale" single "yuppie" guy in New York City in the early 1980s legendary—and notorious. To wit, I'd been awake for almost forty-eight hours, and now a spirited young lady was arriving in short order, fully—and more than justifiably—expecting to spend the next few days sleeplessly and romantically skipping the light fandango to the up-tempo staccato strains of the Big Apple's trendiest boutiques, bars, bistros, theaters, galleries, museums, and exclusive nightclubs.

In sympathy with my still-throbbing head and sensitive eyes, I got up and shut off those painful overhead lights. It was after five o'clock in the late autumn of 1981, and as I returned heavily to my chair I gratefully noticed through my floor-to-ceiling office windows that it was already dark outside. All I wanted was to sleep for a week, but as I buried my pounding head in both hands all I could think was: *My God, what the hell am I going to tell Jeannie?*

My troubles began innocently enough the night before with a surprise birthday party for my assistant, Sheri, who, strange to say, I was also dating on and off at the time. I was living in The Pavilion, a posh building on New York's fashionable Upper East Side, and, as part of her surprise, I filled both bathtubs with ice and stocked them with bottles of Moet & Chandon champagne. Like clockwork for a Thursday night in the city that never sleeps, half of hard partying New York showed up more than ready to mingle, nosh catered hors d'oeuvres, and quaff liquor and free champagne. Then, around midnight, rather than winding down, the party found its second wind when several denizens of some Madison Avenue ad agency injected "toot," or powdered cocaine, into the flagging festivities.

The next thing I remember is stepping out onto my balcony overlooking York Avenue for some air only to be greeted by the first rays of dawn rising over the East River and remorselessly ricocheting down the plate glass front door of a rowdy, preppy bar called Swells directly across the street. Rushing inside, I found Sheri and said, "What time is it?"

Alarmed by the look on my face, she anxiously glanced at her watch and, now equally alarmed, said, "Oy vey! It's 6:20 in the morning!"

"Oh my God, Sher, I got that big presentation to the *New York Times* at 10, and I invited a couple of our top executives to help close the deal. There's no time to wait on a company cab. Here's some cash. Catch a taxi to your apartment, shower and change, and meet me at the office at 8 so we can pull everything together."

Ninety minutes later we arrived at the office still a trifle tipsy and utterly strung out. Somehow my presentation to the *Times* went well, so exceedingly well, in fact, that at noon, Jordan, one of our executives, leaned back in his chair, rubbed his hands together, and said, "Guys, we're making great progress. It would be a shame to stop now. What's say we order in lunch and keep the ball rolling?"

Oh my God, no! I thought. *I'm dying. I barely made it this far!*

We sent for lunch and, against all odds, I managed to hold my own until, sometime after 4, I got back to my office, told Sheri to keep everyone out, closed the door, turned my expensive suit jacket into a trifold pillow and dozed off . . . only to be awakened a few minutes later by Jeannie on the phone.

Precious minutes were slipping away and I had to get moving if I wanted to stop at Zabar's for some gourmet snacks and still beat Jeannie back to my apartment with enough time to straighten up a bit. I rose from my desk with the best of intentions, but instead of heading uptown I put one foot up on the windowsill behind my chair, folded my arms across my chest, and gazed out my 28th floor window at majestic midtown Manhattan, its panoply of skyscrapers all lit up and sparkling like a bevy of diamond-bedecked debutantes dressed to the nines and heading out for a night on the town.

Ordinarily I found this powerful scene intoxicating, but this time I was overcome with wave after wave of melancholy, a melancholy so blackly exhausting that it robbed me of my impetus to rush off to Jeannie. The feeling was depressingly familiar, but before I could muster the energy to probe for its source, I heard a voice so close at hand it seemed to be coming from my own right ear:

"Yeaaaaaah, it ain't easy bein' Augie Turak."

Wrenching my head toward the source, I was greeted by the profile of my friend, colleague, and occasional madcap coconspirator, Mark. He was only inches away and mirroring me to a tee with his right foot propped up on the windowsill and his arms folded identically across his chest. He didn't deign to glance in my direction as he just placidly stared out the window. I was stunned, but before I could wonder how he managed to slip into my office undetected and assume his mimicking pose right under my nostrils, he resumed his speech.

"People look at Augie Turak and see a guy with the world by the ass. Why the hell not? He's a single hotshot, working for the coolest company on the planet, makin' big bucks, livin' it up on the company's dime in the most exciting city in the world. Chicks dig him too. He ain't bad lookin', and all they see is dollar signs, big cigars, and motor cars.

"But what they don't know, can't know, will never know, is Augie Turak is a spiritual guy trapped in exactly the kind of materialistic, superficial, soul-killing lifestyle he is supposed to loathe. No one cares. No one understands. No one suspects the heavy price he's paying as he fritters away his spiritual birthright on this mess of decadent pottage we call MTV: Music Television. He's gradually selling his soul to MTV on a layaway plan, and deep in his heart he knows that someday this devilish debt to the devil will come due. So that's why he's standing here in the dark with a mouth brimming with brimstone-flavored ashes, staring out the window and feeling so damn sorry for himself. Hell, can you blame him? I feel sorry for him too. In fact, if you stop to think about the tragic sacrifice he's—"

"Mark," I roared in mock anger, no longer able to restrain myself. "You dirty bastard! That's incredible. You nailed it perfectly. How in hell did you do it?"

Mark didn't say anything. He just let that impish smile playing on his lips get wider and wider until we both doubled over laughing so hard that in my woozy condition I almost fainted. With effort, Mark gradually regained a semblance of control. He was trying to say something that, try as I might, I couldn't quite make out.

* * *

I opened my eyes. The tall, flickering candle flames were still frantically dancing to the silent rhythms of their own secret rhapsody. I couldn't tell whether I'd been gone for a few seconds or half an hour. I also had no idea whether I'd been asleep and dreaming or whether my flashback to my time at MTV was one of those reveries or "waking dreams" Father Christian told me about.

Regardless, yet another damn prophet, Mark, had just conclusively answered my question: I now knew exactly *when* the bottom fell out of my spiritual tub. It was at MTV that I finally let down, sold out, and decisively lost my longstanding argument with the world. It was at MTV that I gave up, gave in, relaxed my grip, surrendered, let myself go, and betrayed my solemn promise, to the man who gave me *Isis Unveiled*, to "never forget." It was at MTV that, overcome by worldly fatigue, I fell spiritually asleep only to be roughly reawakened fifteen years later by the sharp crack of my ankle being compound-fractured. Only this time, as Rose had so deftly foretold all those many eons ago, I woke up screaming.

Now, as Mark prophesied on a dark November evening in 1981, it was time to pay back the devil for the David-like sin I considered unforgivable, the grievous and irredeemable sin of lost years and lost time. The devilish debt of lost years, lost time, and lost innocence that I knew in my heart could *never* be repaid.

Overcome with guilt, I jumped up and stumbled outside. It was still pitch-dark and deathly quiet and, heedless of the bitter December cold, I staggered out through the breezeway toward the Luce Gardens

299

and the Luce family cemetery. As I did, my painful litany of self-reproach and self-contempt gave way to white hot rage fueled by self-justification and self-pity.

Sure, I thought as I sat down on one of the polished limestone walls framing the long row of Luce family gravestones. I now knew how, where, and when the bottom fell out, but what about the *why? Why did I do it? Why did I ignore Mark's admonition when I knew damn well he was right?* Ignoring his prophetic warning, I instead just accelerated my headlong, hedonistic plunge into a lifestyle of power, pleasure, and privilege in a desperate and ultimately doomed attempt to blot it all out. Why?

When I first arrived in New York, my partnership with Mobley's protégé quickly fell apart. Lonely and broke, I wandered the City's streets, accompanied only by the plaintive "Going out?" proposals I coolly elicited from dark doorways sheltering forlorn street walkers whose icy affections I couldn't afford even if I was so inclined. Eventually, as they got to know me, even the dismal doorways ignored me as I sank deeper into despair.

So when, out of nowhere, I got the chance to join the nascent company that later launched MTV, I jumped at it and held on for dear life.

So yeah, I angrily told myself, *I surrendered all right. But for a host of damn good reasons.* I sold out because I was sick and tired. Sick and tired of being poor, sick and tired of celibacy, sick and tired of being alone, sick and tired of being a stranger in a strange land, sick and tired of watching everyone get on with their lives while I was nothing but a prodigal son. A lost soul, an outcast, a wastrel wasting away in a godforsaken wasteland, a latter day Ishmael wandering around in a Rosean wilderness of ever-decreasing concentric circles like some asinine donkey stubbornly pursuing a spiritual carrot I was obviously not good enough to ever taste.

Most of all I was fed up with an adamantine God who was either implacable, non-existent, or, most probably, simply no longer interested in a loser like me.

But I couldn't keep raging for long. Soon the freezing cold welling up from the seat of my limestone-seated pants chilled my anger as well. By the time I got back to my cozy room behind the cloister wall, I knew damn well there was nothing and no one to blame but myself for my weakness and spiritual failure.

Chapter Eighteen

A MENTAL MELTDOWN

Descend lower, descend only
Into the world of perpetual solitude,
World not world, but that which is not world,
Internal darkness, deprivation
And destitution of all property,
Desiccation of the world of sense,
Evacuation of the world of fancy,
Inoperancy of the world of spirit;
This is the one way, and the other
Is the same, not in movement
But abstention from movement; while the world moves
In appetency, on its metalled ways
Of time past and time future.
—T.S. ELIOT[39]

By any sane assessment my initial reluctance regarding Meredith's
pedagogical opportunity at Duke University was sound. When I re-

turned from Mepkin in January 1997, I was far too fragile to be taking on the added pressure of teaching a course for credit.

This became abundantly clear when, a month into the course, Meredith arrived unannounced at my office in Raleigh. It was Valentine's Day, and I thought it was just like her to drive over to hand-deliver a valentine. However, Meredith didn't even mention Valentine's Day. Instead, after awkwardly fidgeting for a few moments in one of my mismatched office chairs and self-consciously clearing her throat, she told me the course . . . was blowing up in my face. Several disgruntled students were about to drop out, she said, and one, whom Meredith's deep throat refused to identify, was threatening to take their complaints to the administration. I was devastated by the news and the thought of letting Meredith down, but I covered it up by angrily threatening to preempt the student cabal by pulling out myself. Meredith said nothing. She just stared at me wide-eyed and then left.

Closing my office door behind her, I sat down heavily at my desk and anxiously tried to figure out what to do. Deep down I knew from the very first class that I was in over my emotional head, but I was either too scared or too depressed to admit it. Instead, I overcompensated for my vulnerability and waning self-confidence by falling back on a drill sergeant, martinet mentality. I adopted a strict, no-nonsense approach for the course, heavy on reading, testing, Socratic questioning, and little else. I quickly realized some of the students were disappointed and slightly miffed at my heavy-handed methods, but I rationalized it was just the grumbling in the ranks that every good boot camp engenders.

Now things were spiraling out of control, and as I sat slumped behind my desk, a wave of utter exhaustion hit me so hard it knocked me flat. Once again, as with Rose, I felt woefully unappreciated and unfairly maligned. Besides facilitating the regular SKS meetings and teaching the course pro bono, I was driving to Duke every Saturday to meet each student privately to get to know them better. Now, rather than gratitude for my Saturday sacrifices, I was facing a rebellious disaster instead.

I began going over these private conversations looking for instigators, and the prime suspect was Mary Anne. Going into the class I knew very little about Mary Anne beyond the perpetual scowl she wore that seemed to be inspired by her cordial dislike for me. She never spoke in SKS meetings, sat as far from me as she could, and treated me with such chilly disdain I avoided her whenever I could. She was so pitifully thin and pale she seemed chronically ill, and when I mentioned this to Meredith, she told me Mary Anne suffered from such a wide variety of allergies that her doctors had her on a vegan diet of little more than dry grains and raw vegetables. I eventually decided the only reason she attended SKS meetings was because she worshiped Meredith, but then, for reasons I couldn't fathom, she signed up for the house course as well.

When it was her turn to meet with me one Saturday, I dreaded the encounter. So, apparently, did Mary Anne. After barely saying hello, she threw herself into one of four plastic swivel chairs surrounding a blue Formica table in the crowded student union cafeteria, sullenly wrapped her arms around her chest and, with an arched eyebrow, practically dared me to start the conversation. Without thinking, I blurted, "Mary Anne, why are you so angry?"

For a second or two she just looked at me in stunned surprise. Then she launched into a bitter denunciation—not of me, as I expected, but of her father. Mary Anne hadn't spoken to her father, a doctor, since her parents' divorce. Now, she said, he was retaliating by refusing to cover her college tuition. Consequently, it looked as if she would have to leave Duke for a less expensive school back in Ohio. On and on she went, breathlessly excoriating her father for a plethora of pusillanimous sins but especially her parents' divorce. As she did, I sat utterly shell-shocked by how much venomous vitriol was lurking behind such a soft voice nestled in such a frail body. Then, after wiping away a few wayward strands of brown hair with the back of her wrist, she derisively polished the old man off.

"Worst of all, during the divorce he just sat in the living room crying like a baby night after night. He was so pathetic; I utterly despised him. It served him right, and I'm really mostly angry with myself because I still don't have the guts to tell him exactly what I think of him."

During her torrential tirade I never said a word, and when our time was up, she slung her Duke Blue Devil backpack over one shoulder and stood up. "Thank you so much," she said as her fingers danced excitedly on the seatback of her chair. "This has been so good. I feel so much better. Now I know what I have to do. I have to call my dad and tell him how angry I am with him."

But just as she said "how angry I am with him," I spontaneously superimposed the words *"how much you love him"* right on top of hers. For a moment or two we stared at each other in mutual astonishment. Then Mary Anne flushed beet red, her gray eyes flashed, and she stormed out of the cafeteria.

I had no idea where my unauthorized redaction of her final sentence came from or how I managed to time my "love" to so perfectly overlap her "angry." As soon as she left, however, I immediately regretted my verbal virtuosity. Though I felt I inadvertently blurted out the right advice, I was also convinced that Mary Anne came to our meeting irritated with me and left stone cold furious: she confided in me, but rather than the sympathetic encouragement she was counting on, I betrayed her confidence by confronting her instead.

Replaying this incident in my head as I sat stewing in my office, I decided Mary Anne was the student most likely to take the complaints to the Duke administration. Our next class was the following evening, and I frantically explored my options. Should I bring things to a head by revealing what I now knew? Just ignore the student complaints and forge ahead? Pull out?

Suddenly I was too depressed to think about it. Besides, I was running late for my appointment with Paul at his office several miles away.

Paul was a blond-haired, blue-eyed, six-foot-six giant of a man. Four or five years my senior, Paul was a bit of a hero for me. He was happily remarried with two grown sons from a previous marriage and, as a serial entrepreneur, he'd built and sold a number of technology businesses. He owned a couple of horse farms and only worked half-time so he could spend the other half stalking grizzlies in Alaska, hunting elk on horseback in the Colorado high country, or crisscrossing the country on high end Harleys with his sons. While I had no interest in hunting, Paul seemed to balance his vocation and avocations in just the way I wanted to.

Besides, Paul was my beau idéal of a man's man who exuded self-confidence, was always in control, and never gave himself away. He was famous throughout the Research Triangle Park business community for his poker face and tough negotiating skills, and I was deeply flattered when he offered to invest in a joint venture with RGI. While Paul and I never discussed personal matters or met socially, we liked each other, and I always looked forward to our meetings as a way to get out of the office for an hour or so as we discussed our joint venture, Paul's latest outsized adventure, and all the local business gossip.

However, as soon as I walked into Paul's spacious office on that bleak February day, I knew something was wrong. Instead of rising to greet me, he sat listlessly staring out the window for such a long time I became uncomfortable. Finally, he turned to me and, without any preliminaries, told me he recently discovered his wife was having an affair. She was stealing money from the family for her lover and her wayward son from a previous marriage, and for the next hour he added so many other sordid details his litany of betrayal seemed endless.

As I listened, I was shocked by the change I saw in Paul. His poker face was gone, replaced by so much raw anguish I half expected him to melt down at any moment. At first I tried to comfort him but then, without warning, the room began to swim, and I became terrified I was about to melt down instead. Not only was I shocked to find my hero was only human, my empathy for him seemed to open me up to the suffering of the entire world, and this collective sorrow locked my head in a vise so tight I felt as if I couldn't breathe. I felt so much absolute pain and absolute helplessness it threatened to overwhelm me.

The next thing I remember is staggering back into my office at RGI with the world still spinning crazily all around me. On my desk was a valentine. Without thinking I opened it hoping for distraction. It was from my ex-girlfriend in New York: a young woman I was madly in love with but who eventually called off our relationship because I wasn't Jewish. She subsequently married, and we'd spoken only a few times in fifteen years. Besides the normal Valentine sentiments, she asked me to call as soon as I received her card.

I called, and before I knew what was happening, she was telling me how unhappy she was and offering to leave her husband if I would take her back. While infidelity was not involved, her story was even more upsetting than Paul's because I still had feelings for her, and she was so desperate and so desperately lonely. Somehow, I gently told her I was not interested and managed to calm her down a bit, but when I hung up the phone, something snapped.

Moments later I was standing in front of my desk. My business partner, Jay, was apparently trying to tell me something but, try as I might, I couldn't seem to make out what he was saying. His face was a swirling blur, and his voice was floating in and out like a radio station gradually drifting out of range.

Suddenly Jay stopped dead and said, "My God, Aug. Are you all right?"

I shook my head. Then I broke down. Jay rushed out of my office and came back with Dave Gold, but no matter what they said or did I couldn't stop crying. Dave grabbed me by the arm and said, "Let's go to the gym." I meekly followed him out the door.

For a while we silently lifted weights together. Dave finally smiled and said, "Well, your bench press sucks, but you look a helluva lot better." Then he put his hand on my shoulder and, softly imitating Rose's West Virginia idiom and accent, said, "Aug, I think you're all wore out. You're just all wore out." This trivial diagnosis delivered with so much kindness struck me as the most beautiful thing anyone had ever said to me. I threw my arms around him and shocked myself by saying, "Dave, I love everybody. I love everybody—and I just can't stand it."

The next morning I woke up a broken wreck. I was supposed to teach at Duke that evening, but the very thought of facing hostile students in my shattered condition terrified me. When I got to the office, I reached for the phone to call Meredith and cancel the class. But then I hesitated.

Sure, I can cancel this class, I thought as I slowly returned the phone to its cradle. *But what about next week? If I don't feel better, will I cancel again? Then cancel the course? Then what, cancel my life?*

A realization hit me so hard it sent my head spinning: I was *committed.* There was only one direction left for me: forward. It was as if my entire life was one gigantic V lying on its side stretching out over time, and now all the million and one options I explored and choices I made had irretrievably funneled me to this one microscopic point at the base of the V. It all came down to *this* day, *this* class, *this* decision. I felt compelled to show up for class no matter what.

I spent the rest of the day trying to prepare something to say, but all I managed to do was barely beat back incipient panic. When I arrived for class, I was only sure of one thing: I was about to break down in front of these kids. I was certain that if any of them still nursed any lingering doubts about reporting me to the administration and getting me kicked off campus, I was about to dramatically remove those doubts once and for all.

I sat down heavily in a chair and watched the students silently file in and take seats in the circle. Mary Anne came in and, without a word, took the chair right next to mine. *Oh, shit,* I thought. *She's clos-*

ing in for the kill. She doesn't have the guts to tell her father off so she's planning to tell me off instead. Then, just as class was about to begin, I startled myself yet again by leaning over and whispering, "I hope I don't remind you of your father tonight, Mary Anne."

Then I took a deep breath, turned to the class, opened my mouth, and waited for what would come out. Within seconds my voice was cracking. Then I was openly weeping. I told them I'd been coming apart ever since my skydiving accident. I told them I didn't know what was happening to me. I told them I was terrified for myself and terrified of them. I knew I was letting them down, letting Meredith down, letting my friends in the SKS down, letting everyone at RGI down, and in a way I couldn't understand, letting the whole world down. I begged them through tears to forgive me. I told them about panicking in the hospital; about Hugh's baleful prophecy at the gym; about Vespers at Mepkin and how Elijah drove me reeling from the church only to be confronted in the parking lot by a ghostly monk with haunting blue eyes. I told them about *David and Bathsheba*, about Meredith's shocking visit the previous day, and Paul's gut-wrenching story. I told them about my ex-girlfriend in New York, about going to pieces in front of Jay, and about Dave Gold's touching diagnosis. I told them I loved everyone, that my heart was broken, and that my father never told me he loved me. Then I marveled out loud that all this heartache came to a head on, of all days, Valentine's Day. I told them dozens of other things I can't remember while insisting that everything happening to me was not just meaningful, but so incredibly meaningful it was turning my life into a crazy hall of mirrors made up of endless worlds within worlds within worlds threatening to swallow me up.

On and on I rambled, weeping uncontrollably. There was no chronology, timeline, analysis, or attempt to link cause with effect. I never finished a thought, sentence, or story before leaping to another or retracing my steps and, as I listened to my own half-mad acid rap, I was buffeted again and again by the feedback loop of my own horror.

But I was committed. I couldn't stop even if I wanted to, and I was too damn tired—and too damn tired of faking it—to want to.

Then, just as suddenly as it all began, it was over. I just sat there, my chest heaving with my eyes on my lap. Eventually I looked up and was amazed to see the students still there, wide-eyed and staring at me. Not one had fled from shame, horror, or disgust, as I was certain they would. But I couldn't tell what they were thinking either. For a full two minutes we just stared at each other as something hung in the balance by the thinnest of threads.

Then Ed, a freshman from Pittsburgh, of all places, began speaking. He told us about his father's drinking, his mother's depression, and how, in the face of all this, his younger sister was becoming ever more remote and unavailable to him or anyone else. Soon he was gushing through tears that he loved his family so much, but there didn't seem to be anything he could do, and he felt so helpless and guilty about it. Finally, he stopped speaking and just sat there sobbing.

> Like a tongue of Pentecostal flame, it hovered over each student in succession, bestowing as it went its gift of tongues: the universal language of human suffering.

Then, as if on cue, another student picked up where he left off, and when she broke down, another stepped up.

I suddenly realized the spirit, or "voltage," of a Rosean experience was swirling around the room. I could almost see it as, like a tongue of Pentecostal flame, it hovered over each student in succession, bestowing as it went its gift of tongues: the universal language of human suffering. For the next ninety minutes, time stood still as one student after another told his or her story.

There was so much honesty and courage in the midst of so much raw pain that it took my breath away. All I could do was weep along with them.

Then the clock restarted, the class was over, and students were hugging me and thanking me as I was thanking them while everyone was hugging and crying and thanking each other. The whole room seemed lit up with a supernatural glow of joy, peace, gratitude, and indescribable relief. Eventually I collapsed in a chair from sheer exhaustion. As I did, Mary Anne shoved a folded piece of notebook paper into my lap and rushed from the room. She was dry-eyed, and only then did I recall that only she had not spoken up or hugged any of her classmates. Fearing the worst, I opened her note while trying to imagine how I was going to explain everything she just witnessed to some stuffy, chronically risk-adverse, college administrator.

"Aug, you did remind me of my dad tonight—because of your sincerity. When my dad cried, he cried out of so much pain and disbelief that his life was crashing down around him. I had to create something—some blindfold so I wouldn't see that and recognize that that is what I am hiding from myself. I'm going to call him tonight and tell him I love him—because I FINALLY, FINALLY, know I do. Thank you. Mary Anne"

* * *

I once saw an episode of the sci-fi TV show *The Twilight Zone* where an ordinary man on his way to work tosses a nickel into a paperboy's box for the morning paper only to watch it inexplicably land on its edge and stay that way. Soon all sorts of supernatural things start happening until, on his way home, he tosses another nickel for the evening paper and knocks over the first nickel the paperboy had been carefully guarding all day long. When the first nickel falls, everything reverts to normal.

In some strange way my chaotic speech at Duke was a nickel tossed by a desperately ordinary man into a room full of kids, a coin that somehow came to rest on its edge. After that extraordinary evening, the course just took off and swept us all along with the power of its own momentum. Acting on intuition, I threw away the syllabus and asked the students to write up a short paper to be read in class. I told them to write whatever the spirit moved them to write. The results were astonishing: each week the class went deeper and became more intense. The spirit, or voltage, showed up every time we met, and it was as palpable to the students as it was to me. This psychic manifestation gradually became so familiar that, bizarre as it sounds, I think we all took it for granted. However, it did present one difficulty: the students found themselves at a loss when peers and family members asked them what the hell the course was "all about."

For the rest of the term, it was as if we were all living in a magical slipstream or in Eliot's "still point of the turning world." Every hunch or idea anyone suggested was not only spot-on but came prepackaged with all the skills and enthusiasm needed to be flawlessly, effortlessly, executed. For example, some of the students started a musical group called The Zen Pickers. Meredith came up with a couple of university vans, and I took the class to Mepkin Abbey for a retreat. Then the students decided to perform Thornton Wilder's *Our Town* for their parents and the campus at large, and in three short weeks they rehearsed, promoted, and presented *Our Town* with so much poignant intensity that the audience, too moved to applaud, reacted with stunned silence.

Then, as if this unusual audience reaction was not only anticipated but scripted, the students spontaneously sat in a circle on the floor, held hands, and wordlessly led a packed house in an impromptu meditation. Only afterward did the applause come, and when it did, it was deafening. Meredith, of course, played the lead as Emily, and as I sat with her mother, I don't know which of us was prouder.

When the semester finally wound down, I hosted a party to celebrate all we went through together. Mary Anne arrived with a mystery guest: her father flew in just for the party! After watching The Zen Pickers perform, I went into the kitchen to prepare some food, but I was soon drawn back to the living room by the beautiful singing of an a cappella duet. There I saw Mary Anne and her father, arm in arm, singing "Amazing Grace."

Later I was alone in the kitchen when Mary Anne's father walked in. Through tears he said, "I just want to thank you from the bottom of my heart for what this class has done for my daughter, for me, and for all these kids."

Just after the party, Mary Anne's allergies disappeared, and within six months she regained all the weight she needed and looked great.

In the end, so much happened in and around that course that I couldn't see how the students stayed in school, but when I occasionally asked about it, they just smiled and told me that their other courses were going "just fine."

* * *

Yet despite all this, when the course ended and that edgy nickel finally fell over, I was more hollowed out than ever. I was utterly drained. I'd been crying or fighting back tears for months, and somewhere along the line I forgot about eating. I lost twenty-five pounds during the course, and it left me looking gaunt and haggard. I was useless at RGI, and my guilt was exacerbated by the fact that I recently began taking a small salary to cover my living expenses. It was as if the incandescent spotlight of the house course just made everything else seem that much darker.

One day toward the end of the course, I received an email from a student asking if she could have some time at the next class to thank everyone. Just as I was succumbing to her warm, uplifting gratitude so beautifully expressed, I read this:

What I never told you or anyone else is that for the last two years I've been constantly thinking about suicide and came close to it twice. And because of this class, I no longer am. That's the real reason why I want to thank everyone.

Suddenly the golden glow of gratitude I was leaning on was kicked out from under me. The thought that this lovely young woman and straight-A student was suicidal, and I didn't notice, was so painful I couldn't separate my horror and remorse from my joy that she no longer was.

Several weeks later this same student invited me to her violin recital at Duke. Sitting with her parents and siblings, I was astounded by how radiant she looked in her short blue dress and how well she played. But when I glanced over at her ecstatic parents, I recalled they had no idea their daughter had been suicidal. Their happy, loving faces beaming so proudly at their imaginary daughter playing her violin like an angel fingering her celestial harp was almost more truth than I could take. I didn't blame her parents; in fact, I liked them very much. I was even grateful they would now never have to know the truth. But in her parents I also saw myself—I saw us all—blindly living lives full of so much willful self-deception and delusion that even our most joyous times rely on purposeful ignorance. Watching her parents watching her play her violin, I found their blissful lack of awareness almost more tragic than her suicidal ordeal, and this crazy juxtaposition was excruciating.

The house course generated so many of these heart-rending combinations of joy, gratitude, and anguish that I came to describe the course as "awful": it was so terrible and yet so full of awe.

By the end of the course, if it occurred to me, I would have described my reaction to it and my own prospects in much the same way a young woman from South America described hers in this two-paragraph essay called "Popping Amaranth" that the "spirit" moved her to write and read to the class.

When this class first began, I didn't take it seriously. I observed it like a child examining a new toy. However, I am truly impressed with the heat this class has produced, the pressure it subjects upon itself. Perhaps I may still seem like an unattached observer, but it is no longer true. I walk home after every class with tears streaming down my face, touched.

One time I tried to pop amaranth, an ancient Aztec grain, at my friend's house. Amaranths are the tiniest little grains, and we poured them into the popcorn popper. It was so incredible to hear the first kernels popping and then watch them bounce all over the kitchen. We laughed so hard; it was just so beautifully unexpected. A couple of weeks ago this memory came to me, and I realized that this is how I feel about this class. It is so incredible to watch people turning inside out, revealing their rippled white core, breaking out of shells. But the question still remains: Have I popped? Or am I a lone kernel, left at the bottom, unsuccessful and unpopped?[40]

Rather than alleviating the darkness and providing a resolution, I came away from the course feeling as if I merely survived an immediate crisis. I was enjoying a momentary reprieve like a storm-tossed ship that finds temporary sanctuary in the pacific eye of an Atlantic hurricane. Baffled by these persistent feelings of dread and dark foreboding, I shared with the SKS adults one Friday evening the metaphor I related to Father Francis.

"I feel like I'm stuck in a free-falling elevator plummeting toward God knows what," I said. "Once in a while, this tomblike elevator 'catches' on something like Mepkin Abbey or the house course and screeches to a stabilizing halt. But then, just as I start thinking maybe the worst is over and begin climbing unsteadily to my psychological feet, the elevator breaks loose and, *whoosh*, I plunge again."

Chapter Nineteen

DEMONS AND A NEAR DEATH EXPERIENCE

The dove descending breaks the air
With flame of incandescent terror
Of which the tongues declare
The one discharge from sin and error.
The only hope, or else despair
Lies in the choice of pyre or pyre–
To be redeemed from fire by fire.

Who then devised the torment? Love.
Love is the unfamiliar Name
Behind the hands that wove
The intolerable shirt of flame
Which human power cannot remove.
We only live, only suspire
Consumed by either fire or fire.

—T.S. Eliot[41]

"The house course was fantastic," I told Dave Gold one day at the RGI office. "But I'm still terrified. Before I was vainly trying to swim against the current, but during the course something snapped. Now I'm passively being swept downstream. But I still have no idea where the current is taking me, and I know there are still deadly waterfalls just up ahead."

The waterfall was not long in coming. I just didn't expect it to be an actual waterfall cascading into a designer swimming pool.

Anxious to carry the mood of the house course into the summer, a student named Diane invited us all down to her parents' place in Florida for their annual Fourth of July party. Most of the kids signed on for the expedition, but I initially refused. I was too worn out, and besides, I'd just be out of place. But Diane and the others begged me to come. They said it was a great chance for some well-deserved R&R, and, touched by their concern, I finally relented.

The students were caravanning by car to Florida, but I drew the line at joining them and flew down on my own. I also rented a car and motel room rather than bunking at Diane's parents.

Diane's mother and stepfather were both fortysomething doctors, but I soon decided their true vocation was partying. They lived in a sprawling two-story house, and their oversized pool, boasting a ten-foot waterfall, was guarded by an outdoor, outsized refrigerator stocked with plenty of beer for anyone who might stop by. And stop by they did. People from all over town seemed to have a key to the house, and at all hours they would plop down beside the pool and crack a beer whether the owners were home or not.

Diane's stepfather, a cardiologist, worked incessantly while her mother staffed an ER two days a week. The rest of the time she apparently spent bar-hopping in her bright red, open air, two-seater Jeep Wrangler. Along the way she'd accumulated an assortment of blue-collar male friends, including some rough-looking customers. I'd done my share of hard partying, and I could still enjoy a few beers once a year or so, but there was something about the whole fraternity house vibe that made me uneasy and sad. I tried to write it off to my own fatigue and melancholy, but even though I can usually mix gregariously with anyone, I found myself avoiding Diane's parents and their friends and spending most of my time with the students or just reading a book by the pool.

On the Fourth of July, I arrived late for the party. Ed, the student from Pittsburgh, and I had become close, and we spent the day sitting around the pool at my motel talking about our shared passion for golf. When we finally got to the party, it was already in full swing. Most of the students were busy inhaling the vodka Jell-O shots they playfully manufactured the night before. Then, around eleven or so, Thomas, Meredith's boyfriend, rushed up to me.

"Augie, come quick," he said. "Meredith is crying hysterically, and we can't get her to stop."

"Has she been drinking?"

"No, she hasn't been drinking at all."

Ed and I rushed to her side, but she wouldn't let anyone touch her, and she was crying so hard I was alarmed. Finally, she gushed, "There was this guy . . . he dove into the pool naked . . . and I thought it was you!"

She eventually realized it wasn't me, and besides, the man was actually wearing a flesh-colored bathing suit, but, she stammered, she still couldn't stop crying. Baffled, I lamely suggested she had me up on a pedestal. Maybe seeing a guy she thought was me pulling such a stupid stunt was just her way of bringing me back to earth. But this analysis, rather than providing the fig leaf of comfort I hoped for, only made her cry harder. Then, suddenly, she said, "No, no. Can't you see? They're going to strip you *naked*!"

By now I knew better than to ask for an immediate explanation for one of her oracular outbursts, so we all just waited around for her to calm down, which eventually she did.

Later I was sitting by the edge of the pool, listening to the waterfall and chatting with a woman whose daughter was off dancing with

Ed. I heard voices behind me, and swiveling my head skyward I saw two of Diane's parents' rough-looking friends looming over me. They were very drunk, and I asked them what they said. "You heard us, you pedophiliac motherfucker," one of them sneered. "You have about five seconds to get your pervert ass out of here or we're gonna' carry you out feet first." At first I thought they were drunkenly joking, but when it became clear they were not, I told them I was a guest of Diane's parents.

This only produced malevolent laughter, and the other one said, "Shit, man, you must be fuckin' hard of hearing. It's Diane's father who wants your pervert ass out of here, and he sent us to get it done. Now we ain't askin' you. We're tellin' you for the last fucking time: Get your sicko ass outa' here! *Now!*"

I staggered to my feet in a haze of disbelief and stumbled toward my rental car parked in front of the house. My familiars followed, one on either side, cursing me as a "fucking sicko, pedophile, pervert" at the top of their lungs. When I got to my car, five or six other men, including Diane's stepfather, were waiting, their drunken, sallow faces hideously distorted by the halogen halo of a single streetlight. The verbal abuse from the first two men was now abetted by cruel, sadistic laughter from the others. I felt like I was surrounded by demons from Dante's lowest circle of hell—except rather than pitchforks, a few of these infernal creatures were sporting baseball bats. It was something right out of a redneck movie, and I was quite certain that if I threatened to call the cops, one of these drunks would stagger forward and flash his badge.

I just wanted the hell out of there, but then I remembered that Ed drove my rental car to the party and still had the keys. Looking around, I saw one of the students and sent him off for Ed. As I waited, one of my original tormentors repeatedly danced up to within inches of my face bobbing and spinning like an oversized imp.

"Please," he slurred as spray from his drunken lips splattered my face, "I'm beggin' you. Take a swing at me! Just give me an excuse to kick your mother-fuckin' pedophile ass!"

Apparently frustrated by my reluctance to take him up on his offers, he told me if I ever stepped foot across the Florida state line again, he would kill me and feed me to the local alligators, a murderous threat that seemed to strike the others, including Diane's stepfather, as the funniest thing they ever heard.

Just then Ed came rushing up out of the darkness. Taking everything in at a glance, he whispered, "Well, whataya' say, Aug? Do we fight?" This unexpected show of support against such long odds from a kid I knew for a fact was never in a fight in his life hit me harder than anything that had happened so far. But I also wasn't going to put his life at risk defending me.

Shaking my head, I managed to grunt, "No. Let's just get the hell outta here."

I was too shattered to drive, and when we got back to my motel, Ed insisted on staying the night just to keep an eye on me. The next morning, I booked the first flight back to Raleigh. By the time I got to the airport, I felt so fragile and violated I remember anxiously thinking if anyone so much as bumped into me, I would melt down and vanish.

When I got home, I stayed in bed for two whole days, utterly depressed.

* * *

For the next week I just wandered around in a stupor trying to catch my emotional breath. Beyond the obvious reasons for my shell-shocked reaction, there was so much shame. Until Ed volunteered to fight, I felt nothing: no fear, no anger, no indignation. Just a horrifying, bottomless *nothing*.

I tried to chalk up my cowardly paralysis to good sense and self-restraint in an impossible situation, but I couldn't pull it off. Ed was willing to fight, and I used to be the kind of man who, without hesitation, would've waded into those bastards even if I was killed in the process. But I was obviously no longer that man, and I felt so ashamed I was almost sorry they didn't kill me.

But the guilt and shame were so overwhelming that even cowardice couldn't account for it. So I continued to replay the incident until one day I was sitting in my office when suddenly all those redneck allegations of sexual deviancy somehow hit a nerve. Their false accusations tripped a trigger, and in a single instant the shame and guilt from every sexually illicit thought, fantasy, dream, and one-night stand, as well as my tryst with a friend's wife, came raining down on my head.

Yet, in that very same instant, I felt betrayed: something sinister used the magic of the house course to rip me wide open just so I could experience all this shame and guilt without a single defense mechanism to buffer it.

That's it, I thought. *I was stripped of most of my defenses by the house course just in time for those guys in Florida to finish the job.* Then I remembered Meredith's crying jag and her prophetic warning: "They're going to strip you naked!" And this realization on top of everything else hit me so hard that, for a moment, I thought I was going to pass out.

After recovering a bit, I instinctively picked up the phone, called Mepkin Abbey, and asked for Brother John.

"Brother John, I'm in trouble. I need to come down."

"When?"

"Right now."

"That's fine, Augie," Brother John replied without hesitation. "That's what we're here for. You get here as fast as you can and stay as long as you need to. We'll be waiting, and I'll have your room all ready for you."

* * *

When I told my partners at RGI I was leaving immediately for an indefinite stay at the Abbey, they were extremely supportive. Dave Gold, in fact, took one look at me and insisted on driving me there. I was incredibly moved by their kindness. Throughout this dark period of my life the members of the SKS and my partners at RGI stepped up time and again, and no one ever complained about what even I eventually saw as the bottomless pit of my neediness.

At Mepkin I threw myself into the monastic routine like a drowning man clinging to a buoy. I also volunteered for extra work intent on filling every waking moment and driving every thought from my mind. Besides working in the egg house, I talked Brother Edward, the groundskeeper, into letting me mow grass, and I asked Brother Stan to assign me kitchen duty. Rather than taking the usual one-hour siesta after lunch, I maniacally shoved a lawnmower around in the 105-degree heat of a South Carolina summer. Then I would dash to my room, shower, and arrive at the egg house just in time for afternoon grading. When we finished work, I rushed to my mower again, quitting just in time to lay out the community's light supper at five o'clock and clear tables afterward, wrapping up barely in time to make Vespers at 6.

I asked Brother Edward to intercede with the abbot so I could mow all day Sunday. Dom Francis agreed as long as I didn't mow near the monastery proper and disturb the community. My ceaseless mowing kept me so continuously covered cap-a-pie with sweat, grime, and grass clippings that I became a source of fond amusement for the monks. One day Brother Nick interrupted my mowing with a grin.

"You look more and more like a human scarecrow every day," he said. "You know in France they have a saying for a hard day's work. They call it 'getting as dirty as a Trappist.' Congratulations, Augie. You're even dirtier than a Trappist!"

While garnering a reputation for hard work among hard-working monks lifted my spirits a bit, my real goal was the mental relief and physical exhaustion that put me to sleep as soon as my head hit the pillow after Compline. Not to be interrupted until the chimes woke me for Vigils at 3 AM.

Father Christian and I had been swapping letters since my Christmas sojourn at Mepkin, and I eagerly looked forward to resuming our meetings. I arrived for our first appointment and was stunned to find his modest office packed floor to ceiling with dozens of bulging cardboard boxes of various shapes and sizes. His office was so jam-packed we ended up sitting knee to knee in a tiny space he managed to carve out among those claustrophobia-creating cartons.

Father Christian didn't seem to notice our cramped circumstances but, allowing my own curiosity to get the best of me, I asked about all the imposing impedimenta. Christian glanced around the room, taking it all in as if he was noticing the boxes for the very first time. Then he quietly said, "There was this bachelor with no family. He visited a lot, and when he died, he left the little he had to us. These boxes contain his check stubs, receipts, electric bills, income tax returns, kindergarten diploma, and God only knows what else. The other monks wanted to burn it all, but I said, 'No. Put them in my office.'"

"Why, Father?" I asked.

Christian gazed almost lovingly at that brown cardboard cordillera looming only inches away.

"My God, a man's *life* is in those boxes!" he exclaimed with so much vehemence it made me jump. "Somebody has to go through it all before it's thrown away. I know it'll

> Aren't we all frantically trying to stuff momentary meaning into this fragile cardboard box we call life in the face of our own imminent and meaningless mortality?

probably take months. I barely knew the man. But I promised myself I'd do it anyway."

I was deeply moved by Christian's compassion but even more so by the paradoxical nature of his mission. On one hand, the man was dead and gone. Neither he nor anyone else would ever know or give a damn whether his lifeless paper trail was inspected or not. On the other hand, Christian was right: A man's *life* was in those boxes, and there was something terrible—even sacrilegious—about consigning them to flames without at least a cursory examination. Besides, it struck me that this same strange paradox of meaningful meaningless-ness was the woof and warp of life itself: aren't we all frantically trying to stuff momentary meaning into this fragile cardboard box we call life in the face of our own imminent and meaningless mortality? This was exactly the issue I was forced to face in the hospital after my sky-diving accident, but I didn't have time to ponder it further because, just then, Father Christian, having wound up his little eulogy, was asking, "So tell me, it's been a while. How are you doing?"

Taking a deep breath, I haltingly began telling him about being at-tacked in Florida. The deeper I got into the story the more agitated he became: clenching his fists, shaking his head, and occasionally pulling rudely at his beard. When I finished, he spat out angrily, "That was a demonic attack!"

Shocked, I pressed him, hoping he meant it only metaphorically. There was nothing doing: He clearly meant it *literally*. On one hand his infernal suspicions matched my own intuitions of that terrible night, but on the other, I wearily thought: *Oh shit. On top of every-thing else, do I now have to factor demons into the mix?*

Father Christian went on to say my tormentors were projecting their own lust onto me.

Seeing me, a fortysomething man like themselves, apparently sur-rounded by adoring young women, drove them crazy with jealousy. Cloaking lust behind a pretense of moral superiority, they justified their violent hostility by displacing their own deviant desires onto me. Valid or not, I liked this purely psychological exegesis much better than hauling in demons as an explanatory model. But Father Christian refused to let me off the hook.

"It's textbook," he said. "Demonic forces used their lust against them while turning your vulnerability against you."

When I told him about the torrent of sexual guilt the incident later triggered, he shook his head in disgust and, grimacing, said, "I am not surprised. The devil always uses a little truth in order to tell a more convincing lie."

* * *

Most of that summer at Mepkin Abbey is just a bottle-green blur of freshly mown grass clippings, but little by little, all the prayer, work, and meetings with Father Christian seemed to stabilize me somewhat. When I first arrived, the very thought of working with students again was enough to fill me with indescribable fatigue, but by summer's end I knew I was going back. The students had a full semester of events planned, including a lecture by me, and I couldn't imagine leaving them in the lurch. Near the end of my stay, I saw Father Francis again. I told him I didn't want to leave, but I felt guilty about shirking my responsibilities with RGI and the SKS. He urged me to return to Raleigh. He told me he sensed there was something waiting for me out in the world I still had to face.

A few days before I was due to head back, Dave Gold left a message that Meredith would be picking me up. My reaction was mixed. On the surface I was thrilled. Meredith wrote me almost every day while I was at Mepkin and, typical of her sensitivity, she wrote only chatty, upbeat, often humorous letters. Even though I didn't write back often, it gave me a warm feeling to know that a girl her father called "my little pit bull" was busily tugging at my trouser leg just so I remembered to come home. But I also worried I was getting too close to her, and this made me uneasy.

Several months earlier, during the house course, I actually shared my concern. "You know, Mere," I said one day, "I think I'm becoming emotionally dependent on you."

"Well, what's wrong with that?" she smilingly retorted, pleased by what she took for a compliment. I didn't have the heart to explain what I really meant.

Somehow our friendship seemed doomed, and this made my dark forebodings about the future even more personal and painful. It was as if the closer Meredith and I became, the more I already missed her.

* * *

Mepkin's stabilizing effects were short-lived. Within weeks I was spiraling downward again, and as more and more anxiety mixed with depression, I became querulous with my long-suffering friends. I felt like a man sunk in quicksand up to his chin, and I couldn't understand why everyone seemed to be just standing around instead of pulling me out. I realized how unfair and absurd my attitude was, but I couldn't seem to stop whining.

By December 15th I was back at Mepkin counting on another respite. But this time even Mepkin couldn't halt the slide. Father Christian was obviously concerned. One time he asked me, "Don't you ever get consolation? We can't survive without God's occasional consolation." When I realized even he was beginning to worry, I became all the more frightened.

* * *

I returned to Raleigh in January, and a few days later Meredith came to see me. Haltingly, she told me she was going abroad for a semester in Bolivia and leaving the SKS. I was devastated. While she didn't bring it up, I knew her disenchantment wasn't with the SKS; it was with me. I'd been smothering her for months, and now I finally drove her away. It was all my fault, and I tore at myself mercilessly for overwhelming her with my emotional weakness. When Mepkin failed me and Meredith walked away, the last two stable pillars in my collapsing universe gave way and my downward spiral accelerated.

Shortly after Meredith left for Bolivia, I accompanied a large group of SKS students from all three universities on a field trip to the Monroe Institute in Virginia. Robert Monroe wrote a book I enjoyed as a young man called *Journeys Out of the Body* about his "astral projection" experiences, or what psychic researchers prefer to call "remote viewing." He started the Monroe Institute to teach others his techniques. When he died, his daughter, Laurie Monroe, continued his work. Some months previously I reached out to the Monroe Institute, and Laurie graciously offered the SKS students a free weekend seminar.

Throughout the weekend I was too exhausted and depressed to say anything as two psychologists, a man and a woman, facilitated the seminar. They were both about 40 and the man handled himself and the students very smoothly. A little too smoothly, I thought, whenever I managed to muster enough energy to think at all. Despite his athletic body, thick black hair, and rugged good looks, I pegged him for one of those soft, treacly New Agers; he spent the entire weekend nodding vigorously and cheerfully repeating "Thanks for sharing!" to any damn thing anyone happened to say.

The seminar ended on a high note and the students and other adult chaperones headed for the parking lot to take pictures prior to departure. Instead, I followed the male psychologist into a little office adjacent to the main meeting room. He'd been too busy to join us at lunch, and I found him standing with a plate just about to bite into a hamburger. I told him I was going through some tough times and asked if he knew a psychologist in Raleigh he could recommend.

Putting his still untouched hamburger down, he said he didn't know anyone in the Raleigh area. Then he strode up to me until he got far too close for comfort and stood there gazing effortlessly into my eyes until I winced. "If I wasn't moving to California next week, I'd work with you myself," he said quietly. "I've been watching you all weekend, and I think we could have a lot of fun together."

Then he launched into a rapid-fire version of everything Hugh told me at the gym over a year ago. And much more. Barely stopping to breathe, he said my heart was "opening up," and even though I'd been through plenty of hell there was still more to go. He said I was refusing to "surrender" because I was terrified of losing my "power," my sense of "egotistical control," and my "precious individuality." He went on to say my fears were just a pile of stubborn nonsense and my exhaustion symptomatic of my counterproductive struggling. However, during this critical time, he gravely cautioned, I must not give away too much psychic energy to others because I would need everything I had for the final crisis coming very soon.

During the minute or so it took to make his staccato speech, I was too amazed to say anything. He finished up by suggesting I try some "body work" like Rolfing, Reiki, or some other form of holistic massage. But as he did, something that conveyed my long-standing low regard for "body work" must have crossed my face because he instantly seized the few remaining inches between us by jamming four fingers up under my rib cage until I gasped in pain.

"Do you feel *that*? That's the Manipura, the stomach chakra. You don't like that idea, do you?" he shouted straight into my face. "That's the reason why you should try it. You're so fucking smart, your body's the only place left that isn't perfectly defensed. If anyone is going to get anything through that thick skull of yours, they're going to have to bypass it all together by starting right *here*." With this, he jammed his entire hand even further into my solar plexus until I lurched over choking for air.

Suddenly I was weeping, but that didn't faze him or even slow him down. "I'm really not like this at all," he shouted without relaxing his grip. "I'm actually a loving guy, but you've spent your life arrogantly walking all over loving people because you think they're weak. You have me figured for some New Age wimp, so if I'm going to help you I gotta' show you you're damn well not going to walk all over me!"

During the last minute or two of this lopsided exchange, the other facilitator walked into the room and stood there watching him work me over with a pained look on her face. He finally removed his hand from my stomach while flashing a warm smile that felt like a good-natured football opponent yanking me to my feet and patting me on the rump after damn near knocking me senseless. Then he headed back for his orphaned hamburger.

As he did, I heard the other facilitator say, "My God, don't you have anyone in your life who understands? Who loves you? Someone you can turn to?"

"I did, but—" I began, thinking of Meredith.

Before I could utter another word, the male facilitator tucked a bite of hamburger into one cheek and loudly interrupted, "It's not your fault! You blame yourself, but it's not your fault! She's young and she's afraid she'll let you down. She has her own issues. She has her own path. You did what you could for her, and it was just her time to go."

Without waiting for a reaction or reply, he went back at his hamburger in such a deliberate fashion I knew my time was up.

Chapter Twenty

PSYCHICS AND MYSTIC PSYCHOLOGISTS

Whatever we inherit from the fortunate
We have taken from the defeated
What they had to leave us – a symbol:
A symbol perfected in death.
And all shall be well and
All manner of thing shall be well
By the purification of the motive
In the ground of our beseeching.
—T.S. Eliot[42]

Taking the psychologist from the Monroe Institute at his word, I started a regimen of Rolfing, but while I enjoyed my sessions with my affable Rolfer, his muscular ministrations didn't make me feel much better. One day my Rolfer recommended an "amazing" psychic, a Japanese woman who worked strictly by referral. My opinion of psychics was even lower than my erstwhile opinion of body work, but I was ready to try any damn thing, so I took him up on his offer.

The psychic lived in a ranch house in the suburbs of Durham, and overcoming some last-minute hesitation, I thumbed the doorbell. The psychic was a tiny, well-mannered woman of about sixty. Her greeting, in heavily accented and occasionally broken English, was precise and forceful. She had clear, penetrating brown eyes that were so sure of themselves I found it mildly intimidating. I tried to introduce myself in turn, but putting a finger to her lips she hissed, "Please, say nothing! I must know nothing!"

I expected an interior neatly subdivided by bamboo-embossed Shoji screens, but other than a small golden gong on the fireplace, the décor was decidedly middle American. As she led me to a white sofa in the living room, she softly said she wanted only my age and first name.

Proffering paper, she told me to jot down the first names of other people I wanted a "reading" on. She then pulled up an armchair, took both my hands, closed her eyes, took a deep breath, and began.

"August, I see you climbing stairs. You climb these stairs all your life. Now you near top, but step you must now take is very big, and this step missing."

Opening her eyes, she gazed straight into mine. "Now you must leap! Must leap! You know this, but afraid to fall. You very powerful man and afraid to lose this power. Risks, of course, are real, there is much danger—but is no other way."

She told me there were many people depending on me I was pushing away.

"You feel guilty, but is necessary. You must be alone to take leap, and for this leap you need all energy for yourself."

Once I made this big leap, she added, "You will return to share everything with others."

The only other readings I remember were Meredith and my mother. When she came to Meredith, she became physically agitated, ringing her hands and squirming in her seat.

"Who is this?" she sternly demanded, opening her eyes.

"One of my students . . . " I began tentatively, startled by her change in demeanor.

"I know you have feelings," she interrupted. "But you must let her go! You no longer can help her. Let her go!"

She then described Meredith with uncanny accuracy without any help from me while insisting, "She has own path. That is why she go. Now, *you* must let her go!"

Later the psychic told me my deceased mother was trying to contact me, and she urged me to set aside some daily quiet time to try to receive her crucial message.

Back at my car, I idled the engine while going back over the session. Her description of me as a lifelong stair climber running out of steps, of course, struck a scary chord. There was also little doubt my irritable, argumentative, even whining behaviors were driving people away, and I felt guilty about it. Finally, her take on my fears, her admonition about hoarding my energy, her insistence on letting Meredith go, all neatly echoed that hamburger-eating psychologist from the Monroe Institute. Despite being impressed by this psychic's apparent powers, I drew the line however at holding solo seances on the off chance of contacting my mother. I wasn't about to spend precious time and dwindling energy trying to raise the dead.

* * *

When I wasn't Rolfing or consulting psychics, I kept searching for a psychologist—and finally found one. David was a lean, mild-mannered, sensitive-looking man, a few years younger than me. Though a practicing Catholic, he was spiritually eclectic and very well-read. His single-story, redwood-veneered office park was a rabbit warren of boxy units set back in a bucolic tree-covered space choked ankle deep with pine needles and old leaves. The open center was bisected by a boulder-strewn artificial stream that seemed to make the silence all the more palpable by adding its burbling song to the setting's sooth-ing effect.

David's office was bright and airy with a large window that in-corporated the peaceful, sylvan surroundings into our sessions. His methodology was strictly talk therapy, and he combined this with the annoying habit of occasionally and melodramatically interrupting me mid-sentence with a raised index finger. As I obediently fell silent, he would take off his glasses, fold his hands on his lap, close his eyes, drop his chin, and contemplate what I was saying as I sat there feeling like one damn fool watching another meditate at my expense. At the oddest of times he would also catch me off guard by breaking into a shrill, mirthless, almost hysterical laugh that stood my hair on end as I labored, usually without success, to see the humor or get the joke. I often felt like we were merely jogging in place, but just as I was about to pull the plug, David would say something so insightful I would end up reluctantly revisiting his therapeutic hutch the following week.

One time, for example, I exclaimed, "David, why does it have to be so hard?" Without looking up from his notes he replied, "Because we insist on playing our games until the pain becomes so great we can't take it anymore."

One day I told David I never married because I couldn't bear the thought of a woman letting me down. Whatever my other flaws, I argued, I was an honorable man who would nev-er break his word to his wife and let her down.

This stunning rebuke from such a mild-mannered man sent me staggering back in time to an incident with my mother shortly before she died.

This triggered an index finger and yet another long meditative moment that had me squirming in my seat. His chin finally rose from his chest.

"Let me tell you something as a mar-ried man," he said, his blue eyes blaz-ing. "You *will* let your wife down. You'll let her down *again* and *again* and *again*," he shouted, banging both fists on the arms of his chair for emphasis. "And you'll do it mostly because you're *thoughtless*."

This stunning rebuke from such a mild-mannered man sent me staggering back in time to an incident with my mother shortly before she died.

* * *

I loved and respected my mother, but I only realized after she was gone that she was the best friend I ever had. My mom was my confidant, my life coach, my full-time cheerleader, and the one person I could always count on.

One day, while working with Rose, I made a mad dash from Washington, D.C. to Cleveland to head off some incipient group disaster or another. Speeding west along the Pennsylvania Turnpike, I saw the sign for Pittsburgh and decided to make a detour and surprise my mom. As I noisily burst through the door, she sprang to her feet with a happy squeal and threw herself into my arms, just as I was counting on. I was on a tight Rosean schedule, and ten minutes later I clambered back into my white Ford van parked in the street. My mother suddenly appeared on the top of the steep, grassy slope leading to our front door. Cupping both hands, she shouted at the top of her Irish lungs, "Augie, you got chutzpah!" At the time I didn't know what *chutzpah* meant, and I doubt the startled neighbors did either, but the sense was so obvious I became a tad verklempt as I kvelled with delight.

By the fall of 1984 my mother became terminally ill with cancer that, at only 61, would soon take her life. I was visiting for a few days, and one morning, after sleeping late, I headed for the kitchen and met my mother coming through the front door.

"Mom, it's not even ten o'clock. Where've you been?"

"I've been to see a psychiatrist who is also a priest," she said quietly.

"What did you talk about?" I asked, thinking that, considering her prognosis, her thoughts were turning to her immortal soul and its prospects in the afterlife.

"I needed to talk to someone because I feel so guilty about what I'm putting my family through."

In light of my own selfish spiritual aspirations, her selfless answer was the last thing I expected. She just stood there looking like a lost little girl, and I knew all my mom wanted from life, the universe, and God himself was for her firstborn son to take her in my arms, tell her I loved her, tell her I was there for her, and tell her she didn't have to feel that way. But I didn't. The poignant intimacy the moment required terrified me, and after a few awkward seconds I broke the tension with some banal remark and turned away.

In her hour of greatest need, I let my mother down. And so, as I sat suffocating in shame from David's savage reproach, I knew if I could redo anything in my entire life, I would undo my thoughtless, deathbed betrayal of the best friend I would ever have.

* * *

Several days later I started typing Father Christian a casual note. Soon I was pouring my heart out.

Father, so much has happened these last couple of years. Things are opening up that a few years ago would've been unthinkable. Yet so much of this has occurred in the midst of great suffering. This suffering is compounded by intense guilt because I know how fortunate I am and how blessed.

I was speaking of my suffering with an adult member of the SKS when I flashed on a scene from college when I was in great pain with a misdiagnosed case of abscessed tonsils. In desperation I called my mother, and she insisted I come home into her care.

Father, as I told this story, I was flooded once again with intense feelings of relief. The feeling from Julian of Norwich that 'all shall be well, and all shall be well, and all manner of things shall be well.' Suddenly I blurted: 'Now I know after all these years of seeking what I'm really searching for. I want my mom. I just want my mom. Philosophy and theology are so cold. I just want my mom!'

Father, even as I wept, I knew my longing for my human mother was just the surface of something so much deeper. She symbolizes the transcendence I really yearn for. I want so desperately to know always that God does love me, He is looking out for me, and when I do reach the end of my strength, He will pick up the slack for me. I want to know I'm not alone.

*Yet I can't stop stubbornly trying to use my intellect to bring all this about. I strain to understand why so much of life makes no sense to me. I know I **don't** understand. I know I will **never** understand. But I can't stop making super efforts **to** understand. Efforts that have drained me so utterly I fear for my sanity . . .*

While folding my typewritten letter, I grabbed a pen and impulsively scrawled a postscript inspired by Psalm 4 from Compline at Mepkin:

I pray a thousand times a day, Father. Oh Lord, how long will our hearts be closed? Will we love what is foolish and seek what is false?[43]

* * *

Not long afterward, I told David about a disturbing dream. I was standing beside a vast stygian swamp bubbling with putrid excrement. There was a disturbance in the mire, and a lizard the size of a dinosaur came up through the fetid soup. Terrified, I suddenly realized I was holding a long, thin pane of glass. Turning it on edge, I struck the lizard on the back of the neck, trying to sever its head. Unhurt by the blow, the infuriated lizard whirled around and roared at me.

The scene changed. I was in a long alley intersected by an identical alley with a wooden gate. Expecting the vengeful reptile at any moment, I fumbled with the gate, desperately trying to get it closed. The gate and frame were rotten and crumbling, but I somehow didn't consider their shoddy condition an issue. When I did finally close the gate, I noticed another intersecting alley with another rotten gate and after that another and then another. Realizing I would never get all these gates secured before the vindictive lizard arrived to swallow me up, I awoke screaming.

When I finished, David leaned back with his delicate fingers interlaced behind his neck. "You know," he said, "I don't read anymore. I just learn from my clients. In fact, the only book I have is a book on Native American totem animals a client gave me I haven't read." Retrieving the book from an otherwise empty bookshelf nearby, he sifted through it. "Here we are. The Lizard. Why don't you read it aloud and see if anything rings true."

This is what I read.

"Lizard dreaming lizard, will you dream with me? Beyond the place of time and space are visions from afar.

"Lizard medicine is the shadow side of reality where your dreams are reviewed before you manifest them physically. Lizard is the medicine of dreamers. Lizard always helps you see your shadow. This shadow is your greatest fear, the thing you are resisting that follows you around like an obedient dog. If Lizard dreamed in you today, it's time to look at what is following you. Is it your fears? Is it your future trying to catch up to you? Or is it the part of you denying your weakness and humanness?"

When I finished, I anxiously scanned several other entries on other animals, but they bore no relevance to my situation. Giving up, I said, "David, this is spooky. How the hell can this stuff be happening to me?"

David was unimpressed. "Oh, I don't find it strange at all. When the unconscious opens up, you'll find all the answers you need in a Burger King menu."

First, some crazy psychologist at the Monroe Institute, then the psychic, and now I'm channeling dream prophecies from totem animals! Meanwhile, I have an eccentric therapist who thinks it's all in a day's work. And looming over it all was the dark premonition that all that rotting excrement and all those rotten gates meant the worst was still to come.

A few days later I was sitting at my desk at RGI when I decided to call Bill Richards, a Baltimore-based mystic, psychologist, and psychedelic dream weaver of the first rank. A man who offered me refuge once before. A long time ago.

* * *

Back in 1979, while living with Lou Mobley in Maryland, I read an article about a seminar on government-funded research into psychotropic drugs like LSD. One panelist was a local psychologist, William Richards, doing research at the Maryland Psychiatric Research Center. I gave him a call, and a few days later Richards ushered me into his tidy, nondescript office. Bill was in his late thirties, about five-foot-ten with a trim, medium build. His black hair was neatly combed straight back revealing a smooth forehead etched with the thick, uninterrupted hairline of a boy of sixteen. He was wearing a short-sleeved shirt, tie, and khakis, and the skin of his face and forearms was remarkably fair and almost hairless. His large brown eyes were gentle, studious, highly intelligent, and the black horn-rimmed glasses perched on his nose gave him a slightly owlish look. All in all, he looked exactly like a research psychologist should.

After offering a chair and taking one himself, he sat there breathing deeply, smiling gently, and gazing into my eyes. He seemed content to sit forever as he scanned my soul. There wasn't anything intimidating about his demeanor. It was just the opposite. He seemed so open, benign, and comfortable in his own skin it was unsettling. I never felt such an absence of interpersonal tension with a loved one, let alone a stranger. It was as if I was sitting across from an ancient, wise, and loving extraterrestrial who, though humanoid in form, couldn't possibly be human himself.

The next thing I knew I was incoherently rambling on about Rose, Mobley, my parents, Hotchkiss, my self-doubts, my spiritual frustrations, my bouts with depression, and the-devil-knows-what-else to a man who still hadn't said ten words, a man who agreed to see me on the basis of a phone call for a reason I never specified. A man who, for all I knew, wasn't the least bit interested in me or in spirituality. Once in a while I came to my senses long enough to shyly glance at Richards and wonder what he was thinking. Every time, all I saw was a look of shared anguish, as if to say: "Yes, yes, go on. I've been there myself, and being here for you is why I came to earth." Several times he reached out and gently touched my arm, a gesture that moved me more by its naturalness than its evident compassion.

I eventually ran out of gas and regained my composure. Suddenly I was burning with shame at my ridiculous outburst. When I furtively looked at Richards, he was still there, leaning toward me with his elbows on his knees. A few seconds later he burst into a loud peal of laughter and slapped me smartly on the shoulder like I'd just successfully drained a pitcher of ice-cold beer in a single gulp. Then he got up, went out, came back with a glass of water for me, and before I knew it, we were chatting away like nothing happened.

Much to my relief, I learned Richards had been a minister before becoming a psychologist, and he was passionately interested in spiritual experience. His government research into psychotropic drugs was based on their ability to trigger altered states of consciousness that seemed to mirror mystical experiences from all the world's great religious traditions.

Bill took me on a tour of the Institute, and in the basement were the water-filled sensory deprivation tanks John Lilly used for his research into altered states. I read Lilly's bestselling book, *The Center of the Cyclone,* and Richards filled me in on details that never made the book. In the auditorium we watched an episode of *Sixty Minutes.* Hosted by Mike Wallace, it featured Richards's work with terminally ill cancer patients. After several months of standard therapy, he gave the volunteers a dose of LSD to help them come to terms with death. The episode was deeply moving, not only because the therapy seemed so effective but because there was Richards, up on the screen, coaching others in the same silent, compassionate way I had just experienced.

As I was leaving, Bill told me his research funding was running out and he was returning to private practice. I asked him to take me on as a client.

I was early for my first appointment on a bright, sunny Baltimore morning. Richards's office was on the ground floor of his enormous 100-year-old Victorian house, not far from the city center. I parked on the quiet tree-lined street and, following Bill's instructions, took the gate at the far end of the cast-iron fence fronting the house before descending a long series of steps. Taking a stone path to the back, I discovered a magnificent rock-strewn flower garden replete with a wooden bridge over a burbling manmade brook. Veering onto the garden path I came to a deep tree-lined gorge where I could just make out the sound of a much larger stream completely hidden by the dense foliage.

Eventually I made my way to a well-lit waiting room snugly built into the rear of the house. Soon the door to the living quarters swung open and Richards burst in. Taking me by both hands, he stood there smiling broadly and breathing deeply. Then he proffered a huge sigh of satisfaction that seemed to say, "It's so good to see you again. Now, let's have a real look at you."

Still without a word, Richards led me into his thickly carpeted office which felt like a cozy, soundproof cocoon furnished with little

341

more than lamps, plants, a couple of straight-back chairs huddled around a small round table, and a long black couch against the wall. The office was brightly painted, and one wall was lined with books. Half were the standard psychology texts one might expect, but the rest bore the titles of every book on mystical spirituality I ever read or heard of, and quite a few more.

We sat at the table and, after a few pleasantries, he asked, "So, Augie, what are you looking for from our time together?"

"I'm not sure, Bill. I do know this: I'm not interested in being 'adjusted' or 'made normal.'"

Bill nodded but gently persisted. "Yes, but what do you want?"

"I want to be real . . . to be *genuine*," I blurted without thinking.

My words spilled out so emotionally I was embarrassed, but Richards just gleefully rubbed his hands together and said, "I can live with that! Let's go to work."

* * *

Over the ensuing months I met with Richards twice a week, usually for two-hour sessions. Richards said very little, and what he did say had little to do with conventional think/talk psychotherapy. Instead, he introduced exercises designed to short-circuit the conscious intellect and access the unconscious mind. I was soon painting, listening to music, chronicling dreams, and filling page after page with stream-of-consciousness writing. But central to our work was guided imagery, a therapeutic technique invented by the famous Swiss psychotherapist and student of Freud, Carl Jung.

Jung designed guided imagery to produce a kind of waking dream state so the unconscious mind could be more effectively accessed. While I'd never tried it, I read about Jung's first experiments in his autobiography, *Memories, Dreams, and Reflections*.

For our guided imagery sessions Richards had me lie on the couch. Then he produced a blanket and pillows and made me comfortable.

His ministrations were so effective that far from feeling awkward about being physically fussed over by another man, I felt the same way I did when my mother tucked me in. Once satisfied I was not merely comfortable but ensconced, he strapped on earphones and piped in soft classical music. Then, pulling up his chair, we would begin.

"Augie, just relax, close your eyes, breathe deeply, and listen to my voice," he began softly. "Good! Imagine you're back in bed as a child peacefully dozing off to sleep . . . but now, just as your eyes are beginning to close, you suddenly notice a light . . . a magical light . . . emerging from around the closet door."

Hesitating, he allowed his spell to take effect.

"Overcome with curiosity," he began again, "imagine going to investigate. Inside you find a secret trap door with that same warm, benevolent light oozing out around its edges. Now you're pulling the door open only to discover a long golden ladder descending into a deep, dazzling cave. Fascinated, you slowly climb down. Now you are on the first rung . . . that's it, take a deep breath . . . now the second . . ."

Rung by rung Richards led me into these nether regions until, without warning, he would "let go" and ask me to describe in detail everything I saw as I continued my descent.

When we finished, he sent me home to write up everything I experienced.

My feeling that Richards was an exceedingly strange yet wonderful man only deepened as time went on. He continued to say almost nothing, and he was careful to maintain the professional detachment appropriate to our relationship. While I thought he liked me and I knew I liked him, we never became friends. When I realized this, I also realized I had no idea what being friends with Bill Richards would actually be like.

This assessment is not meant to imply that Richards was ever impassive or cold. Instead, he engendered such openness and intimacy that his professional detachment was more like the radiant inaccessi-

343

bility of my guardian angel, an angel who, though utterly committed to my well-being, was by his very nature beyond my ability to ever get to know. There was something otherworldly, even ethereal, about Richards, but I never doubted he was in control, and this made me feel safe. He exercised this control so subtly I felt like a blind man being adroitly maneuvered through a crowded cocktail party by the tiniest of nudges from a devoted wife.

Enigmatic as he was, over time I was able to gather a few things about his life. Besides playing the piano and flower gardening, Richards took great pleasure in singing with the choir in his local Episcopal church. He learned German while studying psychotherapy in Germany under an American mentor he revered. He married his mentor's daughter, and they had two sons before she died young. I no longer remember what prompted Bill to share these details, but I will never forget his face as he spoke of his wife. He loved her very much, and he was obviously still in great pain.

That is all I managed to learn, but at the oddest moments he would occasionally drop his professional guise and say something revealing. One time he suddenly said, "Augie, I enjoy working with you. There's *process* going on inside you. You have no idea how tedious it gets sitting here listening to people who think if they could just get a raise or find a mate, they'd have the universe by the rear end." I was flattered by this offhand comment, but what really struck me was how out of character it was.

Despite Bill's preternatural gifts and my honest effort, our work didn't get very far. I proved such a tough nut that Richards leaned back one day and sighed, "You know, Augie, the problem with working with you is you've read all the same psychological literature I have, and you're unconsciously using it to short-circuit our work together."

I was perceptive enough to realize he was right, but I was helpless to do anything about it. I was as frustrated as he was, and, in fact, the only thing I learned after months of rigorous, expensive, time-consuming work was just how incredibly frustrated I was.

For example, despite strenuous efforts, I couldn't get the hang of guided imagery. I either tried too hard to invoke images I guessed Richards wanted, or, in the rare case when I did go with the flow, it always led to dead ends. Ad nauseum I imagined myself into boxes, coffins, closets, chests, trunks, and one time, I found myself snugly wedged inside a hollow tree.

Besides angry frustration, these imaginary journeys were so coldly devoid of emotional content I didn't even feel claustrophobic.

One day I called Richards and, pleading poor, ended our sessions. He wished me luck, and that was it. I was running out of money, but that had nothing to do with it. I was up against much stiffer odds during my years with Rose, and I never let money stand in my way. It was not money or frustration that led me to part ways with Richards. Instead, it was my fear that we might actually be making progress. As Rose so deftly put it many years previously, I wanted the truth but was terrified by what it might be.

* * *

That was 1980. Now it was 1998, almost twenty years later, and Rose's boy with the burning feet was rapidly running out of running room. As I reached for my office phone, I discovered I still remembered Bill Richards's phone number.

More amazing still, he picked up on the first ring.

I'd barely identified myself before we were chatting amiably as if all those intervening years were merely days. But succumbing yet again to Bill's magical aura, I was soon chaotically spilling my guts about my deepening despair and all the crazy stuff happening to me.

Eventually, my disjointed acid rap settled on an incident at Mepkin Abbey the previous Christmas.

I was browsing the monastic library when I came across *Into Thin Air,* Jon Krakauer's account of two expeditions caught in a blizzard on Mount Everest in which eight people died. It was an unusually cold and dreary holiday season at Mepkin. One night I stayed up long after Compline listening to a winter storm fresh from the Atlantic whip the branches of the towering live oak outside my door while morbidly absorbed in this horrific Everest tale. As I read, the doomed climbers' fatigue, isolation, mountain sickness, confusion, hypoxic psychosis, panic, and crushing despair seemed to mirror my own rapidly deteriorating situation.

"Bill, I was in a stone panic," I said, "but I couldn't stop reading as one by one those climbers 'let go,' 'gave up,' 'gave in,' and finally surrendered to the peaceful sleep of icy death."

I told Richards one of the leaders, Rob Hall, was trapped in the blinding blizzard near the summit. Still in radio contact, his Base Camp colleagues urged him to start down. Exhausted, Hall kept repeating, "I will . . . in a minute." Finally, desperate to get him moving, Base Camp patched in Hall's wife. Seven months pregnant with their first child, she pleaded with him to start down for the sake of their love and their unborn baby. "I love you," Hall whispered. "Sleep well, my sweetheart. Please, don't worry too much." Then he froze to death.

Krakauer blamed the disaster on the hubris of "summit fever." The leaders pushed their expeditions toward the summit despite clear evidence disaster was looming. The summit, according to Krakauer, is only *halfway*. The real trick to Everest is getting down. Almost every death occurs when climbers are too cold and exhausted to make it down *after* reaching the summit.[44]

"Bill," I moaned, "Krakauer was talking to me! I got summit fever back with Rose. I've spent twenty-five years becoming the person I thought I needed to be to reach Enlightenment. Now, in a sense, I've reached the summit. I've become that person I stupidly imagined I wanted to be."

Overcome, I stopped to regain my composure. As I did, I heard Richards say, "That's all right, Augie. Go on. I'm here."

"Now I know," I continued. "Enlightenment, God, Truth isn't at the summit. The summit is only halfway. God's not in the clouds in some never-never land of self-perfection. God's down below; God's safety, home, base camp. Now it's too late. I'm trapped like Rob Hall, but instead of Everest, I'm trapped in this grotesque Frankenstein personality I created. I'm sitting in a snow pit of my own design, slowly dying of exhaustion and freezing cold.

"Bill, everything's so dark, and my mental blizzard is swirling so rapidly, I can't tell which way is down anymore. Even if I could, I'm too tired to think about it, let alone get to my feet and start moving again.

"I'm all alone," I told Richards, "paying the icy price for my arrogance without even a loving wife to be patched through to."

I was weeping almost convulsively, but then I heard Richards say, "Oh, Augie, you've done so much work on yourself. We've got to get you down. Don't worry, we'll get you down."

Bill's heartfelt reassurance had a miraculous calming effect. Eventually he invited me to come back to Baltimore and meet with him daily. In deference to my long-suffering partners, I decided to spend Holy Week with Richards because, between Palm Sunday and Easter, business would slow to a crawl.

A few minutes later I was still slumped wearily at my desk when Dave Gold walked in. I summarized my conversation with Richards as Dave scratched thoughtfully at his neatly trimmed beard.

"When me and you were just starting out with Rose," he said with a wry smile, "you never dreamed in a million years it would ever get this personal, did you, Aug?"

Struck again by Dave's uncanny ability to succinctly put the ineffable into such a few words, I mumbled, "No, Dave, I didn't."

"Yeah, you spent your whole life building a magnificent mansion—only to discover you built it on another man's land."

Chapter Twenty-One

DEATH AND REBIRTH IN BALTIMORE

I said to my soul, be still, and wait without hope
For hope would be hope for the wrong thing; wait without love,
For love would be love of the wrong thing; there is yet faith
But the faith and the love and the hope are all in the waiting.
Wait without thought, for you are not ready for thought:
So the darkness shall be the light, and the stillness the dancing.
—T.S. ELIOT[45]

I crammed a toothbrush and a couple changes of clothes into the car Meredith picked out for me, and on Thursday, April 2, 1998, I set out for my reunion with Bill Richards. The weather was sunny and unseasonably warm and, after a two-hour drive along I-85 through the scenic North Carolina countryside, I merged onto I-95 North toward Richmond, Virginia, Washington, D.C, and ultimately Baltimore. However, I got a late start, and by the time I hit Richmond it became abundantly clear that Washington traffic was going to turn a hitherto halcyon hegira into a hellish bumper-to-bumper ordeal of indefinite duration. In an effort to lift my spirits, I was listening to an audio tape of Mark Twain's humorous classic, *The Adventures of Tom Sawyer*.

Turning it off as traffic slowed to a crawl, I tried to imagine what awaited me in Baltimore.

I was extremely grateful to Richards for rearranging his schedule so we would have at least one, sometimes two, two-hour sessions a day, but I was so damn demoralized I began anxiously trying to cushion my eventual disappointment.

"Whatever you do," I said to myself, "don't get your hopes up. Richards is a good man, but he ain't no miracle worker."

No sooner did this thought cross my mind than I began chastising myself for my self-sabotaging, halfhearted attitude.

*That's your whole damn problem: **resignation**. When you broke with old man Rose you gave up on yourself. You traded that fire-in-the-belly path of reckless abandon for a compromised life of smaller aspirations and smaller victories like working for MTV. Why? Because if you don't aim too high you don't risk the disappointment and humiliation of failure. So, where's twenty years of hedging your bets got you? You're like some wannabe entrepreneur who starts a company while keeping his day job. Now your company's going bankrupt, and you're wondering whether you were smart to hedge or failed because you hedged. All you ever wanted was to go **all in**, to live life at the edge of possibility like that vet and his buddies in 'Nam, but instead you've become what Rose derided as the lowest form of life: a piddler, a wishy-washy, spiritual half-stepper.*

None of this was new territory. I'd been berating myself regularly for similar sins for years. I began working with college students in the 1980s as a way to lower my spiritual expectations and temper my bitter disappointment. I blew my spiritual chance, I decided, but maybe I could avoid utter despair by helping others avoid my fate. Then, in 1996, I fell from the sky, and the shock of reentry brought me face to face with the man I'd become: a hybrid creature unworthy of a berth among the angels and utterly disillusioned with life among men. I awoke from ankle surgery trapped between Heaven and earth, neither fish nor fowl, a grotesque centaur desperately holding onto worldly compensations like running RGI with one hand while vainly reaching for Heaven with the other.

Everywhere I looked I saw only fiendish Failure and her three twisted stepdaughters: Disappointment, Shame, Humiliation. I wasn't even man enough to admit defeat, accept my spiritual inadequacy, and "move on with my life." Meanwhile, despite tons of worldly disillusionment stretching as far back as Mick Jagger wearing my hat at that Rolling Stones concert in 1972, I still wasn't man enough to quit playing David's mundane "games" either.

You've spent the last twenty years, I thought wearily, *with one foot on the spiritual gas and the other on the terrestrial brake. Now, true to form, you're starting to hedge your bets with Richards.*

While going back over this well-plowed ground was an utter waste of time, it did distract me from the brutal Washington, D.C. traffic. I made it to Baltimore just after dark and checked into the small, inexpensive, independently owned motel I chose for its proximity to Bill's office. The glowing VACANCY sign was shy a few bulbs, and my cheap, well-worn, Formica-furnished room, though clean, smelled strongly of moth balls and a surfeit of Pine Sol. The whole motel was tired and dreary, but in fairness to the well-worn matron manning the front desk, I couldn't decide how much of its melancholy mood to blame on faded paint and her fondness for moth balls and how much merely checked in with me and my luggage.

"So," I mused with a wry smile as I bounced gingerly on the bed testing out its testy springs, "Ray's prophecy has finally come to pass. I ended up entombed in the Main Hotel after all. All that's missing is a clanking radiator, a blaring TV, and the fresh smell of stale milk."

Arriving at Richards's office early the next morning, I was stunned by how little had changed in eighteen years. The Victorian house, the garden, the brook, the bridge, the gorge, the poignant silence—it all seemed frozen in time and exactly as I remembered. This forever feel was so striking that, smiling slightly, I couldn't help but wonder whether Bill's urban idyll was actually some kind of therapeutic Brigadoon magically materializing out of the empyrean ether whenever a lost soul like me happens to stumble by every eighteen years or so.

Even Richards seemed impervious to time. Though my hair was thinning and going gray, his thick shock of hair was still jet black, and I had to study his face intently to discover a network of finely drawn lines I didn't notice before. He greeted me so easily I felt like I was returning after a mid-session trip to the restroom in 1980 rather than eighteen years later. The uncanny familiarity of the surroundings and Richards's easy familiarity moved me. I felt like a humbled and broken prodigal son returning to his childhood home and into the arms of a joyful and welcoming father.

We met twice on Friday and once Saturday and, while precariously perched on the leather rim of one of the black swivel chairs now appointing his office, I told Bill about my life during my eighteen-year hiatus.

Richards listened intently but said little, confining himself to all the subtle gestures of encouragement I remembered so well. As I described the intense suffering I was going through since my skydiving accident, his face gradually contorted and, leaning in, he occasionally reached out to gently stroke my arm.

When I finally finished my tortuous tale, Bill leaned back in his chair, clasped his hands loosely behind his head, and gazed thoughtfully at the ceiling.

"You know," he finally said wistfully, and apparently to the ceiling, "I just wish we hadn't hit that lizard."

I eagerly waited for more, but as I swiveled anxiously in my seat it gradually dawned on me that the Richardsonian Sphinx had now spoken and that was it. I couldn't believe it! I just spent almost six hours telling him about my skydiving accident and my nightmarish hospital experience; about Hugh at the gym and his baleful prophecy; about Meredith, Mepkin Abbey, Father Francis, Father Christian, and my eerie encounters with the prophets Elijah, Nathan, and King David. Taking to my feet, I described in gory detail melting down in front of my students at Duke and barely surviving Father Christian's "demon attack" in Florida, all while pacing back and forth in front of Bill's chockablock bookshelves like a caged cat. I wrapped up my disjointed soliloquy with the hamburger-eating psychologist from the Monroe Institute, the Japanese psychic, and my sessions with David. But all I earned in return for my six-hour, often lachrymose effort was a laconic eight-word sentence about that damn lizard!

Deeply disappointed, I eventually asked for an explanation.

"Freud said dreams are the royal road to the unconscious. I agree," Bill began while methodically cleaning his glasses with a Kleenex he deftly plucked from a box on a glass end table at his elbow. "That rotten gate in your dream symbolizes the gateway, the nexus, between your conscious ego and the unconscious mind. Its crumbling condition means your ego's last line of defense is disintegrating, leaving the door wide open. The unconscious tends to treat the ego in the same way the ego treats the unconscious," he continued, holding up his glasses to a few strands of errant sunlight trickling through the partially closed blinds, inspecting his work. "When you struck that lizard in your dream you set up an adversarial relationship with the most fundamental part of yourself and the universe, and I'm afraid we're going to catch hell for it. Listen, I know you're scared. You would be going insane if you weren't," a now re-spectacled Richards added with a gentle smile, "but try to remember as we move forward that love begets love, anger begets anger, and hate begets hate."

He then asked if I was taking antidepressant medication or considering suicide. I was shocked by this question; not because he asked, but because, as I reassured Richards, I never, even in passing, considered either alternative despite my suffering. Why? The only explanation I can offer is that even in my darkest hours the Rosean vector I forged through millions of tiny decisions over so many years—that same vector that against all odds sent me staggering without hope to the house course at Duke when I was falling apart—was still faithfully operating. Like a highly disciplined soldier whose legs automatically keep moving long after his head and heart have given up, my training, my character, my *formation*, drove me forward in the face of despair just as Rose predicted it would.

But I didn't have time to ponder this mystery at that moment because Bill was already saying, "I don't have anything else planned for today, but we still have a few minutes. I am interested in anything you might add to your Mount Everest allegory. I understand your exhaustion, but why do you feel so stuck?"

"I blame it all on Søren Kierkegaard and Charlie Brown," I offered in a weak attempt at humor while inching my chair over a few degrees to avoid another shaft of sunshine stinging the side of my face.

"OK, I'll bite," Bill said with a smile. "I'm familiar with both, but what's the connection?"

"Well, if I got my Kierkegaard right, he said the tragedy of human life is we prefer *possibility* over *actuality*, and as a result we never really live. That's why I feel so stuck. I'm afraid to trade possibility for actuality either spiritually or physically."

"How so?"

"Well, that's where Charlie Brown comes in. Are you familiar with Charlie Brown and the Little Red-Haired Girl from the comic strip?"

"Yes, of course," Bill said with a wide grin, leaning forward in his chair until his khaki-clad knees almost brushed mine. "It's a recurring motif in *Peanuts*. Charlie Brown sits on a bench eating his brown bag lunch all alone. As he does, he promises himself that one of these days he is going to head out onto the playground and befriend the Little Red-Haired Girl. Then he'll never have to eat alone again."[46]

"Exactly!" I fairly shouted, startling Richards and slightly embarrassing myself. "But he never does, does he? Why? Because he's terrified that if she rejects him, he not only loses her friendship in *actuality* but he loses the *possibility* of ever having her as a friend as well. It's a potential double dose of disappointment that destroys his comforting fantasy once and for all. So rather than risk losing both her actual friendship as well as all *possibility* for her future friendship, he passively settles for half a loaf of unfulfilled hope instead. According to Kierkegaard, Charlie chooses his imaginary life over a real one, and that's why he's failing to truly live.

"But it goes even deeper," I excitedly continued after gathering a knowing nod from Richards that he was still with me.

"It's not just losing the girl that's terrifying Charlie and keeping his procrastinating butt forever glued to that lonely bench. It's losing *all hope* in life itself. It's finding himself stuck on Mount Everest with only that searing, burning, all-consuming question—*Now what?*—for company that Charlie can't face. It's utter despair he really fears. So instead of risking it all through decisive action, he passively clings to his quixotic dream, a dream he knows in his heart will never come to pass. Hell, even an impossible dream is *something* to cling to, and any damn something, Charlie thinks, is better than the bottomless *nothing* of abject despair."

"So, you're Charlie Brown?" Bill said with a pained look on his face.

"Absolutely!" I exclaimed with something akin to masochistic joy at finally having a captive audience for these half-mad recriminations.

Stunned by my own admission, I stood up and retraced several stray shards of scattered sunlight back to the window overlooking Bill's magnificent flower garden behind his office.

Finger-spreading a couple panes of partially closed, tan-tinted blinds, I watched his vast array of particolored tulips hypnotically swaying in time with the ambivalent early April wind like an ocean of eavesdropping ears straining to overhear my comic strip-inspired confession.

"Bill, what's the name of the stream at the bottom of that gorge out there?" I asked, glancing back over my shoulder. "You told me once, but I forget."

"Gwynn Falls. There's a park down there with trails. If you want, we can check it out sometime."

"Cool. Me and some SKSers go camping in Linville Gorge every year. We hike for miles prattling philosophy the whole time. It's great.

"For twenty years," I said, picking up the thread without turning around, "I've been passively sitting on a lonely spiritual park bench promising myself 'one of these days.' One of these days I'm finally going to put my back against the wall, go all in, and, as Father Christian said, find out what it must be like to give myself totally to God. But I never do. Why? Because what if my everything is not enough? What if there *is* no God? What if God doesn't want me? What if my best just ain't good enough? *Now what?* What will I do with myself then? So, like Charlie, I cling to my futuristic fantasy instead.

"It's spiritual possibility, that same one-of-these-days syndrome," I continued while retaking my chair across from Richards, "that's also keeping me from accepting defeat, getting married, and moving on with my life. So I'm stuck on Mount Everest unable to summon the faith to go all in or the humility to admit defeat and head back down."

I hesitated, mesmerized by my fists now slowly opening and closing in my lap before again meeting Bill's steady gaze.

"You know, Bill, Father Christian once told me, 'We can't live without hope.' In one sense he's right. But future hope becomes deadly poisonous when, like poor Charlie and me, it keeps us from taking the action we need to take right here, *right now*. This is the giant leap the psychic told me I have to take—but I just can't do it."

Once again I anxiously awaited Bill's reaction and, once again, I was disappointed. He just sat there placidly staring at me with a half-smile on his face until I finally realized he was waiting on me instead. His gentle brown eyes looming large behind freshly cleaned glasses seemed to be saying: "I know there's more. If you're ready, I'm here for you."

After squirming uncomfortably for a while, I took a deep breath and awkwardly broke the tension.

"Well, speak of the devil, there's another Freud connection too," I said, smiling weakly in an attempt to hide my embarrassment.

"There always is," Bill said with a nod and another reassuring smile.

"Freud said it all goes back to sex, and that's true with me too. If I'm really going all in spiritually then I should be celibate as well. If I can't be celibate, then I should get married and productively channel my sexual energy into a family. But my Kierkegaardian dilemma is controlling me sexually as well. I'm stuck on Mount Everest unable to either be celibate or commit to a woman. Instead, I'm sitting in my freezing snow pit all alone, passively clinging to an impossible dream, and masturbating. It's just so utterly unmanly, pathetic, and humiliating.

"Masturbation epitomizes my utter disappointment in myself and life itself. It promises something in *possibility* it never delivers in *actuality*. I always feel let down, used, and disappointed in myself, yet I keep rising to the bait over and over again. Masturbation is so futile, and yet its utter futility is the perfect symbol for all my efforts. It's a constant, glaring reminder of just how utterly impotent, how powerless, I've become both spiritually and physically."

By now I was completely choked up. Bill took me by both hands and, pulling me to my feet, gave me a huge hug.

As he did, I heard myself say, "Bill, I'm so ashamed. I'm just so ashamed."

* * *

The next day was Palm Sunday, and with no sessions planned, Bill invited me to attend Mass at St. Bartholomew's Episcopal Church, where he sang in the choir, followed by brunch afterward. The church was only about 10 miles from my motel, and with the benefit of great weather, sparse Sunday traffic, and Bill's careful directions I made good time. Baltimore was part of my territory when I was fervently spreading the gospel of video music for MTV back in the early

1980s, and as I drove along the city's tree-lined streets and eventually through Gwynn Park all ablaze with spring blossoms, I was soon reliving many fond Baltimore-inspired memories—like spending a romantic evening with my girlfriend sipping chilled champagne and noshing freshly caught Chesapeake Bay blue crabs at one of the Inner Harbor's finest waterfront restaurants.

Or, better yet, that sun-drenched weekend we spent with two other couples on a lavish oceangoing yacht owned by one of my clients, a Baltimore-based, cable television tycoon who took a shine to me. While we lounged around the deck sipping margaritas and testing our sea legs, our host was expertly fishing for the tuna and mahi-mahi he later expertly cleaned, cooked, and proudly had his chef serve us for supper.

These Palm Sunday reveries drawn from far palmier times managed to cheer me up a bit, and I was soon pulling into the overflowing church parking lot. St. Bartholomew's was a small, picturesque, Gothic edifice hewn from stone blocks of various shapes and earth-tone colors. Over the main entrance was a massive circular window subdivided into eight teardrop-shaped panes outlined in thick cement with a similarly encircled glass cross at the center. Mass was about to begin, so I discreetly took a pew toward the back. The choir in their electric-blue robes, with Richards prominently in back, was accompanied by a small orchestra.

I was caught up in the service, and the celebrant was just beginning the Eucharistic Prayer when a 10,000-megawatt flashbulb seemed to go off in my face. This single prayer was suddenly revealing the truth behind all prayer, which was revealing the truth behind the liturgy, which was revealing the truth behind all liturgies, and the truth behind all liturgies was revealing . . .

Instantly I was enveloped in a rippling chain reaction of *truth* cascading backward from that single prayer. Each receding link was so much more powerful and all-encompassing it sucked up the preceding one even before it could completely take shape, let alone be taken in. In less time than it took my heart to beat, these surging, overlapping waves of truth filled me to capacity and then overcapacity with so much pure glory my legs buckled. Seconds later I came to my senses on my knees convulsively weeping, just in time to be ripped apart by an aftershock of wordless anguish. It was as if my remorse for having lived forty-six years in darkness, my heartfelt agony for a long-suffering humanity still lost in darkness, as well as my despair at finding myself back in darkness, hit me all at once.

I have no idea what impression my shell-shocked condition was having on the other people in my pew because when I did finally surface for air, the only thing I remember was almost comically cursing myself for failing to bring a stupid handkerchief. The service was coming to a close, and the choir retreated down the main aisle toward me led by a blonde, bespectacled woman with a round, cherubic face rhythmically banging on her tambourine. As she did, the orchestra led the congregation in a recessional hymn I never heard before: a hymn I later learned is called "What Wondrous Love Is This."

> *What wondrous love is this, O my soul, O my soul!*
> *What wondrous love is this, O my soul!*
> *What wondrous love is this that caused the Lord of bliss*
> *To bear the dreadful curse for my soul,*
> *To bear the dreadful curse for my soul.*
>
> *When I was sinking down, sinking down, sinking down,*
> *When I was sinking down, sinking down,*
> *When I was sinking down beneath God's righteous frown,*
> *Christ laid aside His crown for my soul, for my soul.*
> *Christ laid aside his crown for my soul.*
>
> *To God and to the Lamb, I will sing, I will sing;*
> *To God and to the Lamb, I will sing,*
> *To God and to the Lamb Who is the great "I Am" . . .*[47]

This hymn was so beautiful it seemed celestial, and the words were summing up everything I was going through and everything I longed for. But I couldn't take any more. Forgetting all about brunch with Bill, I rushed from the church, staggered to my car, and sped away with that hymn still ringing relentlessly in my head. Taking hard lefts and rights utterly at random, I was soon wandering aimlessly with no idea where I was going or what I would do when I got there.

It was then that I saw a Catholic church, hit the brakes, and abruptly pulled to the curb.

Catholics hold many services during Holy Week, I thought to myself. *If what I just went through is any indication of what's ahead, I'll need somewhere to go besides that depressing, Pine Sol-soaked motel room when I'm not hanging out with Richards.*

I assumed the church would have a vestibule where I could unobtrusively pick up a bulletin with a schedule of Holy Week services and be on my way. But the heavy oak door opened directly into the church, and Mass was just beginning. I was initially startled, but then I thought, *This is great. I'm a wreck. Attending another Mass will calm me down and give me a chance to focus on something besides that hymn.*

I was just taking the last seat in a crowded pew when the organ came to life, and with one voice the congregation began to sing the entrance hymn:

What wondrous love is this, O my soul, O my soul!

I couldn't believe my ears! I was a choir boy in grade school. I sang a hymn a day in compulsory chapel for three years at Hotchkiss. I sang hundreds of hymns during my extended stays at Mepkin Abbey. Yet I'd never heard this hymn before. Now I heard it twice in fifteen minutes. First going as a recessional hymn, and now coming as the entrance hymn. I felt hounded, cornered, cut off front and back, both "going" and "coming" by something that was much too much for me.

When Mass ended I still didn't have anywhere to go. So I knelt in front of the altar trying to pull myself together. As I did, I recalled kneeling in much the same way as an altar boy when I was seven or eight years old. I gradually realized one part of the Mass always moved me, even as a child. Just before communion the priest raises the Eucharistic host and leads the congregation in the The Centurion's Prayer of Humility.

"Lord, I am not worthy that you should enter under my roof, but only say the word and my soul shall be healed."[48]

I began repeating this prayer over and over, and it made me feel much better. I then began wondering why this prayer moved me so much as a boy and why I never realized it before. Instantly, the answer came to me: I knew even as a child that someday I would find myself in Baltimore fighting for my sanity and, when I did, I would need this prayer. So, I unconsciously filed away The Centurion's Prayer for just this emergency. This idea rocked me to my core. It was so preposterous, the very fact I was thinking it terrified me. But I was also overwhelmed with compassion for myself.

"My God," I said almost audibly, "what a burden for an eight-year-old boy to carry! No wonder I never let it reach my conscious mind. No wonder I closed myself off from the truth. The truth was all too much to know, too much for a child to face. I've been pushing the truth out of my mind ever since because it's always been way too much for me."

Then it struck me that the compassion I was now feeling was the first and only love I allowed myself to feel for myself in my entire life, and this was so gut wrenchingly sad I audibly moaned, "O my soul, O my soul."

I don't know how long I knelt there repeating The Centurion's Prayer, but when I finally left I ran into a knot of middle-aged women just outside the main door holding a meeting about preparing the church for Easter. My sudden appearance so long after Mass startled them, and as I was excusing myself, I noticed one of the women openly staring at me with so much amazed compassion in her wide brown eyes I was moved. For a moment our minds seemed to meld, and I realized every religion and the entire human race is undergirded and stitched together by her and countless women like her selflessly laboring away in relative obscurity. I was deeply grateful for her compassionate eyes and selfless service, but I was also deeply ashamed: I was always so busy self-importantly working on so-called "more important things" I never noticed her before in any of her myriad incarnations.

That night I dreamed I was looking at the cutaway of a glass house. Inside the house a sour-looking, middle-aged man was sitting in a solitary easy chair staring at the door. On the other side of the door was a young boy on his knees, weeping and pleading with the man to let him come inside. The man never moved a muscle, and I knew he was not only indifferent to the boy's suffering, he was enjoying it too.

* * *

On Monday morning I told Richards about my dream and everything that happened on Palm Sunday. He listened attentively but didn't raise an eyebrow. Without comment, he suggested I move to the couch for some guided imagery therapy. Once again, he bundled me up in a blanket, attached headphones softly playing classical music, and drew up a chair so close we were almost touching. He told me to relax, close my eyes, and tell him what I saw.

In 1980 our previous guided imagery experiments yielded almost nothing, and what they did felt hopelessly contrived. This time, as soon as I closed my eyes, all hell broke loose. Goddesses, saints, angels, whirling golden disks covered with strange writing, grotesque landscapes, vortices, swirling comets, heavens, hells, and God-only-knows-what-else appeared in 3-D and living color. I had no control over these visions, and whether they were uplifting, depraved, or just marvelous to behold, they all seemed determined to swallow me up. I couldn't tell where I ended and where these visions began. Sometimes I was sucked right in like stepping into a dream and forgetting you're dreaming. All of this was terrifying enough, but far worse was the emotional content. Wordless realizations unlocking the mysteries of my entire life poured down on me, and each inarticulate epiphany seemed to pack more than enough wallop to drive me over the tiny piece of edge I still had left.

After that first session, separating fact from hallucination was not only impossible but impossibly irrelevant. The onslaught was so unremitting I didn't have the time or tools to make such fine distinctions even if I cared to. The boundaries between inside and outside, objective and subjective, myself and the universe collapsed, revealing the terrifying fact that Reality is, and always had been, seamless and all of one piece.

I ate almost nothing, spoke to no one except Richards, and when I slept at all I slept so fitfully I remembered every detail of every increasingly bizarre dream. I was in a constant panic. All I could do was cling to The Centurion's Prayer with a feverish intensity. I said this prayer so relentlessly I fell asleep saying it and awoke with it on my lips.

As the week progressed, my visions and experiences became darker and even more intense. When I returned to my motel on Holy Thursday after my morning session with Richards, the whole world was dizzily pulsating, and the walls of my room seemed to be breathing in and out. I was supposed to write down my experiences immediately after each session, but this time, as I began writing, some power took over and I automatically began filling page after page after page. When I realized what a dark, crazy turn these writings were taking, I tried to stop—only to discover I was unable to. This is a fraction of what I wrote.

At some point in the vision this morning the whole bush became one gigantic flower with four shimmering red petals, and in the center was a swirling black vacuum inviting me in. Even now that symbol seems like a vast woman's mouth inviting me to oral sex. I feel revulsion yet I am fascinated by the idea of just letting myself be sucked into the vacuum and finding release. Release? Or would it be followed by the inevitable shame and self-reproach of giving in to anonymous sex with something not even human? Giving in?

Giving in? This seems to be the theme of the entire week so far. I try to give in but in vain . . . can I think of one time when giving in has been rewarded? When shame and self- hatred have not been the wages of that sin? This is why I'm so afraid. The terror.

All my visions tempt me with their half-audible promise that if I would only give in I would find peace. They are the devil! Setting me up, setting me up, setting me up, for more disappointment. And my heart is so broken I can't stand any more disappointment. I realize now that so much of my motivation for my spiritual quest was to live my life in such a way that I wouldn't end up playing life's fool.

Now, even now, I feel the way I've always felt about terrestrial life. It is the goddess Kali, the Hindu temptress. I see her now swaying back and forth in front of me—my God, so many arms! Hypnotic, hypnotic, hypnotic. Life is a hypnotic dream. Kali is playing a drum just like the woman keeping time to "Oh my soul, Oh my soul." She never tires and she is relentless. "Rest," she is singing so persuasively, "and come to me. Your strivings are useless. Worse than useless. They tire you to no avail. You belong to me. I am your source. I am your mother, and to me you shall inevitably return. Why make it so hard on yourself? Come to me now."

No matter what I do, I can't make her stop. Oh God, won't you make her stop?

My whole life has been one great attempt to resist her call, to never rest, to struggle on. Once I prayed that there was a place of purity where I could truly rest and be refreshed but . . .

At this point Kali disappeared, the motel floor opened up under my feet, and I saw Hell yawning beneath me. Hell was an ocean of putrid, bubbling excrement with millions of arms reaching up out of it. I was aghast, but I was already so panic-stricken that after a few moments there seemed to be nothing else to do but just keep writing.

Hands reaching up from Hell. I see their hands. Filthy hands clenching and relaxing and motivated by one thought: the mad desire, the will, to add my soul to their number. These hands, their grip, could be broken if only I could reach the sky. But I will never get there. There is only night, and these cries of the damned are deafening—crushing my skull.

I am in mourning. I am mourning because I can never hope again, never trust again, never allow myself to be loved. Love, I know, is all around me, but I can't let it touch me. Because if I did, I might rise to the bait again. And oh my soul, oh my soul, I am so utterly weary of rising to life's bait!

I am terrified by everything that is happening this week. I know I will find myself back in Raleigh perched on my crag with nothing but my plight and my flaws made even clearer and with even less energy to do anything about it. There will be nothing left to do but scream and scream and scream and SCREAM!

When I finally stopped writing it felt like waking up from a trance. I began reading what I wrote like I was snooping at a stranger's private thoughts.

"Who is this person?" I said to myself. "Who wrote this? What was I saying? What does it mean? Am I *insane*?" I grabbed the wastebasket next to my motel desk and vomited repeatedly, even though there was nothing in my stomach.

* * *

Two hours later I was back in Richards's office for our afternoon session. As I read my journal entry, he listened attentively but didn't show the slightest hint of alarm. He told me my tirade was another example, like the lizard dream, of the unconscious fighting me because I was fighting it. He said my ego was superimposing all the darkness and despair through its frantic resistance. When I finally surrendered, he calmly said, the darkness would become light, and I would find my fears groundless.

In my deranged state this was not what I wanted to hear. Instead of helping me resist the demons, he seemed to be parroting their Siren's song, helping them bring me to my knees once and for all. I felt as if my one ally left in the universe had been co-opted. Richards had been duped by the darkness and all those filthy hands reaching out for me. Overcome with anguish and rage at this apparent betrayal, I lashed out at the top of my lungs.

"You're one of them! You're in league with the devils!"

Richards didn't even blink. He just sat there smiling at me with so much innocent benevolence I soon felt even more ridiculous than my ridiculous accusation.

"My God, Bill, I'm coming apart!" I screamed.

"You're coming together," Richards calmly replied.

"But Nietzsche went insane!"

"Your name's Turak."

With nothing left to say, I just sat there trembling as rage and terror drained away in tears. Richards leaned over and took me by both hands.

"Listen to me, Augie," he said in an urgent whisper. "You can't fall out of the universe. Trust the process. You have plenty of ego to get through this. God won't abandon you. Trust the process."

Then he led me back to the couch for another session of guided imagery. I was sitting on the edge of the couch waiting for Richards to retrieve his pillow, blanket, and headphones when I said, "Bill, there's a woman in black standing at the window with her back to me."

"What is she doing?"

"She seems to be doing some kind of slow, sexually provocative dance."

"How does that make you feel?"

"Sexually stimulated, but something is very wrong. It feels icky."

"Why don't you go over and see what she's up to?"

This suggestion frightened me, but Richards said, "Trust me, Augie. If you approach her in an open and loving way, I know she'll react in the same way."

Finally, like stepping into a 3-D virtual reality, I approached the window and the woman without ever physically leaving the couch. I was about to tap her gently on the shoulder when she suddenly whirled around. *She was my mother.* I screamed in shock and almost fainted. But in less time than it took for this reaction, she morphed into the woman, glasses and all, she was just before she started to waste away from cancer at 61. Her face was radiant, and she seemed overjoyed to see me. She told me she was fine, that she loved me, and she was very proud of me. She told me not to worry because every-thing was going to be all right.

Then she vanished.

* * *

When I got back to my motel room there was no way I could write in my journal. Though my mother's comforting message ended the session on an uplifting note, it had been a long, intense Holy Thursday. I was exhausted. I was sitting on the small, black, Naugahyde-covered couch in my room absently going over my encounter with my mother when I suddenly remembered Meredith's cryptic prophecy two years earlier: "Can't you see? It's all about your mom!"

I then recalled my letter to Father Christian pleading, "I just want my mom," about telling David how I let my mother down before she died, and finally I flashed on the psychic's admonition that my mother had a message for me. A message that despite my derisive skepticism at the time had apparently just been delivered. Meredith's oracular in-tuition now seemed to make perfect sense—even if only by the crazy, phantasmagoric standards that were passing for "making sense" these days.

"But I still don't know," I mused, "why she first appeared in such a sexually provocative way."

Giving up, I absently reached for the only book I brought with me: *Moby Dick: An American Nekyia,* by Edward Edinger. The Duke SKS students gave it to me for Christmas because they knew *Moby Dick* was my favorite novel. I'd picked it up as an afterthought, still unread, on my way out the door in Raleigh one week earlier. I began reading and discovered that *nekyia* is a term Carl Jung borrowed from the Greek epic poets for the hero's trip into hell, or the underworld. In Jungian psychology, a *nekyia* is a metaphor for a mystical journey into the universal unconscious in search of the Ground of Being, the Numinous, the Absolute, or God.

Edinger explained that such a journey is usually precipitated by some kind of psychological shock, a shock portrayed in various myths and religious traditions by the hero's violent death or physical injury. Captain Ahab, for example, lost his leg; Dionysius was devoured; the Egyptian hero Osiris dismembered; Christ crucified; and Oedipus severely injured his ankle. (In fact, Edinger said, Oedipus means "swollen ankle" in Greek.)[49]

My mind raced. Like Oedipus, I severely injured my ankle, and this was the shock that sent me plunging into the nether regions. Oedipus unwittingly married his mother and was punished for this sin despite his innocent mistake. But I never had sex with my mother or even thought about it, so how? Instantly the answer came in an explosive epiphany that went something like this: By the time I was twelve, my mother was deeply depressed, estranged from her husband, and isolated in a tiny house full of children. With no emotional outlets, she turned to me, confided in me, and treated me like her best friend. I was just entering puberty, and somehow I conflated my mother's strictly emotional overtures with sexual overtures. Horrified by these sexual feelings, I buried it all in my unconscious mind. There it remained a festering knot of repressed guilt subtly poisoning all my relationships with women until I finally faced it on this very day in my session with Richards. So much of my guilt was sexual, and so much of that sexual guilt, I now realized, was related to these repressed sexual feelings toward my mother.

Like all my realizations that terrible week, this epiphany came to me wordlessly and in a flash. What's more, these revelations seemed to come from the deepest part of me, or even from somewhere else. Every time I or anyone else posed a question, I was immediately knocked flat by an emotionally charged, all-at-once, experiential answer so powerfully delivered it seemed more like a divine fiat preceded by the heavenly fanfare, "Thus says the Lord!"

Before I could catch my breath, I was overcome with sadness for my mother's hopeless plight and my own innocent yet emotionally crippling mistake, and this released all my long-repressed mourning over my mother's death. These powerful epiphanies one on top of another were so overwhelming I once again began to panic. I hurled Edinger's book into a Pine Sol-caked corner of my dismal motel room, grabbed my jacket, and headed for my car trying to get some distance from my superheated mind.

A few minutes later, I was aimlessly driving around obsessively repeating The Centurion's Prayer when I remembered *The Adventures of Tom Sawyer* still in the tape deck. I turned it on, hoping for distraction, only to discover that Tom and Becky were lost in an endless labyrinth of dark subterranean caves with their last candle stub slowly guttering out.

Somewhere in the enveloping darkness their worst nightmare, Indian Joe, was lurking, ready at any moment to burst from his hiding place and gobble them up.[50]

I shuddered and flipped off the tape.

* * *

When I arrived for my morning session on Good Friday, Richards met me at the door. He suggested we take the day off and hike the trails behind his house instead. For several hours we worked up a considerable sweat climbing up and down a series of demanding trails straddling Gwynn Falls. While we did, Bill told me he would be observing Good Friday by attending a novel version of the Stations of the Cross, and he invited me to come along. A liturgical reenactment of Christ's passion and death, the Stations of the Cross is usually conducted in church, but in the version I attended with Richards, an interdenominational group of clergy led us on a walking tour of a run-down Baltimore neighborhood. Poverty and the crack cocaine epidemic had left Baltimore a far darker city than the one I nostalgically recalled on Palm Sunday. Every deserted playground and crack house had a story of murder and mayhem to tell, and at each of these "stations" a different clergyman would relate this story and link it in a meaningful way to Christ's passion and death.

While the service was painful, it was also very powerful, and by the time I got back to my motel room I felt calmer than I had in days. I decided to use this interlude to check in with my colleagues at RGI. As I dialed the phone, I felt strangely detached. Raleigh was a million miles away, and RGI and the SKS seemed like things I once dabbled with in a previous incarnation. One of my partners answered the phone, and before I knew what I was saying I blurted, "Eric, I won't be coming back on Monday like we planned."

"OK," Eric said with obvious concern, "so when will you be back?"

"I won't be coming home at all," I heard myself calmly say. "I'm going to die or be institutionalized."

Thus says the Lord! Moments later the emotional content of what just came out of my mouth hit me and I broke down. This was too much for Eric, and he hastily put Dave Gold on the line. I just kept repeating I was going to die or go insane. This seemed to panic Dave and, groping for something to say, he stuttered, "Tr--try not to hold back!"

"Dave, it doesn't matter. When God puts his shoulder to the door, you can hold back all you want. He's coming in."

"What do you know for sure?" Dave said, almost comically falling back on that standard Rosean icebreaker.

Thus says the Lord!

"I know this. Last night I dreamed Richards told me I was so beat up I should go home and rest up before continuing. In my dream, Dave, I turned him down. I just came from the Stations of the Cross and Christ's last words were, 'It is finished.' It ends here, Dave. If I die or go insane no longer matters. I just can't live the way I've lived my life, in fear and ignorance, anymore. It ends here, Dave. It ends here."

A few moments later I was sitting on the bed still weeping and trying to understand why I just linked God's arrival with death and insanity. Again, wordlessly and from somewhere else, it hit me. All my life I thought my angst stemmed from doubts about God's existence. Now I knew the truth: I always knew God did exist and that's what was terrifying me all along. I was afraid that if I ever did meet God face to face, He would see right through me, be disgusted with what He saw, and, turning on His heel, abandon me . . . forever. God was knocking at my door all my life, but I kept screaming "in a minute!" as I vainly tried to make myself presentable. All along I thought I was running toward God when actually I was running away. My whole life was self-deception. My whole life was a lie. My whole life was *wrong*.

Oh my God, I thought with the only words I could muster for this head-pounding realization. *I've spent my entire life trying to clean up for the maid and never realized it. I psychologically locked myself away in a tiny, dingy, claustrophobic motel room just like this one because I was afraid to face what was waiting for me out on the street.*

But God was no longer patiently waiting out on the street, on the stairs, or even in the hallway. He was hammering down the door. My whole rotten house was shaking, the door frame splintering, and I was still not ready to face Him. I now knew what Hell was. Hell was God turning on His heel in disgust in the face of all my flaws. To be eternally alone, unloved, unlovable, abandoned by God—that was Hell. The clock was striking midnight, I was out of time, God was coming in, and I was doomed.

Then I must have passed out.

Just before daylight I dreamed I was forcing a young boy of about six to dress up as a girl for some sexually sadistic reason. While I never touched him, in my dream I enjoyed this spectacle and found it sexually stimulating. I awoke, it was daylight, and I was physically ill from revulsion and self-loathing. This dream was the sickest thing that ever occurred to me, and it finished me. In an hour or so I would be in Richards's office. I would tell him about this dream. He would ask me to relive the dream through guided imagery. And reliving this horrific dream would prove more than I could stand. There would be nothing left to do but call 911.

I drove to Richards's office like a condemned man being carted to the gallows by a force he can no longer resist. When I related my dream, Richards's face contorted.

"My God, Augie, we got to stop torturing that little boy!"

Moments later, I was on the couch, and instantly the boy appeared. "What is he doing?" Bill asked.

"He's scared. He doesn't understand what's happening."

"Why don't you walk over and comfort him?"

Following Bill's instructions, I began virtually walking and, as I did, I was filled with love and compassion for him. Even though he was staring at the floor in shame and confusion, I suddenly thought he looked like Mr. Jim, my ex-girlfriend's little boy who I still loved and missed so much. I picked the boy up and he threw his arms around my neck and put his head on my shoulder—just like Mr. Jim did so many times.

A few seconds later he pulled his head back and looked me right in the eyes. It wasn't Mr. Jim.

It was me.

This shocking encounter triggered an irresistible energy of unimaginable intensity. The world disappeared and there was a radiant young woman standing in front of me. She took me by the hand and in rapid succession showed me three overlapping visions. The first was the women of Jerusalem weeping for a Jesus I couldn't see as He passed by on His way to His crucifixion. The second was a vision of the women closest to Jesus weeping at His tomb. The third was a magnificent vista. I seemed to be standing on a mountaintop overlooking an infinite landscape of staggering beauty. It was real, surreal, unreal all at the same time and seemed to include multiple dimensions beyond time and space.

Wordlessly, my radiant guide told me I could see or have anything I wanted. I told her, "I only want God."

Instantly, she disappeared and I was enveloped in darkness. I scanned this darkness expecting more visions to appear, but there was nothing but perfect peace and tranquility. Then this dazzling darkness began pressing against my eyes, shutting off my sight. Then it gently pressed against the field of my mind, pushing my thoughts back toward their source until my mind was silenced.

The last thing I remember thinking before my mind went dark and seemed to tip over backward was: *My God, this is what I've been searching for all my life!*

Chapter Twenty-Two

THE RETURN

We shall not cease from exploration
And the end of all our exploring
Will be to arrive where we started
And know the place for the first time.
—T.S. ELIOT[51]

My experience in Bill's office was so cataclysmic that the next thing I remember is standing outside St. Bartholomew's Church after Easter services with Bill and his 25-year-old son, Brian, home on leave from graduate school. It was warm and sunny, and the bells of St. Bart's were joyously pealing all around me. I was so exhilarated I felt as though all that Baltimore-burnished sunshine was pouring down through the top of my head and streaming out the soles of my feet. The reborn world was now a marvelous place, so marvelous in fact I couldn't decide where to focus my attention next. All this was utterly disorienting but in a beautiful, surrealistic, "trippy" kind of way. Things like this were only supposed to happen to mystics and saints but—*mirabile dictu*—they were apparently happening to me.

I once saw a documentary about a comet that hit the earth with such incredible force it not only wiped out the dinosaurs but left a thin layer of rock that geologists now use to separate the age of dinosaurs from the age of mammals. On that Easter Sunday in Baltimore, I felt like a spiritual comet had struck me, leaving in its wake a paper-thin layer of opaque, impenetrable, psychic stone. In an instant, the old Augie, the dinosaur, was wiped out and a new Augie—the mammal—took his place.

Try as I might, I couldn't remember what the old Augie was like.

I remembered every detail of old Augie's ordeal, but I could not place the genesis of all that suffering. What was all the fuss about? That "soul hole" Hugh described so perfectly at the gym was now so utterly filled with joyful gratitude I couldn't remember where it was, let alone what it felt like. Hugh's prophecy was so completely fulfilled I couldn't recall what a broken heart was like.

* * *

Early Easter Monday I arrived for my session with Richards. For several minutes we sat silently staring at each other. Then we started laughing hysterically like a couple of high school boys who just made off with the principal's pants. Eventually we calmed down, but still all we managed to do was grin at each other in mutual astonishment.

"Bill," I finally said with a tad of regret at marring such a marvelous mood, "I know this must sound incredible, but I don't have a single thing left to say."

"I know," Richards responded with a broad smile. Then, loosely interlacing his hands behind his neck, he leaned back in his chair and softly said, "Time to head home, don't you think?"

I was stunned. I couldn't believe I went from telling Dave Gold on Good Friday I would never be coming home to heading home three days later without a care in the world. I told Richards how grateful I was for his help. Then I asked if he ever went through anything similar with anyone else.

"Oh, bits and pieces," he laughingly said. "But I can't say I ever had that much fun before," he added while gleefully rubbing his hands together.

I was eager for an after-action report, but Richards was typically reticent, though I did manage to coax a few things out of him.

"Well, for starters," he said while ambling toward the window to open the blinds and bathe the office in some early morning Maryland sunshine, "that book on Native American totem animals said our friend the Lizard was trying to get you to accept your vulnerability and human nature. Did you notice," he continued while resting both hands on the back of his chair before retaking his seat, "that every significant figure or symbol we encountered was female?"

"No, I guess I was too busy to notice," I said, laughing. "But you're right. The woman outside the church on Palm Sunday, Kali, the Hindu goddess, my mother, and of course the radiant woman who acted as my guide."

"Yes," Bill said with a nod. "And what did your guardian angel show you?"

"The women of Jerusalem and the women weeping at Christ's tomb."

"Exactly, but aren't we forgetting one? The most important feminine figure of all was you. When you finally faced yourself, you were dressed like a girl, and this was the catalyst that produced the breakthrough."

Richards reminded me that in every myth or religious tradition, the Eternal Feminine, the Great Mother, the Goddess, the Virgin, was identified with the earth, with life, with God immanent, with fertility, with our human nature as well as with wisdom.

"It's the feminine with all its humanness, its physicality, its vulnerability, its sensitivity, and even its earthly mortality you were repressing, refusing to accept. That's why you continually associated terrestrial life in your dreams with excrement. God's waiting in the last place we're willing to look, and that means our very brokenness as human beings."

He paused and said, "By the way, how about a cup of tea?" Bill had apparently anticipated the informal nature of this final session because there was a wooden tray boasting an electric kettle and all the fixings gracing the top of a gray filing cabinet just a few steps away.

Handing me a piping cup black and taking a lightly sweetened one himself, he went on to say that we love children not because they're perfect but because they're so vulnerably imperfect, and yet we find it impossible to think God could love us for much the same reason.

"God doesn't love us despite our flaws, but in some mysterious way because of them as well," he said. "Think of Hugh's prophecy. He predicted two years of hell and told you God would be waiting in the midst of it—and so He was."

"Yeah," I added, shaking my head, "it's been almost two years to the day."

As Richards wrapped up his reluctant post-game analysis, I realized he had been on to me all along.

"You son of a gun," I said, "you knew all this back in 1980. No wonder you picked up on the first ring when I called from Raleigh: you were expecting my call! You even knew that boy I was torturing was me all along." Richards just smiled. "Why didn't you tell me?"

"Ah, c'mon, Augie. You've read the same books I have. You know all this mumbo-jumbo as well as I do, maybe better, and what good did it do? We have to make the trip ourselves, and you couldn't make it until you were ready. There are no shortcuts. All those years of prep work were necessary. The suffering too. The shock of surprise is critical as well. It knocks the ego off balance and opens us up. Besides," he continued, wiping away a wide grin with a paper napkin along with a few stray drops of wayward tea, "I couldn't give away the ending, could I? It would've spoiled all the fun!"

Easter Monday evening, I went shopping and, as luck, or fate, would have it, I found the perfect gift: a handmade, crystal, guardian angel—an ornament left over from Christmas. Early the next morning, I stopped to give it to Richards. Then I checked out of that tomblike facsimile of the Main Hotel once and for all and set out for Raleigh.

Driving home I gradually realized I was still in an altered state. An hour or so would fly by without a single thought arising in my head. I was so utterly absorbed in wordless contemplation of my new condition it stilled my mind completely. Then, somewhere between D.C. and Raleigh, a paradoxical revelation suddenly arose of its own accord: *Everything is already perfect in its imperfection.* "I wouldn't change anything," I blurted half aloud in amazement. "I wouldn't even change my desire to change things. But what now?" Instantly, an answer echoed back with that now familiar force of *"Thus Says the Lord!"*

"Your work is over!"

Stunned, I responded aloud, "But what do I do?"

"Wait in hopeful weakness," the voice instantly replied.

* * *

When I got back, I told the adult SKS group and my students at Duke everything that happened in Baltimore. As I did, I wept, but now with tears of joy and gratitude rather than despair. My Duke students gave me a framed poster of a whale plunging headfirst with only its outstretched flukes visible above the waves. At the bottom were these lines from Scripture:

The waters closed over me,
The deep engulfed me.
Weeds twined around my head.
I sank to the base of the mountains.
The bars of the earth closed upon me forever.

Yet you brought my life up from the pit,
O Lord my God!
JONAH 2:5, 6[52]

* * *

Two weeks later I arrived at Mepkin Abbey. The monastery was even more supernaturally silent than usual. There wasn't a soul to be seen. I walked up the paved sidewalk toward the breezeway entrance to the monastery proper still searching unsuccessfully for any sign of a black-on-white Trappist habit. As I wandered into the deserted refectory, I startled Father Christian coming through a swinging door from the kitchen. Without a word, he grabbed me by the hand, whirled around, genuflected toward the large crucifix hanging behind the abbot's table and, still clutching my hand, softly exclaimed, "Thanks be to God!"

Two days later, Christian arrived for our private meeting proffering Gerard Manly Hopkins's "My Own Heart Let Me More Have Pity On," the same poem he asked me to read at our very first meeting all those many eons ago. Once again I read it aloud:

My own heart let me more have pity on; let
Me live to my sad self hereafter kind,
Charitable; not live this tormented mind
With this tormented mind tormenting yet . . .[53]

When I finished, he once again demanded my exegesis.
"I still love this poem, Father. But it's no longer me."
"I know," Christian said. "I knew it the instant I saw you."

* * *

When I returned from Mepkin, I went to see my mentor and campus advisor at Duke, who was also Dean of the Duke Chapel.

He listened intently to my story and then grabbed me firmly by the shoulder.

"Augie," he said, "there's no doubt in my mind that you have been seized by the hand of God. I'm just so glad He's taken a far gentler path with me."

Minutes later I was all alone in the magnificent and otherwise empty Gothic Chapel, weeping uncontrollably with only one thought in my mind: *He doesn't understand. I'd go through a million times the suffering I went through to find just a tiny fraction of what I found on the other side.*

But as the weeks wore on, I decided that having a spiritual experience and living it out are two different things. Like a stroke patient relearning how to walk and talk, I had to get to know myself all over again—from scratch. I'd never been at peace before and, ironically, I found it mildly disorienting. I was so used to living with a knot of twisted anxiety in the pit of my stomach that I felt lopsided and off-kilter without it. I was like a gangly adolescent in a stiff new suit awkwardly navigating his first boy/girl party while not quite knowing how to act. Even learning itself had to be relearned: before, learning required effort; now effort was counterproductive. Instead, I had to humbly "wait in hopeful weakness" as new ways of being steadily emerged at their own pace of their own accord.

Beyond this, at the oddest of times and without warning, I would be overcome by experiences of pure ecstasy. Lasting anywhere from a few seconds to a full minute, these experiences of what might be called "infinite gratitude," while incredibly beautiful, also felt almost life-threatening. I felt like an ordinary light bulb inadvertently plugged into a 220 line as my heart and head struggled to contain a level of effulgent profundity they were never designed to contain. These exaltations were so explosive and the tearful aftershocks so exhausting it took a day or two just to recover.

All this reorientation left me so utterly detached it was downright disorienting. As Rose so colorfully put it after his own spiritual experience, I too found myself "in danger of forgetting to eat." I spent days in my office in a trancelike condition, wordlessly contemplating my marvelous situation like an inarticulate infant finger-fondling the ineffable wonders of space and time through his toes. Once in a while I would spontaneously surface and notice five or six spiritual books cracked open and upside down on my desk. Reaching for one at random, I would peruse a sentence or two only to resurface sometime later to do the same thing.

One time my partner, Jay, and I were in San Francisco for a trade show. While we were sitting at the bar waiting for a table in a crowded Japanese restaurant, Jay began ticking off our business objectives for the show. The next thing I knew, he was elbowing me sharply in the ribs.

"You haven't heard a word I've said in the last ten minutes, have you?" I slowly shook my head.

"You look like a zoned-out statue. What the hell are you thinking about?"

I had no idea what I was thinking about. So I said, "Dewar's. Blended Scotch Whiskey. A selection of fine whiskies aged in oak casks then carefully blended together." Words that I read straight off a label directly across the bar, a sacred reading which sent long-suffering Jay, God bless him, into hysterics.

* * *

Along with these sometimes humorous adjustments, I was also straining to find words for everything I just experienced. When I returned to Raleigh after my sessions with Richards, I felt like I came home with millions of glittering jigsaw pieces to a puzzle I felt compelled to assemble. But all I had to go on was a picture I saw in its entirety only once in Baltimore bolstered by a few through-a-glass-darkly glimpses I garnered during the previous two years.

So I decided to put my Raleigh therapist, David, to work helping me crack this puzzle.

When I finished my Baltimore story, he let loose with one of his shrieking, high-pitched, maniacal laughs and said, "After all that, what the hell do you want from lil' ol' me?"

I told him I just wanted help "unpacking the experience," and our subsequent meetings did help a great deal. Once, for example, I was weeping with gratitude in his office for the umpteenth time when I suddenly exclaimed, "David, why me? No one could possibly *earn* what God gave me. It's all gift. It's grace. It's *all* grace."

This triggered one of David's all-too-familiar meditative moments. Reemerging a minute or so later, he reached for his glasses on the lamp table at his elbow and said, "Yes, it is all grace. But you *asked* for it. You spent your whole life asking for it. What happened to you doesn't typically happen to ordinary folks on their way to the store for a quart of milk."

* * *

As the months wore on and my floating sense of eerie detachment continued, I began to wonder what I was going to do with the rest of my life. While in some sense this troubled me, it didn't detract one jot from my overall sense of wonder, peace, joy, and gratitude. I was just so blissfully filled to overflowing I didn't know what to do with myself. I needed a way to apply what I'd learned and get my feet back on the ground. For now, though, all I could do was "wait in hopeful weakness."

* * *

On Easter Sunday 1999, one year after my Baltimore experience, I was attending Vespers at Mepkin Abbey. The reading was from the Gospel of John that I'd heard so many times before.

. . . Early on the first day of the week, while it was still dark, Mary Magdalene came to the tomb and saw that the stone had been removed from the tomb.

But Mary stood weeping outside the tomb. As she wept, she bent over to look into the tomb; and she saw two angels in white, sitting where the body of Jesus had been lying, one at the head and the other at the feet. They said to her, 'Woman, why are you weeping?' She said to them, 'They have taken away my Lord, and I do not know where they have laid him.' When she had said this, she turned round and saw Jesus standing there, but she did not know that it was Jesus. Jesus said to her, 'Woman, why are you weeping? For whom are you looking?' Supposing him to be the gardener, she said to him, 'Sir, if you have carried him away, tell me where you have laid him, and I will take him away.' Jesus said to her, 'Mary!' She turned and said to him in Hebrew, 'Rabboni!' (which means Teacher). (John 20:1, 11-16)[54]

But this time at Mepkin, when I heard Mary say "Rabboni!" in the passage, something inside wordlessly cried out, "My Lord and my God!" All at once I relived everything I went through in Baltimore. In that same instant I realized that in Baltimore I'd relived my entire life, but in Baltimore, like watching a video on fast-forward, I finally noticed everything I missed, ignored, misinterpreted, or had been too afraid to look at the first time around.

The following day I was talking to a theologian from the archdiocese of Los Angeles who, as an oblate, was the only official member of the Mepkin community not a monk. I told him about my experience in Baltimore and at Vespers the previous evening. He listened thoughtfully, asked a few questions, and said, "Tell me something. Did you experience a personal God?"

"No," I replied without thinking, and he just nodded his head.

Almost immediately I felt there was something wrong with my answer and, as I drove back to Raleigh, I tried to figure out what it was. It was true there was nothing objectively "there" in my experience.

Nothing I could point to as a "person" or "personal God." In fact, my experiences were so impersonal and dimensionless they reminded me of the apophatic mystics and their description of God as Nothing or "not a thing."

Yet there was also something so intensely intimate, tender, loving, and deeply *personal* about what I experienced in Baltimore and Vespers that it felt like . . . and then it hit me! It felt like God calling me by name! Suddenly it all became clear. I'd spent my life as an amnesiac trying to remember my real identity, my true self, my eternal name. That was why God calling David by name in the movie *David and Bathsheba* moved me so much. God, I now realized, had been calling me by name all my life, but rather than tuning in to it, it terrified me so much I ran away instead.

Why? Because my name wasn't Richard Rose, Captain Ahab, Moses, Huang Po, my father's name, or any of the other heroic, masculine names I always wanted or thought I was supposed to have. No, my name was synonymous with the last person I would want to be: Mary Magdalene. Mary, a poor, brokenhearted woman setting out in the dark in tears of bitter disappointment to visit a tomb. Only to find the tomb is empty and she is apparently to be deprived of even the meager solace she seeks by anointing the body of the one she loved most in the world: Jesus.

This is what terrified me: finding out that I, like Mary Magdalene, would find myself stranded in the dark at an empty tomb, utterly bereft, with nowhere else to turn. Yet even as she turns away in final despair from the man she mistakes for the gardener, turns away without even waiting for his answer, she hears that one word, "Mary!" And turning back, she meets her Lord and her God face to face.

In a similar way, God finally forced me to face the empty tomb of all my egotistical hopes and illusions about life and myself.

In a similar way, God finally forced me to face the empty tomb of all my egotistical hopes and illusions about life and myself. And, again like Mary Magdalene, in my darkest hour, I too was called by name. And when I heard my name, I too turned back from abject despair and cried, "*Rabboni!* My Lord and my God!"

Absorbed by these thoughts as I sped north on I-95 toward home, I became increasingly excited. The word *conversion*, I suddenly recalled, means "to turn back"—just like Mary did. Jigsaw pieces with words attached began tumbling into place. I realized, of course, that I didn't literally hear God call "Augie!" So what name did He use? My *mystical name*, I decided. And what was my mystical name? *It was the same name I shared with every other human being!* In God's eyes we all have the same name even though each of us experiences the sound of our mystical name as something infinitely unique and intimate. And with this realization, a critical chunk of the jigsaw puzzle finally fell into place. I now knew what I was supposed to do with myself. I was supposed to be there for someone else, someone who shared my name.

I was sent back from Baltimore to be an instrument and megaphone for God. I was supposed to amplify His voice, calling out to all of us who, whether we realize it or not, are looking desperately for our Lord and knowing not where they have taken Him. And when God used me to help call someone by name, I wanted that person to turn back and see, not me, the mere gardener of God—but to see Rabboni, their Lord and their God.

* * *

Two weeks later I was scheduled to deliver the Sunday sermon at a local nondenominational church. Even though I knew I would become very emotional in the process, I decided to relay my reaction to the story of the weeping Mary Magdalene and use it as a universal metaphor for the spiritual quest. Twice before my scheduled address, a woman from the church called and asked for my favorite hymn. My favorite hymn was now "What Wondrous Love Is This," the hymn I heard twice on Palm Sunday in Baltimore. But I was afraid to request it. I knew if I heard that hymn, I would become too emotional to deliver my homily. So I told her, twice, "Any hymn will be fine."

Arriving early for the service, I found myself alone in a brightly lit room with a hundred folding chairs with a hymnal on each. I impulsively started to grab one of the hymnals to see if it would open at random to "What Wondrous Love Is This." I quickly checked the impulse. "You better not," I said to myself. "If it does open to that hymn, you'll get too choked up."

Thirty minutes later the seats were full, and the minister introduced me as the guest speaker for the service. Then he said, "But before Augie begins, let's open our hymnals to hymn number 36."

Hymn number 36 was, of course, "What Wondrous Love Is This."

After a very emotional sermon, a number of people came up to thank me or ask a question or two. Out of the corner of my eye, I noticed an elderly man waiting patiently for the others to finish. When they did, he took my hand.

"Five years ago, my only son committed suicide," he said, his voice cracking. "A year ago my only daughter was killed in an auto accident. I just want to thank you. Your sermon today gave me a reason to go on."

This encounter, hard on the heels of hearing "What Wondrous Love Is This," completed the circle. I was filled with compassion, gratitude, and awe. I felt as if God, by means of this man, had just confirmed, in an incredibly moving way, my decision on the way back from Mepkin Abbey to spend the balance of my life just being there for someone else.

This was the sign I'd been waiting in hopeful weakness for since returning from Baltimore.

As I walked out of the church, my feet finally touched the ground. The preternatural absorption, eerie sense of detachment, and occasional aftershocks of exaltation vanished. And to this day, some twenty-five years later, I've never heard that hymn again. Yet my life never reverted to normal. Instead, through my encounter with the man who lost his children, I finally became the man I'd always been.

With that stiff new suit finally broken in, I settled into the ordinary man I discovered in Baltimore. The ordinary man I always was and was always too terrified to be.

CODA

April 2023

Easter is fast approaching. The tolling bells on that joyous occasion will mark twenty-five years since my spiritual experience in Baltimore, and I've not had a single moment of depression or anxiety in all those years. I also sold RGI, bought a farm, won the Templeton prize, and launched a second career as a writer and speaker. I seem to be surfing a magical slipstream of Rosean betweenness, a slipstream of ever-increasing joy, peace, and most of all, gratitude.

Easter will also mark twenty-four years since my spiritual encounter with Mary Magdalene at Mepkin Abbey. The encounter that prompted my decision to spend the balance of my life just being there for someone else. I founded and primarily self-fund a nonprofit organization. Our mission is helping people find higher meaning and purpose in a world that so many find bereft of meaning and purpose. All my book, speaking, and consulting earnings are donated to this charity, which also provides grants to underprivileged children and young adults.

During interviews, I am often asked for my greatest achievement. I invariably relate this story.

One day an elderly man I'd never seen before or since was handing out towels at my gym. I found this strange since retrieving towels from a basket is ordinarily a do-it-yourself enterprise. As I took one from his outstretched hand, he used it to suddenly yank my face toward his. Then he shouted, in a rapid-fire manner, "If you could be anywhere, doing anything, where would you be, doing what, *right now?!*"

"I'd be right here, right now, doing this," I instantly replied.

The old man flashed a grin, released my towel, and sent me on my way. As I walked away, my eyes filled with tears. My answer, spontaneously given, came from the deepest part of me and represented the greatest achievement and greatest blessing I could ever receive.

Endnotes

Title Page

1. T.S. Eliot, *Four Quartets* (Harcourt: Orlando, FL, 1943), from "Little Gidding."

Prelude

2. Andrew Sullivan, *New York Magazine,* "The Poison We Pick," February 19, 2018, https://nymag.com/intelligencer/2018/02/americas-opioid-epidemic.html.

One

3. T.S. Eliot, *Four Quartets* (Harcourt: Orlando, FL, 1943), from "Burnt Norton."
4. Herrmann Hesse, *Demian* (U.S., Bantam Books, 1969). The quote from Nancy's book is a paraphrase. Hesse's actual quote is: "I wanted only to live in accord with the promptings which came from my true self. Why was that so very difficult?"
5. Alan Watts, *This Is It, and Other Essays on Zen and Spiritual Experience* (U.S., Collier Books, 1967).

Two

6. T.S. Eliot, *Four Quartets* (Harcourt: Orlando, FL, 1943), from "East Coker."
7. Francis Ford Coppola, director, *Apocalypse Now* (U.S., United Artists, 1979).
8. Christmas Humphreys, A Western Approach to Zen (Wheaton, IL: The Theosophical Publishing House, 1971). The quote can be found at: https://terebess.hu/zen/mesterek/ChristmasHumphreys-Western-Approach-to-Zen.pdf.

Three

9. Eliot, "East Coker."

Four

10. T.S. Eliot, *Four Quartets* (Harcourt: Orlando, FL, 1943), from "The Dry Salvages."

11. Francis Thompson, *The Hound of Heaven* (New York: Dodd, Mead and Company, Inc., 1925), pp. 45-60. https://www.google.com/books/edition/The_Hound_of_Heaven/tGsGAQAAIAAJ?hl=en&gbpv=1.

12. Herman Melville, *Moby Dick* (New York: Harper & Brothers, 1851).

Five

13. Eliot, "Burnt Norton."

14. Richard Harris and Jim Webb, "McArthur Park," from *A Tramp Shining* (Hollywood, CA: Dunhill Records, 1968).

Six

15. Eliot, "Burnt Norton."

16. Huang Po, translated by John Blofeld, *The Zen Teaching of Huang Po: On the Transmission of Mind* (New York: Grove Press, 1959).

17. Eliot, "Burnt Norton."

18. John Sebastian and The Lovin' Spoonful, "Younger Girl," from *Do You Believe in Magic* (New York: Kama Sutra, 1965).

19. Homer; and Robert Fitzgerald, *The Odyssey* (Garden City, NY: Doubleday, 1961).

Seven

20. Eliot, "East Coker."

Eight

21. Eliot, "East Coker."

22. W.H. Murray, *The Scottish Himalaya Expedition* (London: J.M. Dent & Sons, 1951).

23. H.P. Blavatsky, *Isis Unveiled: A Master Key to the Mysteries of Ancient and Modern Science and Theology* (New York, 1877). Centenary Anniversary Edition; both volumes bound in one book. A photographic facsimile reproduction of the original edition was first published in New York City, 1877.

Nine

24. Eliot, "The Dry Salvages."

25. Carl Sigman and Herb Magidson, "Enjoy Yourself, It's Later Than You Think" (New York: Universal Music Group, 1949).

Ten

26. Eliot, "East Coker."

Eleven

27. Eliot, "Burnt Norton."

Twelve

28. Eliot, "Burnt Norton."

29. Po, translated by Blofeld, *The Zen Teaching of Huang Po.*

Thirteen

30. Eliot, "Burnt Norton."

Fourteen

31. Eliot, "The Dry Salvages."

32. The Cartoon Bank, "Trading Consciousness for Money" [cartoon], *The New Yorker* (New York: Condé Nast, 1977).

Fifteen

33. Eliot, "East Coker."

Sixteen

34. Eliot, "Burnt Norton."

35. Manly Hopkins, "My Own Heart Let Me More Have Pity On" (Chicago: Gerard International Hopkins Association), accessed December 10, 2018, https://hopkinspoetry.com/poem/my-own-heart-let-me-more-have-pity-on-let/.

Seventeen

36. Eliot, "The Dry Salvages."

37. Henry King, Darryl F. Zanuck, and Philip Dunne, *David and Bathsheba* (Los Angeles: 20th Century Studios, 1951).

38. 1 Kings 19:9: *New Revised Standard Version Anglicized Edition, The Holy Bible* (Oxford, England, and U.S.: Oxford University Press, 1989).

Eighteen

39. Eliot, "Burnt Norton."

40. Author name withheld, "Popping Amaranth" (Durham, NC: Duke University, 1997).

Nineteen
41. Eliot, "Little Gidding."

Twenty
42. Eliot, "Little Gidding."
43. From Psalm 4:2. Different versions can be accessed for a near reading to the verse as it was given, as stated here, at the Compline at Mepkin. For a close reading, compare *The Holy Bible: The Good News Translation with Apocrypha* (GNTA).
44. Jon Krakauer, *Into Thin Air* (London, England: Pan Books, 2011).

Twenty-One
45. Eliot, "East Coker."
46. Charles M. Schultz, *Peanuts* [comic strip] (Allentown, PA: Evening Chronicle, 1961). https://www.gocomics.com/peanuts/1961/11/19
47. Anonymous, "What Wondrous Love Is This" (US, S. Mead, 1811; American folk hymn, ca. 1835). This hymn is in the public domain. https://hymnary.org/text/what_wondrous_love_is_this_o_my_soul_o_m
48. The Centurion's Prayer from the Catholic Mass is based on Matthew 8 but is not a word for word quote. Matthew 8:8: *New Revised Standard Version Anglicized Edition, The Holy Bible* (Oxford, England, and U.S.: Oxford University Press, 1989).
49. Edward F. Edinger, *Melville's Moby Dick: A Jungian Commentary: An American Nekyia* (New York: New Directions Publishing Corporation, 1978).
50. Mark Twain and John Greenman, *The Adventures of Tom Sawyer* [sourced as an audiobook presentation], United States, 1876. The work is in the public domain.

Twenty-Two
51. Eliot, "Little Gidding."
52. Jonah 2:5, 6: *New Revised Standard Version Anglicized Edition, The Holy Bible* (Oxford, England, and U.S.: Oxford University Press, 1989).
53. Manly Hopkins, "My Own Heart Let Me More Have Pity On."
54. John 20:1, 11-16: *New Revised Standard Version Anglicized Edition, The Holy Bible* (Oxford, England, and U.S.: Oxford University Press, 1989).

AUGUST TURAK FOUNDATION

Our mission is to bring a transformative message
of higher meaning and purpose to a Western Culture
increasingly bereft of meaning and purpose.
www.AugustTurak.com

OTHER BOOKS FROM AUGUST TURAK

Business Secrets of the Trappist Monks

Published by Columbia Business School Publishing, *Business Secrets of the Trappist Monks: One CEO's Quest for Meaning and Authenticity* uses one thousand years of Trappist business success and Turak's own entrepreneurial experience to demonstrate that Trappist monks are not super successful businessmen despite adhering to only the highest ethical values, but because they do.

Brother John

Brother John: A Monk, a Pilgrim, and the Purpose of Life, combines Turak's $100,000 Templeton-Prize winning story of a magical encounter between the author and an umbrella wielding Trappist monk with twenty-two original oil paintings from award-winning artist, Glenn Harrington. *Brother John* offers a blueprint for higher meaning and purpose in a world that so many find bereft of meaning and purpose.

TURAK'S LEADERSHIP ARTICLES ON FORBES

https://www.forbes.com/sites/augustturak/